*S*UCCESS in
*P*RACTICAL
*N*URSING

PERSONAL AND VOCATIONAL ISSUES

SUCCESS in PRACTICAL NURSING

PERSONAL AND VOCATIONAL ISSUES
Second Edition

Signe S. Hill,
BSN, MA, RN

Health Educator
Lake County Health Department
Two Harbors, Minnesota

Formerly, Instructor, Practical Nurse Program
Northeast Wisconsin Technical College
Green Bay, Wisconsin

Helen A. Howlett,
BSN, MS, RN

Instructor, Practical Nurse Program
Northeast Wisconsin Technical College
Green Bay, Wisconsin

W.B. SAUNDERS COMPANY
A Division of Harcourt Brace & Company

Philadelphia, London, Toronto, Montreal, Sydney, Tokyo

W. B. SAUNDERS COMPANY

A Division of
Harcourt Brace & Company

The Curtis Center
Independence Square West
Philadelphia, PA 19106

Library of Congress Cataloging-in-Publication Data

Hill, Signe S.
  Success in practical nursing : personal and vocational
issues / Signe S. Hill, Helen A. Howlett. — 2nd ed.
      p.   cm.
  Includes bibliographical references and index.
  ISBN 0-7216-6465-2

  1. Practical nursing.   2. Practical nursing—
Vocational guidance.   I. Howlett, Helen A.   II. Title.
[DNLM: 1. Nursing, Practical.   WY 195 H648s]
RT62.H45   1993
610.73'069'3—dc20
DNLM/DLC   92-24339

SUCCESS IN PRACTICAL NURSING:
Personal and Vocational Issues   ISBN   0-7216-6465-2

Printed in the United States of America

Last digit is the print number: 9 8 7 6 5 4 3

To our parents

AMANDA AND HJALMARI HINKKANEN

and

HELEN AND WILLIAM STEPHENS

CONTRIBUTORS

Judith A. Mix,
RN, MSN, EdD

Associate Dean—NURSING
Northeast Wisconsin Technical College
Green Bay, Wisconsin

Michael S. Hill,
MS, CRC, QRC

Rehabilitation Consultant,
Employee Development Corporation
Minneapolis, Minnesota

PREFACE

Dear Student Practical Nurse and Instructor,

In the preface to the first edition, we invited you to write to us to let us know what you found especially helpful as well as to make suggestions for improvement. We also indicated that your ideas would be considered for future editions of this book.

Several of you wrote to us. Others became colleagues in the role of reviewers for the second edition. Thank you, both students and instructors, for taking the time. Each idea has been considered; many have been incorporated into this edition. Some ideas reflected protocols specific to individual states. We refer you to the Nurse Practice Act of your state for clarification of your nursing role. Some ideas were excellent but too comprehensive for a textbook on basic personal vocational issues. We dealt with this problem by expanding the reference lists in several chapters and by adding an annotated bibliography in the chapter on leadership skills.

For the sake of ease in both reading and writing, we referred to the student practical nurse as she, rather than he/she or s/he. In the same vein, we refer to the Licensed Practical Nurse and Licensed Vocational Nurse as LPN rather than LPN/LVN or LP/VN. We are mindful and respectful of your gender and of your states' preferences for use of titles.

The chapter arrangement remains the same. Some instructors liked the order of chapters in the first edition, whereas others indicated a different sequence of use. We welcome instructors to use this book in a manner that reflects their preferences.

The numbering of chapters changes because two new chapters have been added to the second edition. New Chapter 12 addresses "Pitfalls to Success in Practical Nursing." It includes topics such as burnout, abuse of alcohol and other drugs, smoking, personal weight management, fear of occupational risks (such as the acquired immunodeficiency syndrome [AIDS], tuberculosis, and hepatitis B), and codependent behavior. This new chapter makes a good complement to Chapter 10 on "Wellness and Personal Care."

New Chapter 18, "Leadership Skills for the Practical Nurse," assists you in identifying your predominant leadership style, specific skills needed for leadership, how Maslow's Hierarchy of Needs acts as a motivator, introduces you to the Howlett Hierarchy of Work Motivators, and discusses strategies for handling common workplace problems.

Our guest author for Chapter 13 on "Job-Related Communication" is Judy Mix, EdD, who has added new content on communication and the nursing process, caring, trust, territoriality, intonation, and communicating with clients with special needs (elderly persons and children) and has expanded the section on computer communication in nursing to bring the chapter up to speed on the rapid changes in nursing communication.

Chapter 21, "Finding a Job," was written by a new guest author, Michael Hill, CRC, QRC. The chapter reflects his area of expertise and down-to-earth approach used with his own clients.

Questions that stimulate problem solving are found throughout the chapters. Their purpose is to get you actively involved in the learning process, to stimulate thinking, and to support your ability to deal with problems as they occur. A glossary with clear definitions is found at the end of the book. Exercises to help you study and understand are found both throughout the text and in the appendixes.

We continue to focus on you as a student practical nurse, in a personal way, as you grow in nursing. Each chapter presents how-to information to help you learn the process of growth, as opposed to facts only. This textbook is intended for use now in your personal vocational issues course and as a reference after graduation. It is interesting to note that as one continues to grow, successive readings of a chapter take on new meanings.

We continue to invite you to write us in care of the W.B. Saunders Publishing Company to let us know what you found especially helpful, as well as to make suggestions for improvement. Again, your ideas will be carefully considered for future editions of this book.

Signe S. Hill

Helen A. Howlett

An Instructor's Manual to Accompany SUCCESS IN PRACTICAL NURSING is available to qualified instructors. Please contact your local W.B. Saunders textbook representative or call the publisher directly at 215-238-8406.

ACKNOWLEDGMENTS

Making additions and revisions for the second edition was influenced directly and indirectly by numerous persons and we want to acknowledge the following: Ilze Rader, our editor at W.B. Saunders, gave continuing encouragement and support. Marie Thomas, editorial assistant at W.B. Saunders, assisted in organization. Former and present students of practical nursing—it is rewarding to see their growth and problem solving—have proved that if you practice what the authors suggest, success will come. Judy A. Mix updated her excellent chapter on "Job-Related Communication." Michael S. Hill rewrote our chapter on "Finding a Job."

The time and effort of the following reviewers resulted in excellent feedback and suggestions: Donna M. Babao, RN, BSN, MA, MSN, Yuba College, Marysville, California; Frances M. Cirello, RN, BSEd, Warren County Vocational-Technical School, Washington, New Jersey; Mary Ann Cosgarea, RN, BA, BSN, Portage Lakes Career Center, W. Howard Nichol School of Practical Nursing, Greensburg, Ohio; Guadalupe Guzman, RN, BS, Valley Baptist Medical Center, Harlingen, Texas; Hilary H. Hamilton, RN, BSN, Southeastern Technical Institute, South Easton, Massachusetts; Maureen S. Howard, RN, BSN, Sussex County Vocational School, Sparta, New Jersey; Nadine C. Lewis, RN, MS, College of the Redwoods, Eureka, California; Marlene Martensen, RN, BSN, South Central Area Practical Nursing Program, West Plains, Missouri; Shirley D. Miller, RN, BSN, MEd, EdS, Okefenokee Technical Institute, Waycross, Georgia; Judith M. Pelletier, RN, BSN, Massachusetts Bay Community College, Wellesley, Massachusetts; and Bernice Rudolph, RN, BS, Casa Loma College, Lakeview Terrace, California.

Instructors nationwide helped by responding to the survey in preparation for the second edition.

Ginny Trost, Librarian, and Donna Otto and Barb Brandtner, Staff, of the Muehl Public Library in Seymour, Wisconsin helped enormously. No request for information was ever too much trouble, and their efforts on behalf of the second edition are appreciated. Gladys Peterson, Reference Librarian at Northeast Wisconsin Technical College outdid herself tracking down sources quickly and with a smile. Kathy Pletcher, Associate Director of the Cofrin Library at University of Wisconsin, Green Bay, helped us find the most recent statistics possible. Our husbands and adult children continue to support us in our endeavors. Friends and peers helped us with their continuing interest, understanding, and support. And finally, we acknowledge each other, colleagues and still friends after two editions. Although separated geographically, our enthusiasm for revising and our senses of humor remained intact, and we are grateful for the continuing opportunity to work "together."

CONTENTS

part I
WHO YOU ARE

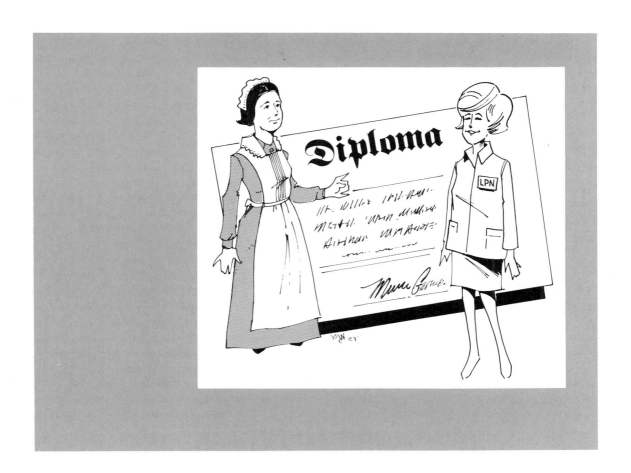

CHAPTER 1

How Practical Nursing Evolved

Learning Objectives

Upon completing this chapter you will
1. Describe the role of self-defined practical nurses throughout history.
2. Discuss four major events that influenced change in practical nursing.
3. Identify the year that the first school of practical nursing was founded.
4. Name the year that licensing for practical nursing first began.
5. Discuss your ideas on the long-range effect that the 1980s movement toward two levels of nursing will have on practical nursing.
6. Present the rationale for your personal stand on entry into nursing practice.

Practical/vocational nursing is defined as performing for a salary, or *compensation*, any simple acts in the care of convalescent, subacutely ill, chronically ill, injured, or infirm persons, or of any act or procedure in the care of the acutely ill, injured, or infirm under the specific direction of a registered nurse, physician, or, in some states, podiatrist or dentist. The length of the course for the modern trained/practical or vocational nurse is approximately one year in most states, with some variation in the actual number of weeks. Historically speaking, nurses had less educational preparation to do their work than do current trained/practical nurses.

In reviewing the varied and colorful evolution of this vocation, practical nurses are being interpreted in a broad sense, as those who from the beginning of time chose to or were appointed to care for individuals who were ill, injured, dying, or having babies. Names used to designate this person included attendant, wet nurse, self-proclaimed nurse, midwife, trained nurse, and practical nurse. Most often, the individual doing this work was someone who seemed to have a "gift" or "touch" for helping others during a medical crisis. Some "nurses" learned from others in an apprenticeship type of setting and yet others extended their "mothering" skill to the care of others. The practical nurse was the original home health nurse and visiting nurse, as much of the care was offered in the home. They were, in essence, on call for the needy. It is worth noting that as early practical-nurse training programs became available, they carefully limited their teaching to what would be known by a good homemaker or a competent maid—information that would in no way compete with the physicians of the time, who themselves had limited knowledge and training. It is also interesting to realize that nursing history does not parallel medical history. When medicine advanced, nursing did not; when medical advances slowed down, nursing progressed.

Nursing has experienced many changes throughout its history and the changes are not yet over. A major change that has occurred in practical nursing history is a gradual increase in the required formal knowledge base and required licensing in order to practice practical nursing. Contrary to the historically untrained or poorly trained practical nurse, who had unlimited, unsupervised freedom to practice, the present practical nurse is now often a hybrid, who is being taught basic skills during the educational program. After graduation the licensed practical nurse (LPN) is permitted to perform complex nursing skills delegated by the registered nurse (RN), and as allowed by the Nurse Practice Act in each individual state, as long as the RN is willing to teach the skill, observe the return demonstration, and document the teaching/learning process for the LPN's file in the place of employment. In addition, most nurse practice acts call for *direct* supervision by the RN for all complex nursing delegated by her.

Reading about nursing history can be enjoyable and can help you see your place among the many centuries of women and men who have given care, relief, and support to the sick. In this chapter we give a broad overview of the role of nursing during different periods of history. By knowing about the changes in nursing in the past, you will be ready to better understand and adapt to possible changes in the future.

Primitive Cultures

Recorded nursing history is about one and one-half centuries old, but it is interesting to speculate what may have occurred before that time. It is known that primitive cultures looked upon illness as being directly related to a personal relationship with their gods. Ill fortune, as it applied to health, was regarded as a sign of disfavor due to behavior not pleasing to the gods. Among these cultures was generally found the wise one (medicine man) who possessed magical powers to get in touch with and deal with the angered gods. For example, some pagan cultures had a shaman (holy man) who would go into a trance; while in the trance he would "slip into a crack in the Earth" to travel down the river to the "valley of the dead." There he would bargain with the gods to find out what was needed from the one who was ill or if indeed he would die. Stories of these customs were passed on through song.

ANCIENT EGYPT

Although no direct evidence exists of nursing in Egypt, written records of procedures used in ancient Egypt were probably those of the attendants (nurses) who assisted the priests in caring for the ill. Temples erected to honor the god Apollo, worshipped as the God of Medicine, became sanitariums where diseased people were treated. It is thought that Egyptian physicians and attendants four thousand years ago had an extensive list of treatments for specific illnesses. It differed rather remarkably from medicines used today. Interesting evidence was found in the tomb of an eleventh-dynasty queen, whose tomb included a medicine chest complete with vases, spoons, medicines, and herbs. "Lizard's blood, swine's ears and teeth, putrid meat and fat, tortoise brains, old books boiled in oil, milk of a lying-in woman, water of a chaste woman, lice and excreta of men, donkeys, dogs, lions and cats are examples of some of the ingredients that were used" (Kalish and Kalish, 1978, p. 3). Egyptian physicians were considered skillful at treating fractures. There is evidence of detailed instructions for daily nursing care, which included recording the pulse, the use of splints and bandages, and the use of hollow reeds for urinary catheters.

ANCIENT HEBREWS

The ancient Hebrews had houses for the sick and homes for the aged and began many practices of personal hygiene and public sanitation. Once again, the close association between religion and medicine was seen, as priests functioned in the role of major health officer.

The Old Testament makes reference to nursing functions: "Many passages refer to wet nurses, and those who nursed the sick or acted as companions. Numbers 11:12, Exodus 2:7, 2:9, II Kings 4:4, Genesis 24:59, 35:8" (Becker and Fendler, 1990, p. 28).

ANCIENT GREECE

In the fifth century B.C., the greatest civilization of all—the Greeks—gave the world **Hippocrates,** *Socrates, Plato,* and *Aristotle* and a system of logical thought that paved the way for rational treatment of illness, rather than seeing illness as god-inflicted. Hippocrates, the "Father of Modern Medicine," translated teachings, once the secrets of priests, into a textbook of medicine and introduced a system of observing symptoms and applying carefully reasoned principles to care. These observations replaced the superstitions and illogical concepts of primitive medicine. However, many of Hippocrates' teachings were discarded because of the previously established beliefs. The Hippocratic oath is the ethical code of modern medical practice. Aristotle provided additional knowledge regarding the heart and blood vessels, but because it was forbidden to touch the dead, his knowledge was not widely used.

Women did not become trained nurses in Greece because they occupied a low position in society. They were not considered worthy to be trained in medicine or nursing. Household nursing and child care was done by domestics or servants. The Hippocratic nursing procedures for the sick were carried out by the physician or the student of the physician.

AGE OF CHRISTIANITY

Greece's power and prestige declined. The Roman Empire became the mighty power about the time of Christ's birth. Rome established military hospitals, and much of the practical nursing of the day was done by relatives and friends. Much of the knowledge of the Greek Era of Power was lost in regard to medicine and nursing, because few could read and understand the works of Hippocrates and other great thinkers of his time.

As Christianity grew and the power of Rome declined, nursing developed as a form of Christian charity. Christian nursing included both men and women, each caring for members of their own sex. St. Paul, of Biblical fame, introduced a woman named Phoebe, an Ordained Deaconess, to Rome about 30 years after the Crucifixion. *Phoebe—a practical nurse—is* known as the *first visiting nurse.* In addition to the Deaconess, other orders were founded who ministered to the sick and the poor.

DARK AGES

The Dark Ages (400–1000 A.D.) were a time of violence and chaos. The Christian church retreated behind the walls of convents and monasteries. It was within these walls that learning was kept alive. The Middle Ages (1000–1450) found both men and women involved in nursing, since monks and nuns continued to do the practical, necessary nursing of that time. One of the more interesting groups of monks was the *Knights Hospitalers,* who were a military order trained to fight as well as to tend the sick and wounded.

MIDDLE AGES

One of the nursing brotherhoods founded during this time was the *Alexian Brothers,* which continues to exist in a dual religious and nursing role. The history of nursing during this period includes stories of highborn women who renounced their heritage to care for the sick. Someone needed to do the nursing, since the Middle Ages was a time of horrible epidemics, among them the infamous bubonic plague that killed millions of people. At the end of the Middle Ages, Europe seemed to be old and worn out. Religious fervor was replaced with cynicism and despair. Religious orders no longer assumed as much responsibility for care of the sick.

THE RENAISSANCE

The Renaissance (1450–1650) was a time for the rebirth of learning. The information of the Ancient Greeks and Romans was sought and put to use.

The scientific method of the Greeks was employed again. Anatomy, physiology, and scientific healing was developed. Nursing declined and was all but forgotten until the nineteenth century. It is thought that the religious reformation, in which the church split into Catholic and Protestant factions, contributed to the decline in nursing. In Protestant countries, such as England and Germany, monasticism nearly ended, and with it, nursing. Greater personal freedom may have been achieved during the Renaissance, but with it the tradition of unselfish service to humanity almost disappeared. It was a cruel age, with neglect of the poor, homeless, and ill. It is worth noting that one man, *St. Vincent de Paul,* almost single-handedly organized the *Sisters of Charity* in France to care for the poor and nurse the sick.

AGE OF INDUSTRIALIZATION

As industrialization became more widespread in the eighteenth century, so did problems with disease in provinces with widespread unemployment. The movement of people to cities, the poor working conditions, child labor, and overcrowding all had an impact on health care as related to the Industrial Revolution. Hospitals did not meet the needs of patients. Hospitals grew in number, as did their mortality rates. Many patients shared the same bed and unsanitary conditions. Medical and nursing knowledge did not include the practice of asepsis. Once inside the hospital, patients frequently contracted more diseases than what they had when they came to the hospital. Home care continued without benefit of training, although chance for survival was probably better in the home than in the hospital setting. During this time, in Vienna, women in labor begged to deliver in the street, rather than in the hospital. To be admitted meant a sure death, as the mortality rate at times was 100%. It was not until 1847 that *antiseptic methods* were first developed and used. **Ignaz Philipp Semmelweis,** a Hungarian obstetrician began to study what was called *childbed fever.* When a physician friend died following a cut on the finger during an autopsy, Semmelweis recognized that his friend had died from essentially the same disease that killed women who had babies. He identified the cause of the childbed (puerperal) fevers as septic materials carried to the mothers on the hands of medical students directly from the autopsy room. As a result, he insisted that medical students and physicians wash their hands in a solution of *chloride of lime* before entering the obstetrics ward. Antisepsis soon included instruments and utensils used in the ward. As a result, the rate of death from childbed fever dropped dramatically in that ward.

SEVENTEENTH AND EIGHTEENTH CENTURY

Meanwhile, back in the colonies, during the seventeenth and eighteenth centuries, hospital care did not exist. (Illustrations in this chapter depict historical nursing settings.) What did exist were almshouses for the poor and pesthouses for those with contagious diseases. The motivation for building the pesthouses was to

protect the public, not to treat the sick person. Medicine in America was less developed than that in Europe. Colonial physicians were poorly trained, except for the few who obtained their education in England. Nursing continued to be done by untrained persons as well as by those in a few religious orders whose mission was care of the sick. The *first real hospital in America* was built in Philadelphia in the mid-1700s at the urging of *Benjamin Franklin*. All of the early American hospitals emulated French and English hospitals and made hospitalization available to the poor for a small fee. Hospitals obtained medical services by permitting teaching on the wards. Medical advances were slow. The treatment of choice for many diseases was brandy, whiskey, emetics, purgatives, and bleeding.

NINETEENTH CENTURY

Early-nineteenth-century American hospitals were a place of confinement and a place to pick up additional disease. The hospital wards were

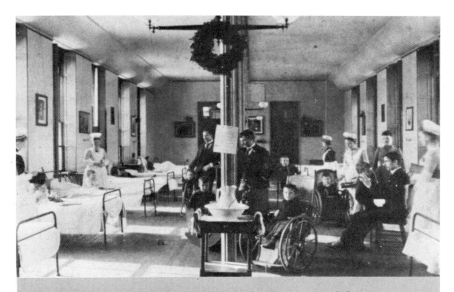

FIGURE 1-1   A pediatric unit under the aegis of the Connecticut Training School (ca. 1878). Note that there are two faculty members supervising three students. (Courtesy of Yale Medical Library.) (From Dolan JA, Fitzpatrick ML, Herrmann EK. *Nursing in Society: A Historical Perspective.* 15th ed. Philadelphia: W.B. Saunders, 1983.)

dirty, unventilated, and filled with patients with discharging wounds. Perfume was used to cover up offensive odors. Nurses of that time used snuff as a way of trying to make their work conditions bearable. Pain, hemorrhage, infections, and gangrene were the order of the day. Nursing was considered an inferior, undesirable occupation. Religious attendants (nurses) were replaced by lay people often drawn from the criminal population. They exploited and abused patients. Supervision was nonexistent and there was little or no nursing service at night, unless a delivery or a death was expected. For that, a "watcher" was hired.

Nurses were often widows with large families. Drinking on duty and accepting bribes from patients and families was commonplace. "Vice was rampant among these women, who sometimes aided the dying by removing pillows and bed clothes and by performing other mor-bid activities to hasten the end" (Kalish and Kalish, 1978, p. 28).

In Europe, nursing in secular institutions had become nonexistent, especially in Protestant countries, where the services of the Sisters of Charity were not available. Typical of the hospital nurse at the time was the ignorant, gin-soaked nurse midwife such as Sairey Gamp and Betsy Prig in Charles Dickens' 1849 novel, *Martin Chuzzlewit.*

Nursing care in America was every bit as ghastly. An extract describing the cholera epidemic in the Philadelphia General Hospital in 1833 painted a picture of overcrowding and demands for increased wages. Nurses drank the stimulant intended for the ill and were seen drunk and fighting over the dead. Finally, an appeal was made to the Bishop for the services of the Sisters of Charity. They came, restored order, and nursed the sick.

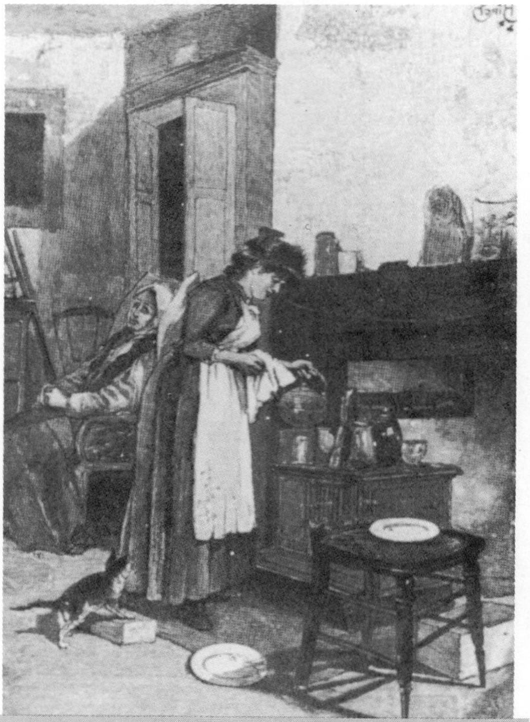

FIGURE 1-2   Caring for a sick person in a tenement house. (From Dolan JA, Fitzpatrick ML, Herrmann EK. *Nursing in Society: A Historical Perspective.* 15th ed. Philadelphia: W.B. Saunders, 1983.)

FIRST SCHOOL OF NURSING

It was not until *1836* that the *first real school of nursing* was founded. In that year a German Pastor established a hospital in his parish in *Kaiserswerth, Germany.* The purpose of the program was to teach the Lutheran Order of Deaconesses principles of nursing care. Many of the graduates of the Kaiserswerth Deaconess Institute settled in other parts of the world and established similar programs. His most famous pupil was Florence Nightingale, Founder of Modern Nursing, who attended the school for three months.

FLORENCE NIGHTINGALE

Shortly after the start of the 1853 *Crimean War* (in which Britain, France, and Turkey fought against Russia for control of the access to the Mediterranean from the Black Sea), information about neglect and poor care of casualties began to reach England. A correspondent for the *London Times* wrote vivid accounts of the deplorable conditions and lack of medical and nursing care for the British Troops. He noted that Russian Troops were tended by the Sisters of Mercy, the French tended by the Sisters of Charity and the wounded of England almost completely neglected. So persistent were his charges that a commission was sent to investigate. As a result, the Secretary of War decided that England, too, should have a group of women nurses to tend to the war casualties. He contacted **Florence Nightingale,** explaining the situation to her. Since she had both nursing and administrative experience, the Secretary of War perceived her as the one nurse in England capable of organizing and supervising care. Florence Nightingale had an unusual background for a nurse of that period. She had wealthy, influential parents, was well educated before pursuing nursing, and had been presented in court. She had to beg her parents to be permitted to take nurses training because they saw nursing as a profession for the Sairey Gamp type of woman.

Being appointed to the task of organization and supervision of nurses during the Crimean War gave Miss Nightingale an unexpected opportunity for achievement. She left England for Crimea with 38 self-proclaimed nurses of limited experience, of which 24 were nuns.

Florence Nightingale and her nurses arrived to find overcrowded, filthy hospitals with no beds, no furniture, no eating utensils, no medical supplies, no blankets, no soap, no linens, and no lamps. The barrack hospital, meant for 1700 patients, packed in 3000 to 4000 patients.

The wounded lay on the floor, in their battle uniforms, in filth. Florence Nightingale took charge, using the supplies she had, and personally raised funds to purchase supplies the doctors could not obtain for the army. She hired people to clean up the "hospitals" and established laundries to wash linens and uniforms. It was not an easy task, and a major prejudice to overcome was that of the medical officers, who considered the nurses intruders. The hours were long and difficult for Miss Nightingale and her nurses. Often after hours, it is said that Miss Nightingale could be seen making additional rounds with her lamp to check on the patients—earning her the name "Lady with the Lamp." By the end of six months, it was obvious that the efforts of Miss Nightingale and her nurses were paying off. The death rate among the wounded

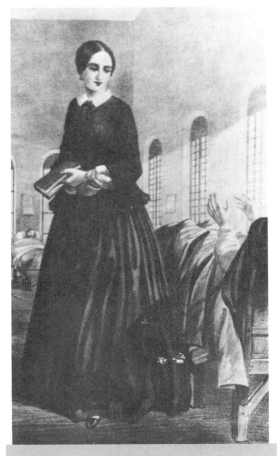

FIGURE 1-3 Florence Nightingale carrying out the "nursing process." (Nursing Mirror Photograph.) (From Dolan JA, Fitzpatrick ML, Herrmann EK. *Nursing in Society: A Historical Perspective.* 15th ed. Philadelphia: W.B. Saunders, 1983.)

dropped from 420 per 1000 to 22 deaths per 1000 casualties. She stayed through the war and was the last to leave. Many of her nurses had become ill during the war and were sent home to recover. Miss Nightingale herself became ill with Crimean Fever and almost died. When she returned home she was decorated by Queen Victoria.

*Santa Filomena**

Whene'er a noble deed is wrought,
Whene'er is spoken a noble thought,
 Our hearts, in glad surprise,
 To higher levels rise.

The tidal wave of deeper souls
Into our inmost being rolls,
　　And lifts us unawares
　　Out of all meaner cares.

Honour to those whose words or deeds
Thus help us in our daily needs,
　　And by their overflow
　　Raise us from what is low!

Thus thought I, as by night I read
Of the great army of the dead,
　　The trenches cold and damp,
　　The starved and frozen camp—

The wounded from the battle plain,
In dreary hospitals of pain—
　　The cheerless corridors,
　　The cold and stony floors.

Lo! in that house of misery,
A lady with a lamp I see
　　Pass through the glimmering gloom,
　　And flit from room to room.

And slow, as in a dream of bliss,
The speechless sufferer turns to kiss
　　Her shadow, as it falls
　　Upon the darkening walls.

As if a door in heaven should be,
Opened, and then closed suddenly,
　　The vision came and went—
　　The light shone and was spent.

On England's annals, through the long
Hereafter of her speech and song,
　　That light its rays shall cast
　　From portals of the past.

A lady with a lamp shall stand
In the great history of the land,
　　A noble type of good,
　　Heroic womanhood.

Nor even shall be wanting here
The palm, the lily, and the spear,
　　The symbols that of yore
　　Saint Filomena bore [22].

---

*Henry Wadsworth Longfellow (His tribute to Florence Nightingale, "Saint of the Crimea." Published in the first number of the *Atlantic Monthly,* November, 1857.)

One of Florence Nightingale's major goals was to establish a school of nursing. An overwhelming number of physicians opposed the school of nursing on the basis that "because nurses occupied much the same positions as housemaids, they needed little instruction beyond poultice making, the enforcement of cleanliness and attention to their patients personal needs" (Kalish and Kalish, 1978, p. 43). Miss Nightingale did establish a school of nursing in 1860 in England and wrote several books on nursing; her most famous book was *Notes on Nursing.* She emphasized high moral character in addition to technical skills. Her philosophy included absolute obedience. She believed nurses should work only in hospitals, not private duty. To her, nursing was a sacred calling, not a business. Miss Nightingale was against licensure, seeing it as being too much like a union. Her major contributions were to eliminate prejudice against a better class of women entering nursing and to generate the push for development of nursing as a respectable vocation.

In the spring of 1989, the Florence Nightingale Museum opened in London, England on the grounds of St. Thomas Hospital, the site of the Nightingale School of Nursing. The Museum is a tribute to this nursing leader despite the fact that Miss Nightingale wrote the following before her death: "I do not wish to be remembered when I am gone" (quote from Nightingale's personal journal as found in museum).

CIVIL WAR

Meanwhile, back in America, when the United States entered the Civil War in 1861, there was no such thing as a trained nurse. In the South, especially, there was a great deal of prejudice regarding women working in hospitals. There was general male opposition, but specifically, opposition from the medical profession. As a southern belle put it, "It seems strange that what the aristocratic women of Great Britain have done with honor is a disgrace for their sisters on this side of the Atlantic to do" (Kalish and Kalish, 1978, p. 49).

Table 1-1 Practical Nursing Milestones

PERIOD IN HISTORY	EVENT
Ancient Egypt	Untrained attendants assisted priests in caring for the ill.
Ancient Hebrew	Wet nurses and attendants who nursed the sick and acted as companions.
Ancient Greece (fifth century B.C.)	Household nursing and child care done by domestics and servants.
Age of Christianity	Both men and women were nurses; each cared for members of own sex. *Phoebe*—The first visiting nurse
Dark Ages (400–1000)	Monks and nuns continued to do practical nursing. *Knights Hospitalers*—A military order trained to fight as well as to tend the sick and wounded.
Middle Ages	Time of epidemics. Highborn women renounced their heritage to care for the sick. *Alexian Brothers* founded—A nursing brotherhood that still exists in a dual religious and nursing role. At the end of the Middle Ages religious orders no longer assumed as much responsibility for care of the sick.
Renaissance (1450–1650)	Scientific methods of Greeks employed again, but nursing declined until the 19th century.
Age of Industrialization (18th century)	Deplorable, unsanitary conditions. Untrained care givers. *Semmelweiss*—Developed antiseptic methods (1847).
17th- and 18th-century colonies	Almshouses and pesthouses. Nursing done by untrained persons.
19th-century America	Nursing considered an inferior, undesirable occupation. Care given by untrained lay people often drawn from the criminal population. Charles Dickens novel *Martin Chuzzlewit* (1849) introduced Sairy Gamp and Betsy Prig as the nurse prototype of that period.

Table continued on the following two pages.

1836	First real school of nursing, in Kaiserswerth, Germany. *Florence Nightingale* attended for three months. Eighteen years later, after start of Crimean War, she nursed wounded with 38 self-identified (untrained) nurses.
1860	*Florence Nightingale* established a school of nursing in England. She wrote several books. The most famous was *Notes on Nursing.*
Civil War (1861)	In the South: Most nursing done by infantrymen assigned to task. Southern women volunteered services. In the North: *Dorothea Lynnde Dix,* a teacher, was appointed Superintendent of Nurses and organized a corps of female nurses (untrained).
1868	*Clara Barton,* a teacher, collected supplies for soldiers. Led to her appointment as Superintendent of the Department of Nurses for the Army.
1881	*Clara Barton* established the first chapter of the *American Red Cross* in Danville, New York.
1892	First class for formal training of practical nursing: YWCA, Brooklyn, New York.
1893	*Henry Street Settlement* founded by *Lillian Wald,* a social worker, who graduated from a nursing program. *Practical nurses* pioneered in this new public health movement. They went into homes and taught to families in New York slums the basics of cleanliness and control of communicable diseases.
1914	*Mississippi* is the first state to pass a law to *license practical nurses.*
1917	*Standardization* of nursing requirements for practical nursing by *National League of Nursing Education.*
World War I	Shortage of practical nurses. Army School of Nursing established. *Smith Hughes Act* of 1917 provided money for developing additional schools of practical nursing.

1920s	Acute shortage of practical nurses. Many did not return to nursing after the war.
1920–1940	Most practical nursing limited to Public Health Agencies and Visiting Nurse Associations.
World War II	At home, practical nurses worked in clinics, health departments, industries, hospitals. In the war, ventured into hardship tours in Europe, North Africa, and the Pacific. Number of practical nurses peaked in 1940 at 159,009.
1941	*NAPNES* (National Association for Practical Nurse Education and Service), the nation's professional organization dedicated exclusively to practical nursing, was founded.
End of World War II	Nursing shortage saw movement of practical nurses into hospitals and gradually increasing responsibilities.
1944	Comprehensive study of practical nursing by U.S. Department of Vocational Education. This was the first time that tasks of practical nursing were agreed upon.
1949	Joint Committee on Practical Nurses and Auxiliary Workers in Nursing Services recommended use of title "licensed practical nurse" and differentiated between tasks of registered nurses and licensed practical nurses.
1952	Approximately 60% of the nurse work force was made up of practical nurses.
1960s	ANA (American Nurses Association) first moves toward two distinct levels in nursing—professional and technical.
1980s	Resurgence of ANA's move toward two distinct levels of nursing. This resulted in some states adopting two levels of nursing and then rescinding their decision because of the nursing shortage.
1990s	The American Medical Association (AMA) initiated and consequently dropped the Registered Care Technician (RCT) proposal. It is hoped the nursing shortage will ease in the near future.

Casualties were high on both sides; many died right on the field; others died because of a poorly trained medical corps. Southern women offered their services as volunteers, but most of the nursing was done by infantrymen assigned to do a task they did not want to do. It was well into the war before the Southern women were recognized by the Confederate government for their contribution.

In the North, women offered their services to the government for nursing. One hundred women were selected to take a short training course from doctors in New York City. **Dorothea Lynnde Dix,** a teacher by profession and a long-time advocate for better conditions for mental patients, was appointed Superintendent of Nurses. Her task was to organize a corps of female nurses. She requested women under 30, plain-looking, wearing simple brown or black dresses and no bows, curls, jewelry, or hoop skirts. Women who did not meet the criteria nursed anyway, but without official recognition or pay from the government. Eventually, through Dix's effort hospitals for the mentally ill were established.

In evaluating the Civil War nursing, doctors decided that the nursing system was defective; they did not approve of the women. However, it was a success in the eyes of the wounded soldiers.

Clara Barton, a teacher by profession, was one of the first civilians in the Civil War to round up army supplies. She rented a warehouse, filled market baskets and encouraged friends to send comforts for the soldiers. Her efforts resulted in her being appointed Superintendent of the Department of Nurses for the Army in 1868. Clara Barton's efforts frequently found her on the front lines, and she nearly lost her life on two occasions. After the war, President Lincoln commissioned her to do what she wanted to do—find missing prisoners of war. Later, while visiting in Europe for health reasons, she met *J. Henri Dunant,* founder of the *International Red Cross.* He asked her help in introducing the Red Cross to America. Finally in 1881, through Clara Barton's efforts, the first chapter of the *American Red Cross* was established in Danville, New York.

As often happens, something good emerges out of something not so good. Many of Florence Nightingale's books and ideas had made their way to America, but had been ignored. The Civil War experience was the impetus to developing nurse training schools. The first training schools were separate from the hospitals, the intent being to educate the nurse. Soon, hospital-based schools of nursing sprung up. In many hospitals, this became a cost-effective way of providing a nursing labor force, that is, free. Being a student nurse in the 1870s was a difficult experience. Living conditions, working hours, and responsibilities required a great deal of physical and emotional endurance. Not only did these students work long hours, but they were required to sign contracts in return for a course of lectures, on-the-job training, and minimal allowances.

FORMAL TRAINING: PRACTICAL NURSING

The *first* class for formal training of practical nursing was offered in *1892 at the YWCA in Brooklyn, New York.* The focus was on training nurses for home health care of patients with chronic illness, the aged, and children. The course was three months in length. The course was considered successful, and because of this, other similar programs were developed. Identified programs included an 1892 program in Boston, under the Massachusetts Emergency and Hygiene Association, the *Ballard School in New York in 1897,* and the *Brattleboro School in Vermont in 1907.* The course of study included cooking, care of the house, dietetics, simple science, and simple nursing procedures.

Until World War I most nursing for the practical nurse was home nursing, primarily because most people were cared for in the home. Even surgery was performed in the home. There is some truth in the way old western movies portray surgery being done on the kitchen table. The nurse's 24-hour schedule included such procedures as cupping and applying *leeches,* preparing *stupes* for relief of abdominal distention, *mustard plasters* for relief of congestion, *poultices* for drawing out pus from infections, and administering *enemas.*

These were often nutritive enemas containing eggnog with brandy or chicken broth. Remember, there were no intravenous solutions then. Some practical nurses also assumed the then-accepted role of midwife and taught to new mothers the basics of cleanliness, diet, and care of the child. In New York City in 1919 approximately 1700 midwives attended 30% of all births in the city.

By the end of the nineteenth century there was a renewed interest in charitable work and concern for the sick. Practical nursing began to extend from home nursing to public health nursing, care of patients in the slums, school nursing, industrial nursing, and well-baby care. Once again, practical nurses pioneered in this new public health movement. One of the best-known centers in **1893** was the **Henry Street Settlement in New York.** It was founded by **Lillian Wald,** a social worker who graduated from nursing and intended to become a doctor. She taught home nursing to immigrants and was so impressed by their need for medical care that she left medical school to begin a nursing service, The Henry Street Settlement. From here, the practical nurses who were members of the Henry Street Settlement went out and taught to families in New York slums the basics of cleanliness and control of communicable disease. There was a decrease in school absenteeism because of reduced spread of childhood illness. School nurses visited schools and new mothers and their babies. They taught mothers the basics of preventing the summertime killer of infants—cholera infantum. It was estimated that their efforts resulted in 1200 more babies than usual surviving the summer heat wave. Another original contribution of the nurses was to develop "Little Mother Leagues" in the slums, in which all girls over eight years old were taught to take care of their younger siblings, including the infants.

TWENTIETH CENTURY: ORGANIZATION/LAW/ LICENSING

By 1903, states began to take steps that ultimately led to monitoring of practical nursing. It was during this period that nursing organizations were developed. Certainly the most influential step was taken by the *National League of Nursing Education* (now the National League for Nursing, or NLN), who in 1917, developed a system for nationwide standardization of nursing requirements for practical nursing.

In 1914, *Mississippi* was the first state to pass a law to license practical nurses. This was an important event, since the public had no way of knowing who was giving them nursing care. Remember, that for centuries, self-proclaimed nurses were responsible for the majority of the nursing that was done. Licensing, however, was not mandatory and by *1938, New York* was the *only state to have mandatory licensure.*

QUESTION: Does your state have mandatory licensure?

At the onset of World War I, there were few practical nurses and few practical nursing schools. Hurriedly "trained" nurses were rushed to the battlefront. An army school of nursing was established to combat the severe nursing shortage and to improve the overall quality of care. Many nurses looking for glamour and excitement found superhuman demands made of them during the war.

The home front was facing a battle of its own in 1917–1918, with a major epidemic of pneumonia in 1917 and a worldwide epidemic of Spanish Influenza in 1918. The mortality rate was high, especially in 1918. The *Smith Hughes Act of 1917* did provide money for developing additional schools of practical nursing. However, the new schools could not supply enough nurses quickly enough to meet the severe shortage on the home front.

After the war, many nurses did not return to nursing. There was an acute shortage of nurses in the 1920s. Many hospitals had schools of nursing attached—their real purpose being staffing. Hospitals without schools were staffed heavily with untrained help.

In the period between the two World Wars, 1920–1940, six states had laws to license practical nurses, but there were few practical nursing schools throughout the country. Much of their work continued to be in public health agencies and in visiting nurse associations.

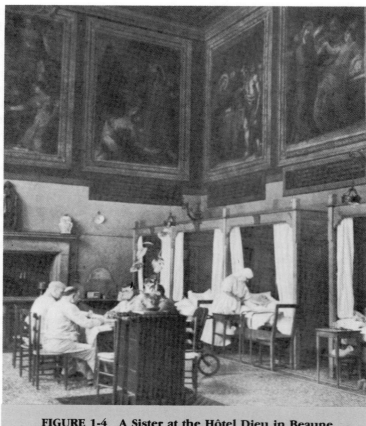

FIGURE 1-4   A Sister at the Hôtel Dieu in Beaune giving care to a patient in a room compartment. Ambulatory patients enjoy meals at the table in the center. Note the works of art. (From Dolan JA, Fitzpatrick ML, Herrmann EK. *Nursing in Society: A Historical Perspective.* 15th ed. Philadelphia: W.B. Saunders, 1983.)

During the depression of the 1930s, many nurses lost their jobs or worked in hospitals for room and board rather than a salary. When it became fairly obvious that America was becoming involved in World War II, nursing leaders began to prepare for surpluses of all kinds of nurses. They did not want to face the nursing shortage experienced during World War I. This was a monumental task, since nursing had decreased in popularity as a vocation. Much of the dialogue then sounded a great deal like that of the mid-1980s. For example, a hospital executive was quoted as saying, "Nurses should either get off their high horses and do the physical work they started out to do or move over and let others do it. There is too much talk about 'high professional standards' and not enough about taking care of the sick" (Kalish and Kalish, 1978, p. 501). In the 1990s, nursing continues to search for its role both as a vocation and as a profession.

Practical nurses played a significant role both at home and in the war. At home, practical nurses worked in clinics, in health departments, in industry, and at keeping hospitals open. In the war, nurses could be found in Europe, North Africa, and the Pacific. One of the most widespread diseases they battled was malaria in the East Indies, the Philippines, and the Southern Asiatic countries. The number of practical nurses in America peaked in 1940 at 159,009 and by 1944 was already experiencing a decline.

NAPNES (The National Association for Practical Nurse Education and Service, Inc.) was founded in 1941. It is the nation's professional organization dedicated exclusively to practical nursing. The multidisciplinary composition of its membership includes licensed practical nurses, registered nurses, physicians, hospital and nursing-home administrators, students, and public members.

This association was the first to be recognized by the U.S. Department of Education as an official accrediting agency for schools of practical nursing. (Accreditation allows students of these schools to be eligible for federal loans and grants.) The Council of Postsecondary Accreditation (COPA) confirms NAPNES as a reliable authority as well as an accreditation agency of practical nursing programs. For the past several years, NAPNES has no longer accredited practical nursing programs.

The end of World War II saw a continuing shortage of nurses. It was this shortage that helped practical nurses play an important part in hospital nursing. Most hospitals gradually increased the responsibilities designated to the practical nurse.

In 1944, the U.S. Department of Vocational Education made a comprehensive study of practical nursing. This was the first time that the tasks of practical nursing were agreed upon. Extensive specific duties were outlined with an emphasis on maintaining aseptic technique and sterilization. The terms "to judge," "to appraise," "to recognize," and "to determine" were often used to describe the scope of the practical nurse's job.

Other important changes followed. In 1949, the joint committee on practical nurses and auxiliary workers in nursing services recommended use of the title "licensed practical nurse." Furthermore, the committee differentiated between the tasks of the RN and the LPN and saw the LPN as being under the supervision of the RN. The committee also suggested that practical nurses organize to make decisions on their salary, working conditions, and employment standards.

Because of the work of the joint committee, many practical nursing programs were strengthened in regard to content, and focus was, for the first time, on the preparation of practical nursing instructors. Up to this point, any graduate nurse was eligible to teach practical nursing.

By 1952, almost 60% of the nursing work force was made up of practical nurses. In many instances, RNs expressed a great deal of bitterness because hospitals, clinics, and other agencies were hiring practical nurses for less money and assigning tasks to them beyond their educational level. They also expressed concern that the public was unable to differentiate between the levels of nursing, since both wore the same white uniforms, caps, and pins. Many practical nurses quickly stopped wearing the practical nursing insignia, which was meant to identify the practical nurse. In many agencies, the pay continued to be poor and the role of the practical nurse vacillated between doing tasks belonging to the RN one day and then being assigned as a nursing aide, for lesser compensation, on other days. Many practical nurses felt trapped in situations such as these because of their need for employment.

In 1961, the *National League for Nursing (NLN),* established a separate department of practical nursing programs. A major breakthrough was developing a system for *accrediting schools* of practical nursing. This was supported by the *American Nurses Association (ANA)* and the *National Federation of Licensed Practical Nurses (NFLPN).* To be accredited by the NLN, a school had to meet standards set by the NLN. With the exception of programs receiving federal funds, it was not, nor is it now, mandatory for schools to be accredited by the NLN, since major responsibility for approval of nursing programs rests with each State Board of Nursing. In some states, responsibility for accreditation is shared jointly with the Department of Education, Vocational Division. It is this accreditation that gives permission for practical nursing programs to operate.

The 1960s brought a move by the ANA to streamline nursing into two distinct levels: the two-year technical and the four-year professional nurse.

In 1975, there were 1337 training programs graduating a total of 46,080 practical nurses. Approximately two thirds of the practical nurses were employed in hospitals, 17.3% in nursing homes, 7.5% in private duty, and 6.5% in doctors' offices, clinics, and dental offices. Admission standards in most schools increased, as did the difficulty of the curriculum.

In the 1980s a resurgence of the ANA movement toward two levels of nursing temporarily gained serious momentum. Some states worked toward adoption of the ANA recommendation.

The professional and vocational nursing organizations took a position for or against the ANA recommendations

- NAPNES went on record as opposing the two levels of nursing

- NLN supported the two levels of nursing and offered their own proposal in 1986. (As in 1989, NLN again supports the practical nursing role and is focusing on how the practical nurse is used in the national health care agenda.)

- NFLPN continued to support maintaining the titles Licensed Practical Nurse and Licensed Vocational Nurse, but recommended an increase in education from 12 to 18 months.

Because a serious nursing shortage developed in the late 1980s, the ANA movement lost momentum.

With the goal to ease the nursing shortage, the American Medical Association in the summer of 1989 proposed a new health care worker, the Registered Care Technologist (RCT). The RCT would be trained in one- and two-year programs. Because this new level of health care worker correlated with existing health care workers, the practical and the associate-degree nurse, the RCT proposal has not been successful. This event is a gentle reprimand for practical nurses to be strong, organized, and vigilant as a group. New efforts to propose new programs and legislation detrimental to the practical nurse role could be initiated at any time (Howlett, 1990).

During 1987–1988, 26,912 students graduated from practical nursing programs in the United States. During 1989–1990, 35,417 students graduated from practical nursing programs—a substantial increase (Nursing Data Source, 1991, p. 40).

As of 1990, 1154 practical nursing programs continue (Nursing Data Source, 1991, p. 23). Employment is available in hospitals and clinics, with nursing homes employing a large number of LPNs. Home health care is once again emerging, because of shortened hospital stays. Difficulty in collecting third-party payments for Medicare patients cared for by practical nurses continues to be a problem in some states. Some agencies are dealing with this by hiring practical nurses as aides and paying them accordingly. Clearly, there is a need for legislative changes.

Practical nurses are also finding employment in insurance companies that handle medical claims, in wellness and diet centers, in veterinarian's offices, as industrial nurses, as private nurses for physicians, and in the armed forces.

What is clear is that the practical nurse continues to be needed, to give skilled, technical care to patients in many areas—hospitals, nursing homes, home care, clinics, etc.—and the country continues to experience a nursing shortage.

*I*MPORTANT INFLUENCES IN NURSING HISTORY

Many RNs influenced the course of nursing and practical nursing history. Table 1-2 identifies some of those registered nurses.

*Y*OU HAVE COME A LONG WAY

As a final note, it may be interesting to compare present practical nursing tasks with those that you would have been expected to perform in 1887. Practical nursing has indeed come a long way.

Table 1-2 Some Persons/Events in Nursing History

Mary Robinson	1859	First visiting nurse
Linda Richards	1873	America's first professionally trained nurse; organized other training schools
Euphemia Van Rensselaer	1876	Introduced first uniform—apron and cap (Bellevue Training School for Nurses)
Mary E.P. Mahoney	1879	First black graduate nurse
Elizabeth Weston	1888	First Native American nurse. Graduate of Training School of the University of Pennsylvania. Came from Lincoln School for Indian girls in Philadelphia. After graduation returned to care for her people on a Sioux reservation in North Dakota.
Emily L. Loveridge	1890	Graduate of Bellevue Training School for Nurses. Went west to establish first school of nursing in northwest at Good Samaritan Hospital, Portland, Oregon.
Isabel Hampton Robb	1893	Wrote first substantial nursing text: *Nursing: Its Principles and Practice for Hospital and Private Use.*
Lillian Wald, Mary Brewster	1893	First visiting nurse service for poor: Nurses Settlement House in slum section, lower east side, New York City. Later moved to Henry Street and name changed to Henry Street Settlement House.
Lavinia L. Dock	1896	First president of forerunner of ANA (Nurses Associated Alumnae of the United States and Canada). Outlined principles on which ANA was founded.
Dita H. Kinney	1901	First nurse Superintendent of Nurses of Army Nurse Corps

Table continued on the following page.

Mrs. Bedford Fenwick (Great Britain)	1901	First president of International Council of Nurses. Proposed state registration of nurses.
Adelaide Nutting	1907	First graduate of John's Hopkins Training School for Nurses. First nurse in the world to hold professorship in a university (Columbia). In 1917 Chair of Committee to Develop National Curriculum.
Lillian Wald, Ella Phillips Crandall, Mary Beard, Mary Lent, Edna Foley, Lystra Greiter, Elizabeth G. Fox	1912	Formed National Organization of Public Health Nurses. Lillian Wald, first president.
Annie W. Goodrich	1918	President of ANA. Became Chief Inspecting Nurse for Army hospitals at home and abroad. Supported formation of Army School of Nursing. Became dean of school.
Margaret Sanger	1916	Spearheaded birth control movement as a response to high maternal and child mortality. A public health nurse. Opened first birth control clinic in America.
Mary Breckenridge	1925	Organized Frontier Nursing Service of Kentucky
Sage Memorial Hospital School of Nursing, Ganado, Arizona	1930	First school of nursing for American Indians
Lucile Petry	1943	Director of U.S. Cadet Nurses Corps
Esther Lucille Brown, Ph.D., a researcher	1948	"Brown" Study: Advocated movement of nursing education to collegiate setting
Mildred L. Montag	1952	Appointed as first Associate Degree Nursing Program Project Coordinator. Project based on Montag's doctoral thesis, "Education of Nursing Technicians." Project located at Queen's College, New York.

The following job description was given to floor nurses by a hospital in 1887 (author unknown):

In addition to caring for your 50 patients, each nurse will follow these regulations:

1. Daily sweep and mop the floors of your ward, dust the patient's furniture, and window sills.

2. Maintain an even temperature in your ward by bringing in a scuttle of coal for the day's business.

3. Light is important to observe the patient's condition. Therefore, each day fill kerosene lamps, clean chimneys, and trim wicks. Wash the windows once a week.

4. The nurse's notes are important in aiding the physician's work. Make your pens carefully; you may whittle nibs to your individual taste.

5. Each nurse on day duty will report every day at 7 A.M. and leave at 8 P.M., except on the Sabbath, on which day you will be off from 12 noon to 2 P.M.

6. Graduate nurses in good standing with the director of nurses will be given an evening off each week for courting purposes or two evenings a week if you go regularly to church.

7. Each nurse should lay aside from each pay day a goodly sum of her earnings for her benefits during her declining years so that she will not become a burden. For example, if you earn $30 a month you should set aside $15.

8. Any nurse who smokes, uses liquor in any form, gets her hair done at a beauty shop, or frequents dance halls will give the director of nurses good reason to suspect her worth, intentions, and integrity.

9. The nurse who performs her labors and serves her patients and doctors without fault for five years will be given an increase of five cents a day, providing there are no hospital debts outstanding.

Summary

The varied and colorful evolution of practical nursing is described with limited reference to roles played by RNs in the course of nursing history. This is an attempt to have the practical nursing student recognize that her vocation began to develop in ancient times, and is not an appendage of professional nursing. Practical nurses can be rightfully proud of their own nursing "roots." Table 1-2 lists some of the RNs who played a major role in the advancement of nursing.

The duties of practical nurses have changed according to the need present at any time in history. Currently, practical nurses are taught basic skills during their educational program. According to some state's Nurse Practice Acts, they are allowed to perform complex skills delegated by an RN. However, in these states, the RN must teach the complex skill involved, be satisfied with the LPN's performance, and document this for the LPN's file. Direct supervision by an RN is also required for performance of complex nursing acts.

In the 1990s practical nurses continue to play an important role in the health care system. The 1980s resurgence of the ANA movement toward two levels of practice was thwarted by the severe nursing shortage during the late 1980s.

If you choose, you can have a voice in the decision for your vocation. Consider the odds faced by these historical figures in nursing:

Florence Nightingale, founder of modern nursing
Clara Barton, founder of the American Red Cross

Lillian Wald, founder of public health nursing

Dorothea Dix, advocate for the mentally ill. First hospitals for mentally ill were built because of her efforts.

No more frontiers you say? Don't you believe that. You can, for example, begin by reading the most current proposals on the levels of nursing and taking a stand through your vocational organization—the local and state Practical Nurses Association.

It has been suggested by some that the history of practical nursing sounds depressing. Not so. Practical nurses have always been on the forefront of doing the real, down-to-earth nursing tasks. They have often done what no one else dared or cared to do. In the beginning most of these "nurses" had little or no training—consider that Florence Nightingale herself left the Kaiserswerth Deaconess Institute training program after three months of training. It is with this in mind that this chapter has focused on figures in nursing history who had limited education and yet, enormous courage to take care of patients—most often without glamour or fanfare. What these nurses did have was the gratitude of their patients and the quiet satisfaction of a job well done. We salute you, the new practical nurses and the nurses who have paved the way for you.

*R*EFERENCES

ANA Report. Trained attendants and practical nurses. Am J Nurs 1944; 44:7–8.

Becker B. and Fendler D. *Vocational and Personal Adjustments in Practical Nursing.* Philadelphia: J.B. Lippincott, 1990, p. 28.

Brown E. *Nursing for the Future.* New York: Russell Sage Foundation, 1948.

Deming D. Practical nurses—a professional responsibility. Am J Nurs 1944; 44:36–43.

Etheridge L. National Commission on Nursing. Written testimony Public hearing. February 1981.

Goldsmith J. New York's Practical Nurse Program. Am J Nurs 1942; 42:1026–1031.

Hill S. *A historical comparison of nursing in England and America* (unpublished paper), 1982.

Howlett H. *History of the Entry into Practice Issue* (unpublished paper), 1990.

Kalish P, Kalish B. *The Advance of American Nursing.* Boston: Little, Brown, 1978.

Kinder J. President NLN. Letter, Nov. 1986.

Nursing Data Source, 1991. Vol. II. *Focus on Practical/Vocational Nursing.* New York: National League for Nursing, 1991.

Philips E. Practical nurses in a public agency. Am J Nurs 1944; 44:974–975.

Spalding E. *Professional Adjustments in Nursing.* 3rd ed. Philadelphia: J.B. Lippincott, 1946.

The Political Works of Longfellow, Cambridge Edition. Boston: Houghton-Mifflin, 1975.

Thompson M. *Cry and the Covenant.* New York: Signet Books, 1955.

CHAPTER
2
Assisting with Nursing Process

Learning Objectives

Upon completing this chapter, you will
1. Discuss what is meant by the nursing process.
2. Explain what is meant by assisting with the nursing process.
3. Describe the practical nurse's responsibility in the following steps of the nursing process:
   a. Assessment
   b. Planning
   c. Implementation
   d. Evaluation

If someone asked you what a nurse does, what would you say? One way to answer would be to describe the *nursing process*. The nursing process is a way of nursing, and is the basis for individualizing patient care. The four steps you would describe would be methodically assessing the patient's strengths, needs, and problems; planning the care; implementing the care; and evaluating the effectiveness of the care that is provided.

Table 2-1 Relationship of Practical Nurse's Role in the Nursing Process to ANA Standard of Practice

ANA STANDARD OF PRACTICE: 1973	NURSING PROCESS
I. The collection of data about the health status of the client/patient is systematic and continuous. The data is accessible, communicated, and recorded.	Step 1—Assessment (LPN role—assisting with assessment)
II. Nursing diagnoses are derived from health-status data.	Step 2—Nursing diagnosis (Formulating the nursing diagnosis is an RN role)
III. The plan of nursing care includes goals derived from the nursing diagnosis.	Step 3—Planning (LPN role—assisting with planning)
IV. The plan of nursing care includes priorities and the prescribed nursing approaches or measures to achieve the goals derived from the nursing diagnosis.	
V. Nursing actions provide for client/patient participation in health promotion, maintenance, and restoration.	Step 4—Implementation (LPN role—assisting with implementation)
VI. Nursing actions assist the client/patient to maximize his health capabilities.	
VII. The client's/patient's progress or lack of progress toward goal achievement is determined by the client/patient and the nurse.	Step 5—Evaluation (LPN role—assisting with evaluation)
VIII. The client's/patient's progress or lack of progress toward goal achievement directs reassessment, reordering of priorities, new goal setting, and revision of the plan of nursing care.	

The registered nurse (RN) has major responsibility for the steps of the process, which includes an additional step to those listed above. That step is Step 2 and is called "Nursing Diagnosis" or simply "Diagnosis." This step is considered to be an RN's responsibility exclusively, because the judgment leading to the diagnosis statement is based upon the RN level of education. Basically, even as a charge nurse in a nursing home, the role of the LPN remains that of a dependent practitioner. Regardless of how remote the supervision or direction, the LPN always works under the direction or supervision of the RN, medical doctor, podiatrist, or dentist. The RN is an independent practitioner in most functions. An example of dependent RN functioning is in drug administration: The doctor prescribes the drug for the RN to administer. This same distinction holds true with the nursing process. As a practical nurse, you are expected to take an active role in four of the five steps of the nursing process, under the supervision of the RN.

Nursing process is a method of organizing care so that the patient will receive the most benefit. Each step depends on the previous step's being completed properly. The steps of the nursing process are as follows:

Step 1—Assessment
Step 2—Diagnosis (RNs only)
Step 3—Planning
Step 4—Implementation
Step 5—Evaluation

It is important to note that the nursing process as currently interpreted, relates to the American Nurses Association Standard for Practice. Table 2-1 shows how each of the eight standards of practice relate to the nursing process steps as presented in this chapter.

The term *nursing process* has been used since the mid-1950s. In reality, organization in delivery of patient care has always been a part of nursing. The most common method used prior to the nursing process was called the problem-solving process. As you will see in Table 2-2, problem solving is a part of the nursing process. Note that here, Assessment (Step 1) is missing. Knowledge of the problem is often assumed in the problem-solving process. Gathering data is most often used to support the problem statement. It is a significant difference that assessment is Step 1 in the nursing process and that diagnosis (defining the problem) is Step 2, based on data that has been obtained in an organized way.

Knowledge of the problem-solving process is a major resource to help you learn the nursing process. You have used it throughout your life to solve problems of daily living. The same is true for nurses whose educational background did not include the nursing process. They too

Table 2-2 Problem Solving versus Nursing Process

PROBLEM-SOLVING PROCESS	NURSING PROCESS
1. Define the problem	Step 2—Diagnosis
2. Decide on the goal	Step 3—Planning
3. Identify alternatives	
4. Choose an alternative	
5. Try out the alternative	Step 4—Implementation
6. Evaluate the effectiveness	Step 5—Evaluation
7. Repeat the process if the solution is not effective	

Based on Bauer and Hill, 1986, p. 188.

can learn the nursing process by building on the knowledge of problem solving.

Each of the steps take practice. Some steps include learning new skills. However, none of the steps are complicated.

QUESTION: How have you used the problem-solving process to deal with a problem during the past week?

ASSISTING WITH ASSESSMENT

Step 1 of the nursing process is assessment. Assessment means gathering as much significant information about the patient as is possible. The practical nurse has an important role in assisting with assessment. What is included in the role varies according to the place of employment and the individual skills of the practical nurse. The practical nurse generally assumes greater responsibility in regard to assisting with assessment in the nursing home, where the patients' condition is considered more stable.

The assessment includes not only gathering data, but also checking it for accuracy and grouping the information to help identify patterns of health or illness. It will be helpful to look at each of these activities separately. First of all, gathering data begins immediately upon admission and continues throughout the patient's stay at the institution. The immediate resource for data, when possible, is the patient. After all, he knows himself and his body better than anyone else. Family members are also helpful in adding to the information. When available, information that arrives with the patient from other agencies adds to the knowledge base, as does the medical diagnosis, doctor's orders, laboratory studies, and progress notes of doctors, nurses, and other health professionals.

Information is gathered by observation, interview, and examination. Observation requires use of all the senses: seeing, hearing, smelling, touching, and yes, sometimes even taste. You observe the patient's general appearance, physical characteristics, personal hygiene, behavior, and more. Each agency has its own format for

information to be obtained during the interview. Again, the LPN's responsibility varies according to the area of work involved.

You are expected to be accurate in gathering information. Avoid asking questions that have been asked before. Be sure that you have looked at the record and know as much as possible before you begin the interview. Make sure the patient is comfortable and at ease and able to participate in the interview. Explain to the patient why you are asking questions and reassure him that he has the right not to answer questions that make him feel uncomfortable. Be a good listener; encourage confidence. There is a difference between listening and hearing. Hearing is physiologic. Listening is the interpretation of the spoken word. Listening will take conscious effort on your part. If the patient is encouraged to talk, he will become more at ease. Question things that concern you—"Pardon me?" "Will you repeat that?" Offer general leads such as "Oh," "Yes," and "Go on." Share observations without drawing conclusions, such as "You are trembling." Acknowledge feelings when appropriate—"It must be difficult." Request clarification rather than pretending that you understand—"I am not sure that I understand what you mean by that statement." Check out what you think you understand—"Am I correct in saying that you are worried about the kind of care you will receive here?" Avoid using reassuring promises that you cannot deliver—"Don't worry, everything will be just fine." Also avoid giving advice, since what may work for you may not be right for this patient. Avoid giving approval—"That's right."—as this may make it difficult for a patient to change his mind. Nursing responsibility involves giving the very best care possible and does not involve judging the patient's behavior, values, or decisions. Finally, avoid showing and verbalizing disapproval and belittling the patient—"You know you shouldn't do that." Chapter 13 on "Job-Related Communication" elaborates on interviewing techniques that will assist you in making the best use of the often limited time that you have to obtain needed data from the patient. Use of therapeutic communication and blocks to therapeutic communication are expanded on. The authors recommend that you read Chapter 13 soon, to enhance your knowledge base for the nursing process. When learning how to check information for accuracy, validating it becomes necessary to learn how to differentiate between subjective and objective data. Subjective data is what the patient feels. Sometimes it will be demonstrated by objective signs. For example, the patient states he feels very warm (subjective); the patient has a temperature of 102°F (objective).

The following patient complaints are strictly subjective: headache, pain, apprehension, dislike. But there can easily be an objective counterpart to each of the above complaints. It is necessary that you look for objective data to corroborate the subjective data, and in this way, assist in checking the accuracy of the information offered by the client. Both subjective and objective data are included in the nurses' notes. Identify the source for subjective data by using "The patient states." There are possible barriers to gathering information about the patient to which you must be alert. They include insufficient time, poor skills in interviewing, communication failure (such as the comatose patient), distractions, a patient who is too sick to want to talk. What can happen readily, if your personal values get in the way, is labeling the patient before the interview is complete, instead of basing decisions on facts. Respectful distancing is necessary for the nurse to remain objective and to use all senses clearly.

The physical assessment is an important part of gathering data. RNs are taught how to do physical assessment of patients as a part of their basic education. Physical assessment for the LPN is a postgraduate course, which some LPNs take and others do not. The additional education, acuity of the patient, and area of employment all determine the extent of the practical nurse's involvement in physical assessment. In acute-care settings the practical nurse is often limited to taking admission vital signs, height, and weight.

When all the data are gathered, you will assist the RN in looking for gaps in information that will need further checking. It is by grouping the information that you assist in beginning to identify patterns of health and illness. Comparing all of the newly obtained data to other information, such as the medical (doctor's) di-

agnosis, laboratory reports, and all other available data sets the stage for establishing the nursing diagnosis. When you are assisting in looking at the total data, remind yourself of the difference between patient problems and nursing problems. Patient problems are unmet needs—physical, psychological, social, financial, spiritual, and so on—which nurses may or may not be able to meet. Nursing problems are unmet needs of the patient, which can be changed by nursing care. And finally, remind yourself that even the best nurse is limited in how much she can change the pattern of illness in some situations.

NURSING DIAGNOSIS

Formulating the nursing diagnosis is exclusively the RN's responsibility. However, you need to have knowledge of what nursing diagnosis is, and how you can make it work for you in order to give the best possible care to the patient.

Nursing diagnosis is an actual or potential health problem of an individual, family, or group that nurses can treat independently, initiating the nursing interventions necessary to prevent, resolve or reduce the problem." Nursing diagnosis is separate from medical diagnosis—the doctors' labeling of the patient's disease condition. Nursing diagnosis is also separate from collaborative problems.

According to Carpenito (1989), collaborative problems are those that may occur as a result of complications of disease, diagnostic studies, or treatments and are prevented, resolved, or reduced by working together (collaborating) with the doctor or other health professionals. Nurses differentiate nursing diagnosis from collaborative problems by asking the question "Can the nurse initiate treatment independently to prevent, resolve, or reduce the problem?" When the answer is "Yes," nursing diagnosis is appropriate. When the answer is "No," the nurse will have to have direction from another health care giver, such as the doctor. Remember the earlier example of the RN's dependent function—that of giving medication. The doctor will order medication to treat a disease condition and the nurse will carry out these directions: A collaborative solution to a problem and a dependent nursing function.

Writing a nursing diagnosis is based on a list of nursing diagnoses. This list is called the NANDA list meaning the list developed by the North American Nursing Diagnosis Association. RNs are encouraged to use the approved list in order to share a common language with other nurses. When doctors use medical diagnosis, all other doctors know exactly what is meant by the terms they use. Nursing diagnosis intends to create a communication bridge for all nurses, so that they will understand each other's terminology.

When you read a nursing diagnosis on the patient's care plan, you will note a two-part statement. The statement includes the *human responses* (how the patient responds to a state of health or illness) and *related factors* (why it is occurring, when known). For example, impaired skin integrity R/T (related to) immobility.

The word *risk* is used to start the statement if the condition described in the diagnosis is not an *actual* problem.

NURSING DIAGNOSIS	OUTCOME
Impaired skin integrity R/T immobility	Mr. Jones will have intact skin over coccyx within _____ days.

Most importantly, how can you make your knowledge of nursing diagnosis work for you? The nursing diagnosis pinpoints the priority problems for the patient and is the key to individualizing patient care.

ASSISTING WITH PLANNING

Step 3 of the nursing process is planning the patient care. You, as an LPN, have major contributions to make in this planning, which includes assisting with setting priorities, establishing realistic patient-centered outcomes, determining nursing approaches to help achieve the outcomes, and documenting the plan of care (charting).

In order for a care plan to be a usable, realistic tool for nursing staff, priorities must be established. It is unrealistic to include on the care plan every problem that the patient has. The most important problems, those that are potentially life threatening, must be taken care of immediately. It is not uncommon to be working on several problems at the same time and to find a relation between problems. Priorities may also change rapidly depending on the patient's condition. There is a great need for you to remain flexible and to recognize the need to shift priorities according to patient needs. The patient, of course, will be far more cooperative with his care if he has been included in identifying priorities of care.

Think back to Step 1, assessment. Did you remember to ask the patient what he expects/wants/needs during the time that he is a patient (important information as you assist the RN in planning the care)? Did you also remember to assess patient strengths—the pluses in his life; what he can do for himself? Strengths are the building blocks for developing a realistic plan. For example, if the patient has the capacity to feed himself, this is a strength to be encouraged, rather than feeding the patient, because it is "faster and less messy."

Specific outcomes provide direction for individualizing the care of the patient. In order to be useful, outcomes must be patient-centered, clear and concise; describe observable and measurable behavior; be realistic and time-limited; and be determined by the patient and the nurse together. The focus of the outcome is on the patient, not the nurse. To get the desired results, an outcome must be set for each priority problem or need. Terminology will vary to some degree. Some agencies use the terms *goals* or *behavioral objectives*. "Regardless of what they are called, the purpose is the same—

they define how the nurse and the client know that the human response identified in the diagnostic statement has been prevented, modified or corrected" (Iyer et al., 1991, p. 122).

If a problem is considered to be temporary, such as a fever or inadequate food and fluid intake, it should be listed as a temporary problem (TP) in the care plan, so that it is not overlooked. Temporary problems are short-term problems with resolution within a brief period of time. As temporary problems are resolved, resolution is indicated on the care plan according to agency policy (Bauer and Hill, 1986, pp. 32–33). The following example shows how the patient's care plan may look at this point now that a nursing diagnosis has been written and realistic, measurable, time-limited outcomes

have been established for a top-priority problem.

Note that all outcome statements are written positively: what the patient will expect to happen within a reasonable amount of time. "Measurable" answers the question "How will I know?" Read the goals again, with that question in mind.

Specific approaches indicate a plan of action that relate directly to the problem (nursing diagnosis) and offers a possible solution. The possible solution offered should indicate movement toward the desired outcome. With every plan of action there should be a rationale or reason given for using that particular approach. As an example, let us continue with the care plan started in the previous example.

OUTCOME	NURSING INTERVENTION
1. Mr. Jones will have intact skin over coccyx within _____ days (list actual time).	1. Turn Mr. Jones every 1½ hours (reduction of pressure).
	2. Massage all bony prominences and up to and around coccyx area (increase circulation).
	3. Use pillows to maintain position.
	4. Position on back for 20 minutes only, four times per day (decrease pressure on involved area).
	5. Use chart at bedside to indicate time and position.
	6. Increase fluid intake to 1000 ml per shift while awake. Likes water and apple juice (increase hydration—promotes healing).

When the date stated arrives, the effectiveness of the approach will be evaluated and adjustments made as needed.

Finally, documenting the plan of care is essential, because legally, if it isn't charted, it wasn't done. Many agencies have advanced into the computer age for documenting on patient records. Whether documenting on the computer or the traditional handwritten progress

notes, the patient-care plan must be the guideline. After all, this is the plan for individualizing patient care, and the flow charts and progress notes show that the plan was followed and indicate progress or lack of progress in following the plan. Ideally, flow sheets have been developed to record all important routine-care items. That means that the progress notes include charting by exception only, that is, those exceptional items that cannot be covered in the flow sheets. If this rule of charting by exception only is permitted in the agency, duplication of charting is avoided and valuable nursing time is released for other nursing tasks.

ASSISTING WITH IMPLEMENTATION

The fourth step of the nursing process is implementation, that is, nursing interventions/actions related to the nursing diagnosis and outcomes. Implementation is putting the plan into action. Again, your responsibility will vary according to the work area in which you are involved. In an acute-care setting your primary responsibility will be to use the care plan as your guideline for giving direct patient care, continuing data collection, giving verbal reports to the RN, and charting. In the nursing-home and extended-care setting, you may be functioning in the role of a charge nurse and have responsibility for managing patient care under the supervision of the RN. The key for all of your activity, regardless of your position and agency involved, is to use the care plan as the basis for your nursing action. For example, as a student, you draw information from the care plan on how to provide individualized patient care. While providing care, you continue to make observations based on your knowledge of the patient's strengths and disease conditions. You chart on flow sheets and nurses' notes, following the priorities indicated by the nursing diagnosis, plus any new observations. You use the care plan as your guideline when reporting to the RN and offer information on any changes you have noted. Specifically, you speak to the nursing interventions outlined in the care plan: Do they continue to be appropriate? What change or lack of change did you observe? In this way, the RN is able to update the plan of care and needs only to validate the data. Your use of the care plan is

similar when you function as an LPN staff nurse, in an acute-care facility. As an LPN charge nurse, in a nursing home, you manage care by directing the other LPNs and aides in the use of the care plan, demonstrating care of more-difficult patients, and checking periodically to be sure that the care plan is being followed. When receiving a verbal report at the end of the shift, you take notes to pass on to the RN for rapid updating of care plans on a daily basis—an efficient cycle.

ASSISTING WITH EVALUATION

Evaluation is the fifth and final step of the nursing process. Have you noticed how heavily dependent each step of the care plan is on the others, and how the steps are often going on simultaneously? Evaluation begins as soon as nursing care is implemented, and the continual data collection helps to make daily evaluation part of the natural flow of good nursing care.

Evaluation involves taking a critical look at how effective the nursing action has been. It involves checking to see if the care was delivered as planned, if the outcomes were achieved, what got in the way, and modifying the plan of care or terminating the care if all involved, including the patient, are satisfied with the outcome. The sources used for information on evaluation include the patient responses, patient's record, daily observations, and input from all members of the health team—this includes you.

In many agencies, a formal, extensive evaluation of patient care, called a nursing audit, is a part of ensuring quality care. A nursing audit team has a specific format, which is used as a guideline to examine patient records for proof of follow-through on the nursing process, patient response to the care that is given, plus legally correct documentation of care.

Summary

The nursing process is specific to nursing and is an organized way of individualizing patient care. The LPN's role is to assist with assessing planning, implementing, and evaluating care under the supervision of the RN. The RN is responsible for establishing the nursing diagnosis. The LPN's role in the use of the nursing process varies according to the personal skill of the nurse and agency policy. The patient-care plans that are developed as a result of the nursing process are guidelines for individualizing daily patient care. Use of the care plans by all health providers ensures continuity of patient care and a greater possibility of reaching the established goals.

REFERENCES

American Nurses' Association. Standards of nursing practice. Kansas City, Mo.: American Nurses Association, 1973.

Bauer B, Hill S. *Essentials of Mental Health Care Planning and Interventions*. Philadelphia: W.B. Saunders, 1986.

Carpenito L. *Nursing Diagnosis*. 3rd ed. Philadelphia: J.B. Lippincott, 1989.

Gordon M. *Nursing Diagnosis: Process And Application*. 2nd ed. New York: McGraw-Hill, 1987.

Iyer P, Taptich B, Bernocchi-Losey D. *Nursing Process and Nursing Diagnosis*. Philadelphia: W.B. Saunders, 1991.

Kozier B, Erb G. *Fundamentals of Nursing Concepts and Procedures*. 3rd ed. Menlo Park, Calif.: Addison-Wesley, 1987.

Taptich B, Iyer P, Bernocchi-Losey D. *Nursing Diagnosis and Care Planning*. Philadelphia: W.B. Saunders, 1990.

Yura H, Walsh M: *The Nursing Process*. East Norwalk, Conn. Appleton & Lange, 1988.

CHAPTER 3

The Health Care Team and the Nursing Team

Learning Objectives

1. Identify the personnel that make up the health care team.
2. Explain, in your own words, the goal of the health care team.
3. Define nursing.
4. Describe the personnel that make up the nursing team according to the following criteria:
   a. education
   b. role and responsibilities
   c. licensing
5. Describe, in your own words, the following methods to deliver nursing service:
   a. case
   b. functional
   c. team
   d. primary care
6. Describe the practical nurse's role in the methods to deliver nursing service listed in 5.

WHO IS RESPONSIBLE FOR MR. JORDAN'S DISCHARGE?

Introduction

Anthony Jordan, age 76, has had a stroke affecting the left side of his brain that resulted in some slurring of speech and weakness in the extremities of the right side of his body. After 7 days in the hospital, he was discharged and went home with some improvement in his speech and increased function of his right side. Sounds like another success story for nursing, doesn't it? We will follow Mr. Jordan as he progresses through the health care system and let you decide who should get credit for Mr. Jordan's condition on discharge.

Mr. Jordan's Emergency Care

Mr. Jordan lives on a 200-acre farm in rural Wisconsin. When he first shows symptoms of a stroke, his daughter calls the ambulance to transport her father to the nearest hospital, located 20 miles away in a city of 75,000 people. The three persons manning the ambulance are EMTs (Emergency Medical Technicians). Each EMT had taken an approximately 120-hour course in basic life support skills, and each had been certified as an EMT by means of a national test. If Mr. Jordan had lived near a larger urban area, paramedics, persons with a more advanced five-month course in life support training and skills, might have responded to the ambulance call. On the way to the hospital, the EMTs monitor Mr. Jordan's blood pressure, pulse, and respirations and level of consciousness (he is awake, but confused), and maintain contact with the hospital emergency room by means of a two-way radio.

Upon arriving at the emergency room, the EMTs provide the registered nurse with a verbal and written report of Mr. Jordan's status. The emergency room doctor examines Mr. Jordan, and on the basis of this examination, the vital signs, and observations of the registered nurse and the EMTs, diagnoses Mr. Jordan as

having had a cerebral vascular accident (stroke) due to a cerebral thrombosis (clot) and admits him to the intensive care unit, under the care of his family physician. In order to be in charge of the medical care for Mr. Jordan, the family physician has had four years of college, four years of medical school (a program that provides the basic knowledge and skills needed to be a medical doctor), one year of internship (a program of clinical experiences to complete the requirements for licensure as a practicing physician), and approximately a three-year residency program (a program for medical doctors, to prepare them for practice in a medical specialty—family practice in this situation. The emergency room doctor has had the same education as the family physician, but took a residency program in emergency or trauma medicine). Both doctors passed their boards, which licenses them as medical doctors. The nurse who receives Mr. Jordan in the emergency room and observes and cares for him until he is admitted is a graduate of a diploma or three-year program in nursing, and has passed a national examination to become a registered nurse. This registered nurse participates regularly in continuing education courses at the hospital and at seminars given regionally and nationally for emergency room nurses. Mr. Jordan is admitted to the intensive care unit.

Intensive Care—A Time of Close Observation

The intensive-care unit (ICU) is staffed by registered nurses who went to school for either two years (Associate Degree Nurses), three years (Diploma Nurses), or four years (Baccalaureate Nurses). Each nurse has taken the same national examination to become a registered nurse. None of these nurses are qualified to work in the intensive care unit immediately upon graduation from their various programs. Most institutions prepare a nurse for the responsibilities of this unit through in-service classes after a minimum amount of experience or a postgraduate/continuing education course. Mr. Jordan's nurse is a two-year graduate and is responsible for care and observation of two patients. The family is unable to answer some questions about Mr. Jordan's medical history, so the family physician asks the clerk receptionist (ward clerk) to obtain his medical records from the medical records department. The clerk receptionist assumes the responsibility for many of the clerical duties that are a necessary part of any patient care area, such as arranging for laboratory and x-ray examinations; transcribing doctor's orders; requisitioning repairs, supplies, old records, and dietary trays; and sending charges for supplies used. The clerk receptionist learns these skills by taking a course that varies in length, depending on the area of the country, and averages about 120 hours of theory and clinical experience. The medical records department is staffed by personnel who have gone to school from two to six years to learn the skills involved in indexing, recording, and storing patient records, which are legal documents. Thanks to Mr. Jordan's old records, which are found and sent to the intensive-care unit very quickly, the family physician has answers to his medical questions. The physician writes admission orders for Mr. Jordan, including an order for an anticoagulant to help prevent further thrombi (clots) from forming, thereby reducing the risk of additional strokes. The hospital pharmacist, who studied for five to six years to become licensed to prepare, compound, and dispense drugs when prescribed by a physician or dentist, fills the order for Mr. Jordan's drugs and intravenous solutions.

Since the drug heparin prolongs the time it takes blood to clot, the laboratory draws a sample of blood and obtains the result of a clotting time before each dose of heparin is scheduled to be given. Lab personnel have varied educational backgrounds, that range from one year for a laboratory assistant, to four plus years of college for a medical technologist (MT), who can be certified by a national examination. Lab personnel are responsible for collecting specimens needed for lab tests, treating and analyzing these specimens, and informing doctors and registered nurses of test results.

The family requests that their parish priest be contacted to give Mr. Jordan the Sacrament of the Sick. The Roman Catholic priest anoints Mr. Jordan with holy oils, prays with him, hears his confession, and gives him Holy Communion.

To be able to meet Mr. Jordan's spiritual needs, the priest has had four years of college and four years of theology before being ordained. The x-ray department is called to take a portable admission chest x-ray in the intensive-care unit, and the radiologic technician brings the x-ray equipment to the bedside. This health care worker has had a minimum of preparation in a two-year program conducted by a hospital or technical school, and is prepared to perform diagnostic and therapeutic measures involving the use of radiant energy. When Mr. Jordan's family physician checks the results of the chest x-ray, the radiologist (a medical doctor with a residency program in radiology, the reading and interpretation of x-rays) informs the family physician that Mr. Jordan has had atelectasis (collapse of some of the tiny air sacs in the lung that exchange carbon dioxide [a waste product of the body] for oxygen). The respiratory therapy department is contacted to evaluate Mr. Jordan's respiratory state and suggest treatment to prevent respiratory problems. The respiratory therapist is an expert in meeting respiratory needs of patients and administering treatments ordered by a physician. The respiratory therapist receives his education in a two-year technical-school program or a four-year collegiate program. Two days after admission, Mr. Jordan is judged to be in stable condition and is transferred to the medical floor.

Medical Floor—An Eye to Discharge

The head nurse on the medical floor at this hospital is a registered nurse who graduated from a four-year program and, as manager of the unit, is responsible for all the care given to patients. Mr. Jordan's team leader is a registered nurse from a two-year program who is responsible for formulating a plan of care for each of the assigned patients and modifying these plans as needed.

The team leader receives a verbal report and the current care plan for Mr. Jordan from the ICU personnel and begins assessment of the new admission. The practical nurse helps put Mr. Jordan to bed and immediately takes his vital signs. The licensed practical nurse is a graduate of a one-year vocational program in nursing and has taken a national examination to become licensed as a practical nurse. Although a patient on heparin is not considered stable, since Mr. Jordan is conscious, his vital signs are stable, and is showing signs of improvement, the practical nurse is assigned to give him bedside care. A referral is sent to the physical therapy department, so that they can assess the level of functioning of Mr. Jordan's right side. The physical therapist assesses the amount of strength and mobility of Mr. Jordan's right arm and leg and begins a program of exercises and treatments that will help restore as much function as possible. The physical therapist is educated in a four- or five-year college program; many physical therapists have a Master's Degree. The physical therapy assistant is educated in a two-year community college or technical-school setting.

Another referral is sent to the occupational therapy department. Since Mr. Jordan is right-handed, the occupational therapist helps him to learn to use his weak right hand and arm so that he will be able to care for himself and be as independent as possible. The educational requirements needed to help patients restore body function through specific tasks and skills includes a four-year occupational therapy program at the college level with some graduates choosing to pursue Master's Degrees in their field. Occupational therapy also has a two-year program to prepare occupational therapy assistants. The third referral for Mr. Jordan involved the speech therapist, a health professional who has been educated with a minimum of a four-year college degree. The speech therapist suggests exercises for Mr. Jordan, in order to strengthen muscles required for speech and swallowing. Soon after being transferred to the medical floor, the social worker visits Mr. Jordan and his family to discuss discharge plans. Unless there is a change in his condition, the family states that they want to care for Mr. Jordan at home instead of having him complete his rehabilitation at an area nursing home. Social workers help patients and families solve problems with the financial concerns of hospitalization. They arrange for community agencies to provide appropriate care and services needed

by patients at home and help the family communicate their health care needs more clearly. Social workers are educated in college programs, obtaining a Bachelor's Degree in four years and a Master's Degree in one additional year of college. Mr. Jordan's social worker talks to the physical, occupational, and speech therapists and they all agree that with exercise and skills teaching, the family can adequately care for Mr. Jordan; the professionals encourage Mr. Jordan's continued rehabilitation at home.

As Mr. Jordan gets closer to discharge, a nursing assistant (nurse's aide) is assigned to assist him with his personal care. Nursing assistants are educated to give bedside care by courses of at least 85 hours' duration. The family physician prescribes a restricted-salt diet, so the dietician comes to teach Mr. Jordan and his wife about this type of diet. The dietician is responsible for planning meals for patients and staff, supervising the preparation of food, and counseling patients and their families about nutritional problems and therapeutic diets. This health professional is educated in a four- to five-year college program, followed by a year of internship in a health agency. Every day during Mr. Jordan's stay, the housekeeper cleans his room and bathroom in an effort to maintain medical asepsis (absence of germs) and provide a pleasant environment. The housekeeper receives training in needed skills by the employing institution or through a short course in a technical school.

Who is responsible for Mr. Jordan's discharge? After reading this scenario, you can see it is impossible to give any one member of the health care team credit for sending Mr. Jordan home.

THE HEALTH CARE TEAM

A primary goal of health care is optimal physical, emotional, and spiritual health for all persons. This goal is accomplished by promoting health, preventing illness, and restoring health when illness has occurred. Because of increases in knowledge and technology, it is necessary for groups of people to work together to provide patients with all the services they need for comprehensive health care. These groups of health care workers are called the health care team. It took a minimum of 85.5 years of education in order for the various health care workers to learn to do their respective jobs, so that Mr. Jordan could be discharged from the hospital. The occupational, physical, and speech therapists; pharmacist; and nursing staff were involved in restoring Mr. Jordan's health and preventing further illness by avoiding complications. The x-ray technician's chest x-ray film pointed out a potential complication that could have been life-threatening, and the treatments by the respiratory therapist helped prevent pneumonia. The dietician's expertise accounted for Mr. Jordan receiving the basic nutrients he needed to maintain his health. Teaching Mr. and Mrs. Jordan about low-sodium diets was a measure to promote health, in an attempt to keep his blood pressure within acceptable limits, thus eliminating one risk factor for additional strokes. As you can see, each member of the health care team, with their specific preparation in a field of study, can increase the quality of health care for a patient. It is impossible for one person to provide the knowledge, expertise, and skills that the health care team as a whole provides.

Each member of the health care team must have good communication skills, so that care can be coordinated for the patient's benefit and fragmentation of care can be avoided. The team must continually strive to keep their care patient-oriented, and realize that a cooperative effort is needed to reach patient goals.

WHAT IS NURSING?

Just what is nursing and what do people on the nursing team do? In 1979, the American Nurses Association (ANA), a national organization and the official representative for all professional nurses in the United States, defined nursing as the "diagnosis and treatment of human responses to actual or potential health problems" (*Nursing—A Social Policy Statement,* 1980, p. 9). Another often-used definition of nursing, which complements the definition by the American Nurses Association, is "the unique

function of the nurse is to assist the individual, sick or well, in the performance of those activities contributing to health or its recovery (or to peaceful death) that he would perform if he had the necessary strength, will or knowledge" (Henderson, 1966, p. 15). The ANA's definition includes the diagnosis of responses to health problems and the second definition includes the ill or well person, both important considerations for nursing in general. It is important for practical nurses to understand their role in nursing. The direction of practical nursing has been channeled by the above definitions. An understanding of the members of the nursing team with regard to education, licensure, and roles and responsibilities is necessary.

THE NURSING TEAM

Members of the nursing team include unit managers, registered nurses, licensed practical nurses, student nurses, nursing assistants, and ward clerks. The members of the nursing team are generally on duty in health care institutions 24 hours a day, seven days a week. Some other members of the health care team are not available at night or on weekends or holidays. Some of these persons are available on an on-call basis.

Registered Nurses (Professional Nurses)

Today there are 1.6 million registered nurses employed in nursing (Moses et al., 1991, p. 27). Although 3% of registered nurses are male, nursing remains a female-dominated profession. The graduates of the three types of nursing-education programs for professional nursing—two-, three-, and four-year programs—currently take the same licensing examination and, upon successful completion, hold the title "registered nurse." Associate Degree programs are found in community colleges, junior colleges, and technical schools. The educational program involves general-education courses, including the biologic, behavioral, and social sciences, in addition to nursing-theory courses and clinical practice. Upon graduation, the two-year (Associate Degree) graduate receives an associate degree in nursing and is eligible to take the NCLEX-RN examination (licensing exam) to become a registered nurse. Three-year programs (diploma programs) are usually associated with a hospital and are conducted by a hospital-based school of nursing. The educational program involves the same general-education courses as the two-year programs, as well as nursing-theory courses. Diploma programs traditionally emphasize clinical experience. The three-year graduate receives a diploma in nursing, and upon graduation is eligible to take the NCLEX-RN examination to become a registered nurse. Four-year (Baccalaureate) programs are found in colleges and universities, and emphasize course work in liberal arts, sciences, and nursing theory. Upon graduation, the four-year nurse receives a Bachelor of Science degree in nursing (B.S.N.) and is eligible to take the NCLEX-RN examination to become a registered nurse.

Graduates of all three programs are prepared for general-duty staff nursing in a hospital or nursing home. Although you may find two- and three-year registered nurses in supervisory and administrative positions, only baccalaureate graduates have been prepared for advancement to these positions. Baccalaureate graduates are also prepared for beginning positions in public health agencies and are the only nursing graduates that may elect to go on to do graduate work in nursing at the Master's and Doctoral level. In 1988, graduates of Associate Degree programs in nursing outnumbered BSN (Bachelor of Science in Nursing) graduates, while the number of diploma graduates continued to decline. This education mix is expected to continue (Moses et al., 1991, p. 27).

All registered nurses function under the nurse practice act of the state in which they are working and use the nursing process to formulate a nursing diagnosis and plan of care for each patient. Frequently, the plan of care is the blueprint that auxiliary personnel use to meet patient goals. The registered nurse delegates routine care and the care of stable patients to auxiliary personnel so that she may have time to carry out the roles of planner of care; coordinator of all the activities of the plan of care;

giver of care that requires more specialized knowledge and judgment; teacher of patients, families, and other members of the nursing team; and patient advocate. The registered nurse functions independently in nursing, initiating and carrying out nursing activities. For example, the registered nurse, in the assessment of a patient on bedrest, will identify the need for a turning routine, deep breathing, leg exercises, and range-of-motion exercises, in order to prevent complications in the respiratory and circulatory systems. Registered nurses will include these nursing interventions on the plan of care without obtaining a doctor's order. Because of her level of education, the registered nurse knows which patients can and cannot have these nursing interventions on the plan of care. When the registered nurse carries out the legal orders of another health professional, for example the physician or physical therapist, she is functioning in a dependent role. Frequently, the registered nurse functions interdependently when decisions regarding patient care are made jointly by members of the nursing and health care team. It is the registered nurses' independent role in decision making that distinguishes them from other members of the health care team. The registered nurse has the ultimate responsibility for care given to patients. Nurse practitioners and clinical nurse specialists are registered nurses who have obtained additional nursing education experience in specialty areas.

Practical Nurses

In 1989, The National Council of State Boards of Nursing, the organization that administers the licensing examination for practical nurses, identified the number of active LPN licenses at 887,802. Remember, some persons may have licenses in several states and some RNs also hold practical nursing licenses (Nursing DataSource, 1991, p. 17). The educational program for practical nurses in most states is approximately 12 months long. The practical nursing program is found in trade, technical, and vocational schools as well as community colleges. These institutions are usually public, tax-supported institutions. Practical nursing programs can also be found in private schools. Theory is offered in the biologic and behavioral sciences and nursing, in addition to clinical experience. Upon graduation, the practical nurse receives a diploma or certificate in nursing and is eligible to take the NCLEX-PN examination to become a licensed practical nurse. Practical nurses must be aware of the contents of the nurse practice act of the state in which they are employed, as their role is found in this law and the law differs from state to state.

Practical nurses are bedside nurses when they are working in health care institutions. Practical nurses give care to patients who are stable and require nursing interventions that do not involve specialized knowledge. These nurses function under the direction of the registered nurse, physician, podiatrist, or dentist at all times. Practical nurses are also caring for patients who are more seriously ill; this reflects the practice of discharging patients from hospitals for continued recuperation in extended-care units and nursing homes—places that are hiring more and more practical nurses. Because practical nurses work under another professional's direction, their role is called a dependent one. Although employers expect practical nurses to problem solve in patient care situations, the registered nurse is available to help in decision making when questions arise during implementation of the plan of care. Refer to your state's nurse practice act to determine the circumstances under which you may function with direct or general supervision of a registered nurse. Practical nurses function interdependently when they offer input to the registered nurse regarding the effectiveness of the plan of care or offer suggestions to improve the patient's plan of care. Since practical nurses are bedside nurses, their observations are valuable in helping meet patient goals. The practical nurse's dependent role is a major criterion in differentiating between the roles of the registered and practical nurses. Practical nurses must realize, however, that although they function dependently, they must function responsibly. That is, practical nurses must function safely and are accountable for their actions; they should assume responsibility only for

nursing actions that are within their role and/or that they feel safe in carrying out. Differences between the LPN and the RN are stated in Table 3-1.

Student Nurses

Student professional and practical nurses come to the clinical area under the supervision of clinical instructors, as an extension of the classroom and to have the opportunity to apply theory to practice. When assigned to patients, the students have the responsibility of giving safe care and functioning responsibly under the supervision of the instructor. Since these students are going to the clinical area to learn and not to give service, it is possible that a clinical instructor can remove them at any time for additional learning experiences. Students, however, are a member of the nursing team and are expected to assist other team members as needed—for example, passing trays, answering call lights, and assisting patients. These activities help students learn how to get along in a team situation. Student nurses are responsible for giving the same safe nursing care that graduates provide, and this is a legal matter. Therefore, the student role demands preparation and supervision.

Nursing Assistants

Excluding home health aides, there are approximately one million nursing assistants in the United States (Rowland, 1984, p. 511). Nursing assistants can be trained for their positions on the job by combining federally mandated classroom instruction with close supervision by registered nurses while in the clinical area. Vocational schools offer programs that last a minimum of 85 hours and that combine classroom instruction with clinical practice. During the course, testing for competencies occurs to meet federal OBRA requirements. When testing is satisfactory, the names of nursing assistants are placed on a registry. Some states have these health-care workers place NA-R (Nursing Assistant-Registered) after their names. Nursing as-

Table 3-1 Differences between the RN and the LPN Using the Five Roles of the Professional Nurse (RN) as a Guide

FIVE ROLES OF RN	RN	LPN
Professional	Belongs to and is actively involved in ANA at state and local level.	Belongs to and is involved in NFLPN at state and local level.
Provider of care	Independent role	Dependent role
Manager of care	Controls decisions regarding staff and care of clients.	First-line manager in nursing home/extended care. Responsible to nurse manager.
Teacher	Initiates all health teaching.	Initiates health teaching for health habits (nutrition, cleanliness, etc.) Reinforces health teaching of RN in all other areas.
Researcher	Theory included in four-year program. All levels interpret and implement research findings. Participates in the research process.	Theory not included in one-year program. Assists in implementing research findings.

sistants who work in hospitals, nursing homes, extended-care units, or psychiatric hospitals assist in providing for personal and comfort needs of stable patients, under the direction of registered or practical nurses. They are assigned routine tasks, often involving housekeeping chores. A large number of nursing assistants are employed by nursing homes. The increasing complexity of care needed by nursing home patients has led to a discussion of the need for more skilled health care workers in these settings. Some nursing assistants receive additional education and are employed in private homes as home health aids. People in some areas of the country refer to male nursing assistants as orderlies.

Ward Clerks (Clerk Receptionist/Health-Unit Clerk/Health-Unit Coordinator)

The job of the ward clerk is mainly secretarial in nature, but the duties vary from hospital to hospital. With the ward clerk performing this job, nurses are freed from much of the paperwork involved in patient care. Ward clerks are trained on the job or in programs of several months' duration in technical schools. Ward clerks prepare, compile, and maintain patient records on a nursing unit. Other duties include scheduling lab tests, x-ray procedures, and surgery; scheduling other appointments for services; routing charts upon transfer or discharge; compiling the patient census; answering the phone; maintaining established inventories of supplies; and distributing mail to patients.

Unit Managers

Some large health care institutions have unit managers to supervise and coordinate management functions for patient units. Some college background and supervisory experience is desirable for this position, and it is combined with on-the-job training for specific duties. Functions include supervision of ward clerks, assignment and evaluation of clerical personnel, inventory of patient's valuables, coordination with housekeeping and maintenance, and clarification of hospital compliance with Medicare requirements (Rowland, 1984, p. 378). If a health care institution does not have unit managers, some of these duties would be given to the ward clerk or head nurse. In some agencies, the head nurse is known as a nurse manager.

*T*HE DELIVERY OF NURSING SERVICE

The nursing team uses several different methods to assign patients, with the goal of providing optimal care. The different methods evolved as a response to changing needs in staffing of nurses. Each of the methods will be discussed in its general form, as it was intended to function. Keep in mind that health care institutions will modify these methods to fit their individual needs.

Case Nursing

At the turn of the century, families hired nurses to meet a patient's special needs in the home. By the 1920s, private-duty nursing was popular, and this case nursing method continued in degrees into the 1960s. Vestiges of case nursing, or a one-to-one relationship with a patient, can be found today as total-care nursing (comprehensive care), a method in which one nurse is assigned to one or two patients and is responsible for the total care of these patients. Today, total care occurs in the intensive care or special care units, as Mr. Jordan experienced when he was first admitted. Nursing instructors frequently use the total-patient-care method when assigning students to the clinical area.

Functional Nursing

In the 1950s, functional nursing was a popular method of patient assignment, because registered and practical nurses were in scarce supply. Functional nursing is task-oriented and the tasks that are needed to be done for patients are divided among the staff. An example would be one person taking all temperatures, another measuring all the blood pressures, and still another making all the beds. This method's emphasis on efficiency and division of labor is based on the assembly-line–production concept found in industry (Rowland, 1984, p. 237).

The nursing home nearest Mr. Jordan's home schedules patient assignments by the functional method. If he had spent some time there, he would have had a nursing assistant help him with his physical care and a practical nurse give him his medications and do his treatments. The charge nurse, a registered or a practical nurse, would be kept busy with managerial and nonnursing duties, in addition to having responsibility for all care given to patients. Functional nursing can easily overlook holistic care, especially the area of psychological needs, and result in fragmentation of care. Although this method is efficient and appears to be less costly to implement, it can discourage patient and staff satisfaction. The functional method could work well in times of critical shortages of personnel.

Team Nursing

After World War II, team nursing was introduced because of the increasing numbers of practical nurses and nursing assistants. Team nursing is more a philosophy than a method. It is the belief that goals can be achieved through group action. The patients on a unit are divided into small groups, and small teams are assigned to care for the patients in each group. Assignments are made based on the needs of each patient and the skills of the team members (who take total care of their assigned patients). The team is led by the team leader. The registered nurse continues to have the final responsibility of planning, coordinating, and evaluating the implementation of plans of care for each patient and supervising the personnel giving the care. In this method, the capabilities of each team member are used effectively, increasing the quality of care for the patient and satisfaction on the part of the team member. An integral concept in team nursing is the team conference. During this conference, which is held daily, information is shared by team members about specific patients, problems identified and solved, and nursing-care plans developed and revised.

The method just described was presented by Thora Kron (1987, pp. 212–219). However, it is rarely carried out in this manner. When busy, the team leader may administer medications and perform treatments and the team conference is often postponed, thereby neglecting nursing-care plans. In this way, team nursing becomes functional nursing. The nurses on the medical floor where Mr. Jordan was assigned used the team method, but frequently the team leader functioned as the medication nurse.

Primary Nursing (Primary Care)

The hospital in which Mr. Jordan was a patient was interested in increasing the quality of care of patients and was seriously looking into the primary-care method of delivering nursing service. This method was instituted in the late 1960s as a result of dissatisfaction of professional nurses with their lack of direct patient contact, and the fragmentation of care that resulted from functional and team nursing. Pri-

mary nursing involves having nurses with a knowledge of the nursing process individualize patient care and accept responsibility and accountability for total patient care. Ideally, staffing for this method requires having a nursing staff composed entirely of registered nurses, with each nurse assigned to a maximum of six patients. There are no team leaders in this method, and each primary nurse is a bedside nurse, having received the assignment from, and in turn reporting to, the head nurse. The major characteristic of this method is the responsibility and accountability of the primary nurse. The primary nurse is assigned to a patient on admission, develops the nursing-care plan after the admission interview, and is responsible for the care of that patient 24 hours a day until discharge. When the primary nurse is off duty, an associate registered nurse continues care by using the nursing-care plan. If any changes are contemplated in the plan of care, the primary nurse must be contacted.

Primary nursing facilitates continuity of care. This method has been shown to shorten patients' hospital stays, improve communication among staff, and attain the goal of holistic care (Schweiger, 1980, p. 109). Some hospital administrators find this method costly because of the number of registered nurses needed. Some hospitals have difficulty recruiting a sufficient number of registered nurses. Practical nurses are utilized in these situations and have performed safely and effectively.

Although the severe nursing shortage of the 1980s is easing, a shortage of nurses at all levels is anticipated through the year 2000. Around 1989, nursing journals began talking about a new system of assigning patients for care. Barnum refers to this system as differentiated practice, although it resembles more restructured practice (Barnum, 1991, p. 171). This system recognizes persons on the health care team with less education than registered nurses as important in reorganizing the delivery of nursing care (Tonges, 1989b, p. 20).

Regardless of the method of patient assignment used by a health care institution, remember that you must accept responsibility and be accountable for your actions.

Summary

Because of changing technology, today it is necessary for many individuals to provide services to patients. The term *health care team* is used to describe a group of persons who provide comprehensive health care. In order to avoid fragmentation of care under these circumstances, good communication skills are essential for anyone on the health care team. The nursing team is a part of the health care team and includes registered, practical, and student nurses; nursing assistants; and the clerical and managerial personnel, ward clerks, and unit managers. It is important for you to be aware of educational background, role, and responsibilities and possible licensing requirements for all levels of personnel on the nursing team in order to understand where you as a practical nurse fit into the picture.

It is also necessary for you to have an understanding of the different methods of delivering nursing service—case, functional, team, and primary care—in order to round out your understanding of your place on the nursing team. In the 1990s, practical nurses are recognized as important members of the nursing team.

REFERENCES

Barnum B. On differentiated practice. Nurs Health Care 1991; 14(4):171.

Ellis J, Nowlis E. *Nursing: A Human Needs Approach.* Boston: Houghton-Mifflin, 1988.

Dugas B. *Introduction to Patient Care: A Comprehensive Approach to Nursing.* 4th ed. Philadelphia: W.B. Saunders, 1983.

Henderson V. *The Nature of Nursing: A Definition and Its Implications for Practice, Research and Education.* New York: Macmillan, 1966.

Kron T, Gray A. *Management of Patient Care: Putting Leadership Skills to Work.* 6th ed. Philadelphia: W.B. Saunders, 1987.

Meyer J. Educator's conference is a success. Pract Nurs 1986; 36(2):6.

Moses E, Rosenfeld P, Yocum C. The Nursing Shortage: Challenging the Myths, Report of the 20th Biennial NLN Convention in Nashville, Tennessee, June 9–13, 1991. The Communique: Quarterly Publication of the Wisconsin League for Nursing 1991; 10(2):27.

Narrow SB, Buschel K. *Fundamentals of Nursing Practice.* 2nd ed. New York: Wiley, 1987.

Nook J. Trends forecast potential crises. The Communique: Quarterly Publication of the Wisconsin League for Nursing, 1986; 5(2):49.

Nursing DataSource, 1991. Vol. II. *Focus on Practical/Vocational Nursing.* New York: National League for Nursing, 1991.

Nursing—A Social Policy Statement. Kansas City, Mo.: American Nurses Association, 1980, pp. 9–13.

Nursing education: a steady shift to the BSN. RN 1986; 49(8):8.

Occupations Handbook 1991–92. Madison, Wis.: Wisconsin Career Information System, University of Wisconsin–Madison, 1991.

PN enrollments show two-decade rise. Pract Nurs 1986; 36(1):6.

Rowland H, ed. *The Nurse's Almanac.* 2nd ed. Rockville, Md.: Aspen Systems, 1984.

Schweiger J. *The Nurse as Manager.* New York: Wiley, 1980.

Tonges MC. Redesigning hospital nursing practice. Nurs Admin 1989a; 19(7):31–38.

Tonges MC. Redesigning hospital nursing practice: The Professional Advance Care Team (ProACT) Model. Nurs Admin 1989b; 19(9):19–22.

CHAPTER

4

The Adult Learner

Learning Objectives

Upon completing this chapter, you will
1. Identify yourself as a traditional adult learner or returning adult learner.
2. Identify personal areas of strength that will help ensure success in the practical nursing program.
3. Identify personal areas that could interfere with success in the practical nursing program.
4. Explain, in your own words, three rights of learners.
5. Describe personal responsibility for learning and active participation in the learning process as learner responsibilities.
6. Identify the purpose of evaluation in the practical nursing program.
7. List 10 learner responsibilities.

Welcome! You are one of thousands of adult learners in the United States who have decided to pursue a formal program in education this year. Every year adults enroll full-time and part-time in educational activities and programs that will help them achieve job skills, increase self-esteem, and generally improve their quality of life. You are not alone.

You are entering school at an excellent time. Because of a decrease in the number of 18-year-olds, schools have put full effort into attracting and keeping adult learners in their programs. The adult learner is a very serious and capable learner. These learners are helping to increase standards in our schools. Schools are looking seriously at the special needs of adult learners and are taking these needs into consideration when setting up educational programs, so that the adult learner can succeed. And to think, all these years you have been saying, "I was born too soon," or "I was born too late." It turns out you were born at just the right time.

THE ADULT LEARNER DEFINED

Who is the adult? Adult learners perceive themselves as adults and have adult responsibilities. They are generally of two types: the traditional adult learner and the returning adult learner. The traditional adult learner comes to an educational program directly from high school or from another program of study. Although a traditional adult learner, according to this description, can be any age, most are in their late teens and early 20s. The returning adult learner has been out of school for several years and many have not taken any courses since high school. Although returning adult learners can be any age, most are in the mid-20s. As which type of adult learner do you classify yourself?

FORMAL AND INFORMAL EDUCATIONAL EXPERIENCES

Generalizations can be made about each of the two types of learners. Keep in mind that gener-alizations are broad, sweeping statements and that characteristics of each type of adult learner are not found in each individual. The traditional adult learner is accustomed to formal educa-tion, which is also known as planned, organized learning, such as entering a nursing program in a vocational–technical school or junior college. Frequently, returning adult learners will say they are rusty and have not been to school since high school. Only the latter part of this statement is true. They might not have been in a classroom for some time, but they have been learning and have had informal educational experiences every day of their lives. Some ex-amples of their informal educational experi-ences are learning to make a new recipe, using a new tool, using a blow dryer, filling out a new income tax form, driving a new car and han-dling a new family problem. Can you list at least five informal educational experiences you have had since high school? Returning adult learners tend to put more emphasis on formal educa-tional experience and underemphasize the value of informal learning experiences. As you read, you will find that these experiences can be helpful to you when learning new material.

GEARED FOR SUCCESS

Both types of adult learners have things going for them that will allow them to succeed in school. Traditional adult learners are generally experts at educational routine. They know how to get through registration as painlessly as pos-sible, to find the fastest way to get from one class to another, the best time to get through the cafeteria line, and how to take a test using a computerized answer sheet. In comparison, re-turning adult learners may feel they have used up the last bit of their energy trying to find a parking space and once they do, may be puz-zled in finding their way to their assigned class-room. Traditional adult learners have been given the opportunity to develop reading, writ-ing, studying, and test-taking skills, are at their prime physically, are filled with energy and stamina, and many times have few out-of-school responsibilities to distract them from their stud-ies. On the other hand, the returning adult learner is a very serious learner who is ready to work. Returning adult learners have had many responsibilities and life experiences that will help them relate well to new learning, help them make sense out of it, and get the point quickly. They are mature, motivated, and self-directed, have set a goal for themselves, and many times have made economic, personal, and family sacrifices to get themselves back to school. Remember, both types of adult learners are geared for success, each having their own strong points. But each group also has some liabilities—things that could stand in the way of success.

LIABILITIES, PITFALLS, AND HIDDEN DANGERS

Hidden Danger Shared by All Adult Learners

One of the greatest liabilities shared by all adult learners is the fear of failure. Fear of anything is a very strong motivator, but in a negative sense. Fear of failure in school is a feeling that usually develops as a result of past negative experiences with learning situations. Perhaps you did not do well in some high school classes. Maybe you did not study, studied the wrong way, or allowed yourself to be put down by teachers in the past. Maybe you allowed yourself to underachieve because of peer pressure. Regardless of the cause, you may look at school in a negative, threatening way.

Well, a surprise is in store for you. Your past is history and you have a clean slate ahead of you! Many adult learners with the same history and fears as you may experience have succeeded in their educational programs. You are not a child in grade school. You are an adult in an adult educational experience. You will do yourself a favor if you begin to picture in your mind the rewards of succeeding in the practical nursing program rather than the failures and setbacks you may have suffered in high school and other educational experiences. Replace your fear of failure with the desire for success. Keep your thoughts positive and practice these positive thoughts continuously. Watch the content and tone of your thoughts and words. Negative thoughts and words can play like a tape. But as surely as you learned this negative script,

you can learn a positive script. But it takes time. Replace all your "I can'ts" and "I never coulds" with "I want to," "I can," "I will," and "I'm going to." Do not dwell on the past, but look to the future. Dominate your thoughts with positive ones. You know, go all the way with PMA—positive mental attitude. If you consistently expect to succeed, and combine it with putting effort into your studies, you will succeed. Did you know your brain believes anything you tell it? Well, if it believes you can fail, it can learn to believe you can succeed. Start today and engage in positive self-talk.

Dangers for the Traditional Adult Learner

Although traditional adult learners have fewer outside responsibilities to distract them from their studies, they may have social events that can compete with school and study time. A serious interference with school responsibilities is a party mentality. Parties and "going out" used to be special occasions for celebrating and getting together, a well-earned and much needed break from work and everyday routine responsibilities. Today, sometimes work and everyday responsibilities in life and at school get in the way of the traditional adult learner's party habit. Another interference is the amount of time the traditional student is employed outside of school hours. Ask yourself, "How much of the time I am employed outside of school is necessary for food, shelter, and other realistic expenses?" Many explanations can be given for this occurrence. Some traditional adult learners may still be working at developing an awareness of who they are and what life is all about for them. They may lack a sense of direction and have no clear goal or idea of what they really want to do in life. These examples of pitfalls for traditional adult learners are good examples of generalizations. They may or may not apply to the traditional adult learners you know.

Dangers for the Returning Adult Learner

Returning adult learners may experience difficulties with academic behaviors. Reading, writing, test-taking, and studying skills may be rusty. Physical changes occur as adults age and can affect learning. The senses of vision and hearing are at their peak in the adolescent years and decline very gradually through the adult years. As the decades go by these adults may notice the need for more illumination when reading, and experience problems with reading smaller print. Socially, returning adult learners have many roles to play outside of school. They can be husbands, wives, daughters, sons, grandparents, employees, volunteers, and generally very busy people. Coming back to school may result in feelings of guilt because returning to school will affect their relationships and routines outside of school.

Because of their many roles, returning adult learners have more demands placed on them. Some families may not support mom's or dad's choice to continue their formal education, and spouses may object to the extra demands placed on them. In many cases, the returning adult learner must struggle with having to learn how to juggle the worlds of learner and head of family.

Regardless of marital status, returning adult learners need to learn how to manage their time, as do traditional adult learners, and learn how to concentrate when time for concentration is made available. Sometimes returning adult learners set unrealistic goals for themselves and have to readjust their game plan. Although past experience can be an asset, returning adult learners will have to rethink and possibly unlearn some things they have learned in the past and have allowed to become habits. When faced with these pitfalls, some adults may decide to throw in the towel and write off school as a bad idea. *This book can help you to avoid this negative way of thinking and to go on to succeed.*

Special Challenges for Practical Nursing Students

Whether a traditional or returning adult student, some students have special challenges to success in practical nursing. Students with a spouse at home may be extremely busy with school and family affairs. Single parents may feel overwhelmed when the student role is assumed

in addition to all their other roles in daily life. It may be good for students with spouses to imagine what it would be like to be a student without a spouse to offer support.

Occasionally, practical nursing students with English as their first language will complain about the difficulty of schoolwork and the amount of time it takes to complete assignments. It may be good for students who speak English as their first language to imagine being responsible for the same schoolwork when English is your second language. Students with English as a second language need to strive continually for understanding of content presented in a language different from their native tongue. This would be comparable to presenting English-speaking students with textbooks written in Spanish or Russian.

The authors have experienced many students facing the above challenges and commend them for the good job they have done, against great odds, in the practical nursing program. They are a testimonial that success is within your reach if you face these special challenges.

LEARNERS HAVE RIGHTS

You must start thinking of some fundamental rights that you have been granted as an American through the U.S. Constitution that will affect you as a learner. The First Amendment gives you freedom of expression, as long as what you want to express does not disrupt class and infringe on the rights of your peers. So, when your instructor asks you to join in a discussion, do not be afraid to do so. Instructors want your input in a class session and have no intention of holding your comments against you. The Fourteenth Amendment assures you due process, which means that if you are charged with a violation of policies or rules, you will be presented with evidence of misconduct and be entitled to state your position. So relax. The institution in which you are enrolled cannot terminate you at whim, nor do they want to. They exist to help you to succeed. A more detailed account of the above two rights can probably be found in your school's student handbook. You did not get one? You lost yours? Hurry to Student Services and get a copy today.

A very important learner's right is the right to have an organized curriculum and a responsible instructor who is prepared. Although your tuition and fees do not pay for all the services you receive at school, you are the most important person on campus, and the reason for the instructor's being hired. Contrary to popular belief, you do not interfere with the instructor's work but are the focus of it. You have the right to know the requirements of each course and how you will be graded for each course.

RESPONSIBILITIES OF LEARNERS

The first responsibility of learners is to learn. The authors want you to test your knowledge about the process of learning before you read any further. Read the following four statements and answer "true" or "false" to them. As the chapter continues, these statements will be discussed and you will be expected to check the accuracy of your responses. Remember, your answers are for your eyes only.

1. The instructor has the responsibility for my learning.

2. If I fail, it is the responsibility of the instructor.

3. If I succeed, the credit for my success should go to the instructor.

4. My instructor has the responsibility to pass on to me all the information I will need to know in my career as a practical nurse.

Teaching versus Learning

A wonderful thing has happened in teacher education, especially in the education of adults. Teachers are more aware of the difference between teaching and learning, and great emphasis is being placed on the role of the learner. The authors feel it is only fair for learners to be aware of the exciting world of learning and the role of teaching and learning in that process. In doing so you will know what is expected of you as an adult learner.

Many of you, including the authors and some of your instructors, have had educational experiences that encouraged dependency and passivity on the part of the learner. Think back to educational experiences you have had. Did they involve sitting in classes where the teacher did most of the talking and you just sat there? Did you view the teacher as someone who possessed knowledge and somehow was going to pass it on to you? And if you did not pass did you say, "The teacher flunked me"? When you think about it, these situations are characterized by the adjectives *dependent* and *passive*.

About the last time you should have been dependent was when you were an infant, but even then you were far from passive. When you became a toddler, you became very independent and began to learn about the world in earnest. You very actively pursued your learning or the acquiring of new knowledge and skills. And you did it with gusto! Now, here you are an adult learner. How unfair of an instructor to expect you to become dependent and passive in your learning, especially when studies have proved that people learn best when they are actively involved in their own learning and have an interdependent relationship with the instructor. Today, instructors are viewed as facilitators of learning. You have already learned it is the instructor's responsibility to set up a curriculum. Your state's Board of Nursing will dictate the content of the curriculum of a school of nursing, but it is then up to the faculty to decide how that content will be included in the nursing program. Instructors have the responsibility to create a learning environment in which learning can take place, by arranging a variety of activities and experiences. Part of that learning environment involves being available to learners when they encounter questions and problems they cannot solve themselves. Instructors also have the responsibility to evaluate learning and do so by testing and observing learners.

To learn is to acquire knowledge and skills. The verb *acquire* means to obtain or gain by one's own effort. Learners must open themselves up, reach out and stretch to gain their knowledge and skills. They are agents of their own knowledge and skill acquisition. Learning is a very active, not passive, activity. Learners have the personal responsibility for acquiring knowledge and skills, and they cannot expect instructors to pour these into their heads. Learners must become self-directed in their learning. Instructors will not hover over you and guide your every step, although they are always there to help you along when needed. Do not expect the teacher to assume your skill for you, be your medical dictionary, or replace Chapter 2 in *Body Structure* because you did not have time to study. Instead, expect your instructor to observe you while you are trying to work through a difficult skill and make suggestions and demonstrate a point here and there to help you along. Expect your instructor to help you put a definition of a medical term in your own words if you are having trouble doing so. Expect the instructor to answer specific questions you have on Chapter 2. These are the roles of teacher and learner and an example of their interdependency.

Remember, if you are to learn and succeed, you must become actively involved in your learning. You say you are too old to learn. You say you cannot teach an old dog new tricks. Be aware that much study has been done in this area, and to date, studies of adult learning clearly indicate that the *basic ability to learn remains essentially unimpaired throughout the lifespan* (Knowles, 1980, p. 55). Now review the answers to your true/false questions on page 48. Any answers you want to change before looking at the key?

1. False. You have the responsibility for your own learning. You must get actively involved in the learning process.

2. False. If you fail, it is your own fault. Adult educational programs are geared for success. You are geared for success. And although you could list many reasons why you might not succeed, the teacher's flunking you is not one of them. Learners sometimes allow themselves to flunk.

3. False. When you succeed (and you are perfectly capable of doing so), only you can take credit for the success, because you were the person who assumed responsibility for your

own learning and became actively involved in the process.

4. False. Although instructors have much experience in nursing, they do not know about all the experiences you will have in your career as a practical nurse. And if they did, there would be no time or way to transfer this knowledge to you. Instructors help learners to learn how to learn, especially important in an ever-changing field like nursing.

If you got none wrong, you should be an expert on learning. Now put your expertise to work for you. One wrong or more, the authors suggest you reread "Teaching versus Learning."

The Role of Evaluation

The second responsibility of learners is to receive and to participate in evaluation of self. Evaluation plays an important role in your education in the practical nursing program and throughout your career. You have set a goal to become a practical nurse. As the year goes on you will be evaluated by your instructors in several different ways as a means of determining whether or not you are progressing in the achievement of that goal. When you graduate, you will be evaluated periodically while on the job, sometimes as a means of determining if you are to receive a salary increase and other times to see if you are functioning well enough to keep your job. Evaluation generally occurs in two areas: written tests that measure your knowledge of theory and performance evaluations that measure your progress in the clinical area. Evaluation in these areas is a learning experience in itself.

Learners and instructors look at test results very differently. Learners focus on the number of items they answered correctly. Instructors focus on the specific items the learner had wrong, indicating theoretical knowledge the learner does not have. Try to arrange time with your instructors to review your tests. Do not just ask for your grades. It is impossible to say grades do not count; you must make the minimum grade established by your nursing program. Try to look at tests as learning experiences in themselves. Be as interested in your wrong answers as you are in your correct answers. Take time to look at the items you got wrong with the goal of understanding why you were wrong.

The most meaningful evaluations you will receive during the year will be your performance evaluations while you are in the clinical area. Since these evaluations present you with the opportunity for career and personal growth, it is important to understand this form of evaluation and the responsibilities you have with regard to it.

In the clinical area, instructors will be observing you as you go about your patient care. They are observing you in order to discover the positive things you are doing to reach your goal to become a practical nurse. These behaviors are to be encouraged, as they indicate learning has taken place and you are growing and progressing toward your goal. Instructors are also observing you in order to discover behaviors that stand in the way of your reaching your goal. These behaviors are to be discouraged. Generally, your instructor will update you daily on your progress, in a verbal or written manner. At the end of a clinical rotation, you will receive a written performance evaluation during a conference with your clinical instructor.

From the start, you should look at performance evaluation as a two-sided coin, with the instructor on one side and you on the other. Although the instructor, as part of her job, has the responsibility of giving you a performance evaluation, you also have the responsibility of being aware of your behaviors. You are responsible for self-evaluation. The National League for Nursing and other nursing organizations have indicated that practical nursing students at the time of graduation should be able to look at their nursing actions and be aware of their strong behaviors and behaviors that need improvement. The development of the ability to be aware of one's behaviors begins with day one in the practical nursing program, including the skills laboratory. It is an important skill to have as an employee. A learner does not graduate and automatically have this skill. Learners must consistently work at viewing themselves objectively; instructors will help in this area. For example, when learning how to make a bed,

ask yourself, "Is the finished product as good as I had intended it to be when I started?" Do not wait for the instructor to identify areas of success or needed improvement.

Do you remember receiving comments about your behavior in grade school and high school from your teachers and parents? How did you feel when you received these comments? Many persons grow up with bad feelings toward these episodes of criticism and even the word itself. Criticism means evaluation, but many persons attach a negative meaning to it and view it as a put-down. The phrase *constructive criticism* evokes negative feelings. The phrase *constructive evaluation* is frequently used instead, and this choice of words may help you look at evaluation of your behaviors in a positive way. It is important to distinguish what is being evaluated. You must separate your behaviors or actions from yourself, the person. Constructive evaluation directed to your behaviors has no bearing on your value as a person. Look at your behaviors as being either positive and helping you to reach your goal or as needing improvement. Behaviors needing improvement must be modified so that you can reach your goal.

As you progress in the nursing program, you will learn about the nursing process, a systematized way of conducting patient care. An important part of the nursing process is evaluation of your nursing actions while giving patient care. If your actions are not helping patients to reach their goals, they must be modified. Knowledge of the nursing process will help you develop your ability to look at your actions and evaluate them. Comments from instructors will help your self-awareness. Remain open with yourself and remember that these comments are directed toward your behaviors and not you as a person.

A good way to start learning self-evaluation is to look at yourself in everyday life. Ask yourself how you look through the eyes of others:

How would you like to be your own spouse?
How would you like to have yourself as a learner?

How would you like to be your own
   mother or father?
How would you like to be your own
   nurse?

If you would not like to be any of these people, identify the reasons why. Another good
exercise is to make two lists, one a list of assets
or strong points, and the other a list of your
liabilities or areas that need improvement.
When asked to evaluate themselves, learners
traditionally rate themselves more negatively
and tend to neglect their strong points. Identifying strong points is not to be thought of as
proud or vain behavior. It is dealing with yourself honestly and openly. After you have identified assets and liabilities, review your assets periodically and make an effort to continue these
strong points while modifying your liabilities.
Pick one liability at a time to work on. If you do
so, your assets list will grow and your liabilities
list will shrink.

A good way to start self-evaluation in nursing
is in the skills lab of your basic nursing course.
Practice becoming very observant of the results
of your actions. Are the corners of the bottom
sheet really the mitered or squared ones you
intended them to be? Are you using the bath
blanket as a drape to avoid chilling and invasion
of privacy? Are you aware of the effect of the
tone of your voice on your instructors and
peers?

Evaluation is an ever-present reality in any
career you may choose. Getting into the practice of self-evaluation early in your program of
study will help you to develop a skill you will
use daily in your career and personal life.

Other Responsibilities of Learners

In addition to assuming responsibility for your
own learning, becoming actively involved in
the process, and receiving and participating in

evaluation, it is necessary to be aware of some
other responsibilities you have as a learner.

1. Be aware of the rules and policies of your
school and the practical nursing program, and
abide by them.

2. Follow channels of communication both at
school and in the clinical area when problems
do develop. The rule of thumb is, go to the
source.

3. Be prepared in advance for classes and clinical experiences. You expect teachers to be prepared, and they expect the same of you. When
you are unprepared for classes, you waste the
time of the instructor and your peers. When
you are unprepared for clinical experiences,
you are violating an important safety factor in
patient care.

4. Prepare your own assignments. But utilize
your peers and the experiences and knowledge
they have and learn from each other.

5. Seek out learning experiences at school
and in the clinical area. Set your goals higher
than the minimum.

6. Assume responsibility for your own
thoughts, communication, and behavior. Do not
give in to pressure from your peers. BYOB: Be
Your Own Boss.

7. Be present and on time for classes and clinical experiences. Follow school and program
policies for reporting absences. Getting into
this habit will prepare you to be a favored employee.

8. Enter into discussion when asked to do so
in class.

9. Treat those with whom you come into daily
contact with respect, always mindful of their
rights as an individual.

*10. Seek out your instructor when you are
having difficulties in class or in the clinical
area.* Many times instructors can tell when students are having problems, but more important
are the times they cannot tell, and only you
know a problem exists. Do not be afraid to approach your instructors; they are there to help
you.

Summary

Adult learners are numerous today on campuses throughout the United States. Adult learners fall into two categories: the traditional adult learner and the returning adult learner. Each category of learner possesses characteristics that can help them to succeed in the practical nursing program. Each group also possesses characteristics that can prevent success from occurring. These liabilities occur in areas where learners have control over their solutions, and are not concrete barriers to success. Although learners have rights, they also have responsibilities. The most important of their responsibilities are the personal responsibility for learning, taking an active part in the process, and participating in the evaluation of their learning and growth.

REFERENCES

Apps J. *The Adult Learner on Campus.* Chicago: Follett, 1981.

Cross KP. *Adults as Learners.* San Francisco: Jossey-Bass, 1988.

Haponski W, McCabe C. *Back to School.* Princeton, N.J.: Peterson's Guides, 1982.

Kidd JR. *How Adults Learn.* Englewood Cliffs, N.J.: Cambridge Books, 1988.

Knowles M. *The Modern Practice of Adult Education.* Chicago: Follett, 1980.

Knowles M. *The Modern Practice of Adult Education.* Englewood Cliffs, N.J.: Cambridge Books, 1988.

Knowles M. *The Adult Learner: A Neglected Species.* 4th ed. Houston: Gulf Publishers, 1990.

Waitley D. *The Psychology of Winning* (audio tapes). Chicago: Nightingale-Conast, 1978.

part II
HOW TO BEGIN

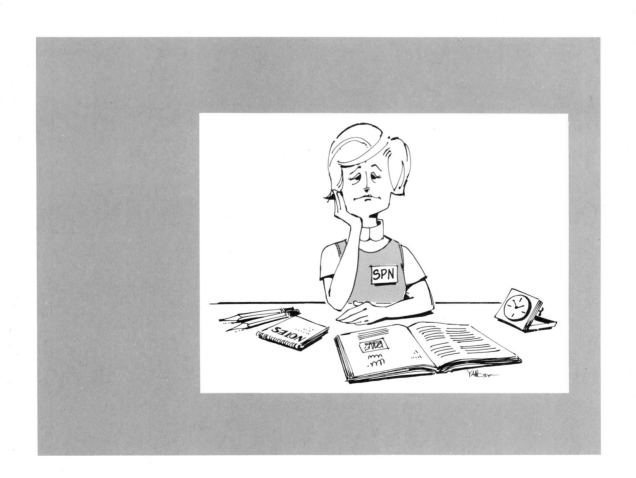

CHAPTER 5
Time Management

Learning Objectives

After reading this chapter, you will
1. Discuss three benefits of time management for an adult student.
2. List the activities of the various roles filled in daily life.
3. Arrange the list in 2 according to high- and low-priority items.
4. Keep, at least, a one-day activity log to determine present time use.
5. Devise a semester and weekly schedule to reflect present time commitments.
6. Make a daily "to do" list.
7. Carry out weekly and daily schedule for two weeks.
8. Evaluate effectiveness of personal-time—management plan, and modify if necessary.

Have you noticed at school and in your personal life that some people seem to get more done than others? Worse yet, some of the busiest people are the ones getting the most done. To add insult to injury, all of us are given the same amount of time, 168 hours a week, in which to get the job done. How can some individuals get the job done and some not? The answer does not lie in the fact that some people have fewer responsibilities and less to do in a week's time. The answer lies in their ability to manage their own time. Time management is a major skill for learner success. It is also a necessary skill for practical nurses so that they can manage their time spent in the clinical area in order to meet patient goals. To start this chapter, it is necessary for you to take a self-test on time management so that you will know how you stand with regard to this important skill. If you are going to be responsible for managing clinical time, you must be able to manage personal time. Answer "yes" or "no" as you read each of the following statements, and apply them to your personal use of time.

▰▰▰▰▰▰▰ Learning EXERCISE ▰▰▰▰▰▰▰

Self-Test on Time Management (Adapted from Cooper et al., 1977, pp. 3–4)

_____ 1. I keep a semester or course calendar to reflect requirements and due dates of work for all my classes.

_____ 2. I keep a written weekly schedule of all things that must be done at school and in my personal life.

_____ 3. I keep a written daily list of things I must do at school and in my personal life.

_____ 4. Daily I list and rank in importance my priorities for using school and personal time.

_____ 5. After listing and ranking my daily priorities for school and personal life, I stick to the list I have made.

_____ 6. I use my best working time during the day for doing my high-priority work for school.

_____ 7. I plan to do lower-priority schoolwork before higher-priority schoolwork.

_____ 8. I start school tasks before thinking them through.

_____ 9. I stop a school task before I have completed it.

_____10. I spend the few minutes before class talking to my classmates about anything other than the class.

_____11. I have trouble starting a major task for school.

_____12. I become bored with the subject I am studying.

_____13. I have a hard time getting started when I sit down to study.

_____14. Sometimes I avoid important school tasks.

_____15. I find myself easily distracted when I study.

_____16. I always try to get everything done in my personal life that must be done.

_____17. I frequently watch television instead of doing schoolwork.

_____18. I manage to turn a short coffee break into a long coffee break.

_____19. I study nightly for my classes.

_____20. I frequently have to cram for exams.

SUGGESTED ANSWERS TO SELF-TEST

1. Yes	6. Yes	11. No	16. No
2. Yes	7. No	12. No	17. No
3. Yes	8. No	13. No	18. No
4. Yes	9. No	14. No	19. Yes
5. Yes	10. No	15. No	20. No

Count the number you disagree with and plug yourself into one of the following categories:

1–5 Disagree with	You deserve the Alan Lakein* award.
5–10 Disagree with	Hang in there! With a little guidance you will get on the right track.
11–20 Disagree with	We know you must be exhausted, but keep on reading, fast!

The answers to the self-test are the ones suggested by time-management experts. Although different time-management techniques work for different people, these suggested answers reflect basic time-management techniques that could help you succeed in the practical nursing program.

BENEFITS OF TIME MANAGEMENT

Time management is a technique to help you do not only the things you have to get done, but also those you want to finish in a definite time period. Time management can put you in control of your life, rather than be a slave to it. Although you will have to give up some of the things you were accustomed to doing before you became a practical nursing student, time-management techniques can help you gain some personal time for family and yourself rather than feeling there is time only for school. Time management can help you work smarter, not harder. It will not give you more hours in a week, but will help you use what hours you have more effectively. Please note that we did not say more efficiently. Time management does not necessarily deal with efficiency, as did the efficiency experts of the 1950s. Efficiency can bring images of robotlike individuals working to get every task done in the shortest time possible in a machinelike manner. Effectiveness, a goal of time management, involves setting priorities among tasks that need to be done and doing them the best way possible. Efficiency takes the thinking out of tasks while effective-

---

*Alan Lakein is a famous time-management expert. In 1973 he first published a very readable book entitled *How to Get Control of Your Time and Your Life*. New York: New American Library.

ness puts it back in. Efficiency can make us a slave, while effectiveness can make us free.

REVIEW OF GOALS

How did you score on the self-test? If you are a typical adult, you are probably reading quickly right now to find out what to do to improve. Take heart. Very few of us get the Alan Lakein* award, and most of us could stand to learn how to use our time more effectively. Ineffective use of personal time is learned behavior, better known as a habit. Any behavior that is learned can be unlearned if you work at it, and new habits can be acquired.

You are already on the right track in time management, no matter what you scored, if you have set the goal to be a practical nurse. This is the bullseye to which you will direct your efforts for the next year. It would be beneficial to write that goal on a recipe card and place it where you will see it frequently. Some suggestions are your car visor, the bathroom mirror, and the refrigerator door. Be sure to include the date of your graduation. There will be some tough days in the months ahead, and the visibility of your long-term goal can keep you going. In order to realize this long-term goal, you must break it down to smaller, more manageable goals. These are called your "short-term goals." Examples of short-term goals are passing each of the courses you must take in order to graduate from the practical nursing program. These short-term goals can be broken down even more to include the individual requirements for each of the courses you must take. For example, for your professional issues course you might have the following requirements to pass the course:

1. Earn a minimum grade on each of a certain number of major tests.

2. Give two oral reports.

3. Write a four-page paper on a selected topic.

Fulfilling each of the requirements will eventually lead to passing the course, and when each of the courses you are required to take are passed you will graduate from the program. While keeping your eye on your long-term goal, you will fulfill requirement after requirement until that goal is reached. Now, let's start learning how to manage your time.

GETTING ORGANIZED

At all levels, nursing has a special way of getting organized, called the "nursing process." You have studied the nursing process and how it relates to you as a practical nurse. The nursing process and its four components—assessment, planning, implementation, and evaluation—will be used to help you get organized as a student and in your personal life.

Assessment

According to *Webster's,* assessment is the act of placing a value on something. To do this, the element of judgment must be brought into the picture. Assessment in time management involves gathering data on how you actually spend your time and discovering what roles you fill in your daily life.

Being enrolled in a vocational–technical program, whether you are single, divorced, widowed, or married, requires change to some degree in the activities in which you were involved before entering the program. Regardless of your state in life, all the roles you fill can be classified in any of five general categories: school, job, family, community, and recreation (Harper-Peterson, 1984, p. 56). The activities involved in going to school are very structured. You must get there, attend classes, and get home. When you are enrolled in a vocational–technical program such as practical nursing, your school day is chock-full; seldom do you even have the choice of when you will take a specific course. The same structure is not evi-

dent in the other four categories. Frequently, you might be involved in activities in these other roles that you either did not plan to do, do not enjoy doing, do not have time to do, or do not feel need to be done. You are encouraged to complete the activity on page 292 of the Appendix in order to gather information about your *personal roles and activities* for the assessment portion of time management. A sample exercise and explanation is on page 291 of the Appendix. You are now ready to document how you actually use your personal time. Ideally, a time log should be kept for about one week to document how you use your personal time. Since time is marching on, a one-day time log can give you a general idea of how you use your time at present. Page 293 of the Appendix explains the exercise entitled "Use of Personal Time." On page 294 of the Appendix, you will find a blank page on which to record your "Personal Time and Activity Log." Now, supply only one more piece of information and your assessment will be complete. After this paragraph, list one activity you wish you had time for. The activity could have been listed under your roles, but maybe was not listed at all. Remember, the sky's the limit as long as your wish is something that is really important to you.

My special wish is _____
_____
_____ .

Planning

In completing the assessment exercises in the Appendix, you are now ready to proceed to the planning stage. The planning phase of time management will result in a blueprint for action. In this phase you will learn how to plan use of your precious 168 hours a week. Planning involves thinking about setting priorities (most important tasks), but to be successful, these thoughts must be written down. You should devise written schedules for yourself so that you can program your time on a monthly, weekly, and daily basis. The schedules should include the activities that are part of all the roles you fill and not just your role as a student. Your schedules should reflect the total you.

Schedules help keep you honest. They reflect the classes you must attend and the studying you must do to reach your long-term goal. With a schedule you will avoid the rollercoaster phenomenon all too familiar to students—falling behind in school and trying to catch up. Schedules help you include time for friends and family. Schedules help you avoid overlooking an important part of your well-being: recreation. And schedules help you avoid the pitfall of allowing extracurricular activities to come before schoolwork, a situation that accounts for more failures in post-high-school educational programs than any other factors (Pauk, 1988, p. 40).

Arguments against Planning

At this point some individuals will say they do not have time to plan and will pass off the suggestion of scheduling. Individuals who are too busy to plan are the very persons that should be planning. They cannot afford not to plan. If you do not plan, you will overlook priorities and possibly miss some available free time. For the small amount of time planning takes, the benefits are great. Some persons who do not have time to plan really do not want to find time to get priority work done and use lack of time as an excuse. Some individuals look at planning and scheduling as leading to inflexibility and loss of freedom. They want to "hang loose" and go in different directions as the opportunity arises. Flexibility of this sort can result in disorganization and the accomplishment of few, if any, important tasks. As imposed deadlines near, guilt, frustration, and anxiety appear. These individuals wind up being a slave to time, instead of being its master. A schedule written with principles of time management will help you be a master of time and not a slave to it. The schedule will be written with flexibility in mind, and you will be able to trade time with yourself when unexpected events come up.

Unlearning old habits and learning new habits is not an easy task. It takes work in the form of self-discipline and determination to drop old, comfortable ways. But it is possible. Be sure to practice the new habit whenever the opportunity to do so presents itself. In doing this, the new habit will eventually become a part of you.

Ah! You say you slipped up and reverted to old habits. Do not give up! Start from where you left off and try again.

Scheduling Time

The only special equipment you need for scheduling is a calendar. Ideally, you should have one that has blank space for each date so that you can list activities. These calendars should be available at the bookstore. You can also make your own monthly calendar by copying a current calendar. In order to schedule your time, you should be able to set priorities and delegate activities.

Setting priorities Page 295 in the Appendix has an exercise entitled "Setting Personal Priorities" to help you decide which of your activities are most important or which things should come first.

Delegating activities. Some of your activities can be delegated to specific persons in your life. Pages 60–61 contain a chart of activities with examples of tasks that can be delegated in this manner. The tasks listed for children are excellent ways for them to learn responsibility, taking their growth and development into consideration.

As in the study of growth and development, these suggested activities apply to the typical child of that age group. The suggestions may or may not apply to your individual child. But do not underestimate your children. Hopefully, you will be able to come up with some ideas that do fit your children and add to the list. At first, it may take some time to instruct your children, but in the long run it will be worthwhile. Have you ever heard of the saying "You have to spend money to make money"? Well, in time management, sometimes it takes time initially to teach persons what is expected of them, but in the long run it will pay off handsomely in time saved. Plus you get the added bonus of encouraging independence. In fact, the very same principle will be used in patient care. It may take time to teach a patient how to master a skill for himself, but in the long run it will save you time once he or she learns, and as a bonus the patient gains independence. These suggestions are a wonderful way to help a child become independent and develop lifelong skills.

Are you having trouble getting your spouse to cooperate? Do not interpret stubbornness as lack of love or laziness. Chances are that your spouse grew up in an environment that divided household chores by sex and now feels that his masculinity or her femininity is jeopardized by being expected to assume new tasks. Gather your thoughts and decide on the areas in which you feel your spouse could be most helpful during this hectic time of your life. The answer lies in communication. Talk to your spouse (and only you know the best time and situation for this). Hopefully, you both agree that you should be going to school and have identified the positive features of this endeavor for both of you. Review these positive features. If you have not identified them, do so together. Then collaborate on solutions to ease your lack of time. While you are at it, establish some precious "spouse-only" time to be honored during your hectic year at school. You do not want to create in your spouse the feeling of being left out during this whole experience.

Page 295 in the Appendix has an exercise entitled "Delegating Activities" to help you decide which personal roles and activities can be delegated.

Chart of Shared Tasks That May Be Delegated

SIGNIFICANT OTHER	PRESCHOOL AND EARLY SCHOOL AGE (4–8 YEARS)	SCHOOL AGE (9–12 YEARS)
Pay bills	Fold laundry	Cook simple meals
Help clean	Make laundry piles	Wash dishes
Take charge of car maintenance	Deliver laundry to correct room	Dry dishes
Mow the lawn	Clear dishes from table (not best china)	Put dishes away
Paint		Start laundry
Do small repairs		Shop for a few food items as indicated on list
Sort laundry		Dust
Transfer laundry to dryer		Run vacuum
Shovel snow		Sew patches on own shirts
		Plant garden
		Weed
		Shovel snow
		Make own bed

Rationale for Activities Chosen for:
> **Preschool and early school age**—Children in these age groups are experiencing muscle development, and notice their psychomotor development; they want to try new things. Make-believe rides high with these kids and they love to play house. Capitalize on this.
>
> **School age**—These children are adults-in-training. Muscles continue to develop and psychomotor skills are increasing. They need tasks of the real world to engage in and should be encouraged to carry them through to completion.

ADOLESCENTS (13–18 YEARS)	FRIENDS	RELATIVES
Run errands with family car if they have a license; use bike if no license	Replace you at bowling the night before a big exam	Substitute for mom or dad at scout meeting, PTA meetings, or school activities
Plan menus	Replace you in car pool (or substitute)	Spend time with children
Prepare grocery list within budget	Feed you occasionally	Holiday baking or shopping
Mow the lawn		
Paint		
Make own bed		

Rationale for Activities Chosen for:
> **Adolescents**—sometime during adolescence, the ability to think as an adult will develop, allowing this age group to budget, apply principles of basic nutrition, etc., to everyday life. One of the tasks of adolescence is to become independent. Help its development by delegating meaningful activity to this age group.

School-age children and adolescents can also do activities in the column to the left of their column, but would probably prefer the specific activities listed for their age group.

LEARNING EXERCISE

Semester Scheduling

Time Involved: Approximately 10 minutes.

On your planning calendar, list the things that must be done that will occur during this time frame. Examples of activities to include here are

• Your class schedule.
• Dates of major exams.
• Dates papers are due.

- Dates of doctors' appointments.
- Dates of club meetings.
- Dates for haircuts, etc.

Include activities that are delegated and indicate them by circling the activity on the calendar and writing in the name of the person who is responsible for it. Post these sheets, one month at a time on your refrigerator for you, your family, and/or your roommate to see. The semester schedule is done only once, in pencil, and additions or corrections are made as needed. This is also a way of communicating your new life to those with whom you live. Keep in mind, if you do live with other people, that your new schedule is something to which they must get accustomed.

Weekly Schedules

Time Involved: Approximately 10 minutes.

The weekly schedule is for your peace of mind. A blank form can be found on page 296 of the Appendix; you can copy this sheet on looseleaf paper. Fill in all your classes and other fixed activities for the week and photocopy as many sheets as there are weeks in the semester or time period of your current classes. Use some time each weekend to plan your week. Be sure to include in your planning your time before and after classes. As assignments are made, add them to your weekly schedule, and your weekly schedule will not only reflect study time, but specify what should be studied when. The following are some suggestions to keep in mind when planning your week.

1. Schedule studying for your prime time. Prime time is the time you are most effective in doing a task. High-priority-A courses should be studied for during prime time.
2. Schedule blocks of time for studying by identifying your personal attention span for various school activities. For example, when reading, note the time you start reading and when you begin to lose your concentration. Note the amount of time that has passed. Do this for several episodes of studying and you will begin to see patterns in your attention span. Take a three-to-five-minute break at this point in your studying, varying your activity.

   Some people may find they have a 20-minute attention span. Others may have an attention span of one hour. The important thing is not to let your break extend beyond a few minutes. Condition yourself to get right back to work, without the need for start-up time.

   It is impossible to tell you exactly how much time you will need for studying for each of your classes. This will vary from student to student and class to class. Does the class meet daily? If so, you will have a daily assignment. The old suggestion of two hours of study for each hour of class will be just right for some classes, too much for others, and not enough for the rest.
3. Identify small blocks of time and make them work for you. They are important sources of time and these minutes can add up quickly to large time losses. These small blocks of time usually occur between classes. Get up and stretch and take deep breaths if staying in the same classroom or walk briskly, while taking deep breaths, to get to your next class. Review in your mind the class you just attended. These activities will get more oxygen into your bloodstream and help it circulate to your brain, resulting in better thinking and a fresher you. One of the worst things to do is to grab a soda or a cigarette. The soda, if nondiet, will quickly elevate your

blood sugar, encourage insulin to be deposited in the blood, and then quickly lower the sugar content, leaving you with a tired, dragged-out feeling. Smoking constricts your blood vessels and will decrease the amount of oxygen carried to your brain. Your brain needs oxygen to help you think and to keep you alert. While waiting for your next class, select one of the following activities.

   a. Review your notes from the class that just finished. This will allow you to fill in any gaps you may have in your notes. You will aid your retention and understanding by reviewing in this way.

   b. Get mentally prepared for your next class by reviewing your assignment if a lecture/discussion class or reviewing your plan of activities for the class if an autotutorial class. School is a social activity, but do not waste time by fooling around during all of your small blocks of free time. The more you get done at school, the less you will have to do at home.

   c. Discuss an assignment with a peer.

4. Write only what is essential on your schedule. Details take too much time to write down and are a real turnoff.

5. Plan for three meals a day, with appropriate snacks, based on the basic four food groups. Doing so will help avoid tiredness and irritability, two things you need to avoid at all costs with a busy schedule.

6. Plan for adequate sleep. Individuals have their personal sleep patterns, so try to get in tune with yours. Do you ever wake up before your alarm? Next time you do, calculate how many hours sleep you have had. Odds are your hours of sleep are some multiple of $1\frac{1}{2}$ hours. Brain research has shown that you will function better if you get up after 6 hours or after $7\frac{1}{2}$ hours of sleep rather than after 7 or 8 hours. Apparently, we repeat a sleep cycle every $1\frac{1}{2}$ hours. If you get up one-half hour into your next cycle, you could be very sluggish. Think of this when you set your alarm. And when the alarm goes off, resist the temptation to set the alarm on snooze.

7. Remember, although some sacrifices must be made, your life is more than just school. Review your sky's-the-limit wish on page 58 of this chapter and include it on your weekly schedule.

Daily Schedule

Time Involved: Approximately 5 minutes

This schedule could prove to be the most important as far as getting things done. Alan Lakein, the time-management expert, calls the daily schedule a "to do" list. He states that successful and unsuccessful persons both know about "to do" lists. Successful persons use a "to do" list every day to make better use of their time, whereas unsuccessful persons do not (Lakein, 1989, p. 64). This is the simplest schedule to make. Use a 3-by-5-inch card and head it "To Do." List the items you have to accomplish. Be sure to list the high-priority activities for school and your personal life. Refer to your weekly calendar to refresh your memory regarding assignments and their due dates. Rank your activities so that you can handle first things first.

   Decide for yourself when your best time of day is for writing your "to do" list. Some persons like to make up their list while eating breakfast as a way to get into the activities of the day. Some persons like to make up their list right before going to bed. These persons may be getting an extra benefit that they are not aware of—your subconscious will be able to go over your "to do" list while you peacefully sleep and renew yourself. Carry your list with you and stick to the activities and priorities you have listed. Cross off the activities when you have completed them. Ah, what a feeling!

Planning takes so little time; it will be fun and not a chore. Just think of all the benefits that come out of taking 10 minutes to plan each month, 10 minutes to plan each week, and 5 minutes to plan each day. What great returns for so little effort. And, by writing your schedules and lists, you have freed your brain from one more source of clutter and saved it for all the learning you must do.

Implementation

This is the part of your time-management program where your plans become action. The only value of a plan lies in its being used. Thanks to the planning you have done, you now have an incentive to get started because you already know exactly where you have to be and what you have to do. Now for some hints on how to follow that plan.

General Hints

As you begin to follow your personal plan, you may notice that some of your peers at school are not planning their time and may even give you static for attempting to plan yours. Have the intestinal fortitude to follow your schedule, even if it means leaving some peers in the shuffle. You paid your tuition and have your own personal-time problems to contend with in order to get full mileage out of that tuition. There may be students who put their efforts into games instead of scholastic pursuits. They think they will look better if others do not succeed. You will recognize these students when they tell you that your efforts will make them look bad. Whose problem is that, anyhow? Make sure you never miss a class, regardless of peer pressure or any reason other than an emergency. When you miss a class, you spend more time than the class would have taken trying to obtain the information from the class, and you may never capture all of it.

In actually carrying out your schedule, be aware of a phenomenon called Parkinson's law (Pauk, 1988, p. 50). In this phenomenon, the time it takes to do a task, whether for home or school, will stretch out and fill whatever time you have assigned to it. So practice setting realistic time limits in which to complete tasks so you do not fall into this trap.

Procrastination

You know what you have to do and when it must be done, but do you ever find yourself putting off high-priority tasks to a time in the future? Take time now and list one task that you have put off this week.

_____

_____

_____

_____

How did you feel about postponing this task? Such action usually leads to tension (just what an adult student needs more of). What is causing your reluctance? Reevaluate the task you have been avoiding. Is it really a high-priority task? Remember, your planning should be flexible and the priority status of tasks can realistically change. But be careful if you find yourself using this explanation too frequently. Other causes for putting off what is important are ill health (you do not have the energy), laziness (you do not have the motivation), and past successful episodes of procrastination (if you did not do it, someone else did or nobody cared). Regardless of the cause, we all procrastinate to some degree, but some persons make more of a habit of it than others. If you look truthfully at the tasks you keep postponing, odds are they are unpleasant, difficult, or time consuming. It seems we never postpone things that are fun or simple to do. In fact, sometimes we avoid high-priority tasks and do a bunch of low-priority ones. This action gives us an immediate and false feeling of accomplishment. For others, fear of failure causes them to put off things to the last minute, thereby providing the individual with an excuse for not doing well.

A sure way to finish those unpleasant, difficult, and time-consuming tasks you have been putting off is to reduce the entire task to a series of mini-tasks. There are two rules for doing this. First, the mini-task must be simple to do and take no more than five minutes of your time. Second, for best results, the mini-tasks should be written and carried in your pocket for quick reference. Many students fear upcoming major tests and put off studying for them. Some examples of mini-tasks for this situation could be

1. Review your notes before and after each class.

2. Write more-difficult information you must know for the test on index cards. For example, write a term on one side of the card and its definition on the other. List causes of, consequences of, prevention of, and differences between items of class content and have these cards handy for quick reference whenever you have a spare minute. One of the authors studied vocabulary for a German final in this way while having a root canal done.

3. Do the same as in mini-task 2 for items you got wrong on quizzes.

4. Talk to a peer about course content.

Now, write some mini-tasks for the high-priority task you identified as having put off.

1. _____
2. _____
3. _____

These mini-tasks will get you involved in starting the task in a less painful way. Just starting a task, even in a minimal way, is a positive force, because getting started takes more effort than keeping going.

Whatever the cause of your procrastination, to be behind in work is to be behind in success. Most times it takes more time and energy to escape the task than to do it in the first place. Start today to keep life in the present and avoid deferring life and all its opportunities to the future.

Hints for Handling the Home/ Apartment

No matter how much you delegate, if you are a spouse and parent or a single parent, you must realize that your house or apartment is not going to be as spic and span while you are a student as it was before. A few hints may help ease the transition. Some of these hints are also helpful for spouses who are helping out while

the other goes to school and single adults on their own for the first time.

- Grandma always said tidy up to make it look like you really cleaned. Pick up papers and magazines as you pass through a room. If you don't have time to wash dishes, rinse and stack them to be done later rather than just collecting them on the counter in the kitchen. Make your bed each morning when you first get up. It only takes a minute and improves the appearance of the bedroom dramatically. In fact, you can teach yourself to smooth out the top covers before you get out of bed and then slither out. Place dirty clothes in a laundry basket in your bedroom or bathroom instead of just heaping them on the floor. Hang up other clothing instead of just draping it over furniture. Clean the tub after using it by soaping up your washcloth and washing the sides of the tub while it is still warm; then the soap and dirt ring will not have to be scoured. (Be sure to put your washcloth in the laundry and get out a clean one.) Put hair dryer, curlers, etc. away after use or collect in a basket to reduce clutter. These suggestions take hardly any time and really help things look straightened up.

- If you live in a two-story home, put a box at the top of the stairs and another one at the bottom for objects that need to go upstairs or come down. There is always something coming or going, and this will save extra trips.

- Having trouble with the family remembering their assigned chores? Draw the shape of a house on cardboard, draw 31 windows on the house and number them in sequence. Cut three of the four sides of each window so that it opens up. Place over shelf paper and write in names and chores for each day. Paste chore sheet in place and tape up windows. The first month takes the most time, but the chore list is a snap after that. Be sure to include a surprise or treat occasionally.

- A fun and fast way to dust for an adult or child is to wear a washed garden glove, spray the glove with furniture polish, and go to it.

The sky's the limit as far as creative ideas for saving time at school and in your personal life. You will come up with some out of sheer necessity as the year goes by. When you do, be sure to share them with your peers.

Evaluation

This part of your time-management program will take place continuously from the minute you start implementing your plan. Evaluation involves determining how well your plan is working and how you are progressing toward meeting your long-term goal. It is a crucial part

of time management. Why continue with a plan if it is not helping you reach your goal?

If it is not working, modify your plan. Ask yourself, "What changes should I make in my plan so that the plan will help me reach my long-term goal?" The best gauge you have for evaluating your plan is your test grades. They will tell you if you are devoting as much time as you need to make the grade in a course.

And how is your daily participation in class? Do you have assignments completed when they are due? Are you even aware that you had an assignment? Did you forget the test was on Thursday because you didn't mark it on your weekly calendar? Are you lapsing into the habit of procrastination? Not only will evaluation help you see how well you are progressing toward your goal, but it will also help you develop evaluation and modification skills you will need as a practical nurse.

Summary

Time management is the effective use of personal time to meet long-term goals. Techniques of time management can help you gain control over your life rather than feel a slave to it, and help you work smarter, not harder. By using elements of the nursing process, you can set up time-management techniques to fit your personal life. Assessment includes gathering data about present personal-time use and the activities included in the various roles you fill. Planning involves writing semester, weekly, and daily schedules to reflect high-priority activities. Implementation involves carrying out your plan. Evaluation is coming to a decision about whether your plan is helping you meet your long-term goal and modifying it accordingly.

REFERENCES

Bliss E. *Getting Things Done.* New York: Scribner Macmillan, 1991.

Building Better Study Skills. Iowa City, Iowa: The American College Testing Service, 1989.

Chenevert M. *Mosby's Tour Guide to Nursing School.* St. Louis: Mosby-Year Book, 1991.

Cooper C, Sullivan A, Shulman J. *Making It in College.* Lansing: Michigan State University, 1977.

Harper-Petersen M. Making time work for you. Nurs Life 1984; 4(5):56–57.

Lakein A. *How to Get Control of Your Time and Your Life.* New York: NAL-Dutton, 1989.

MacDonald-Clark N. Time management for nurses returning to school. Home Healthcare Nurse 1983; 1(1):13, 16, 28.

McNiff M. Getting organized at last. RN 1984; 47(6):23–24.

Pauk W. *How to Study in College.* 4th ed. Boston: Houghton-Mifflin, 1988.

Shepherd J. *College Study Skills.* Boston: Houghton-Mifflin, 1990.

Sotiriou P. *Integrating College Study Skills.* Belmont, Calif.: Wadsworth, 1988.

CHAPTER

6

Discovering Your Learning Style

Learning Objectives

Upon completing this chapter, you will
1. Explain what is meant by learning style.
2. Discuss three learning styles.
3. Identify your personal major learning style.
4. Identify which hemisphere of your brain is more active in learning.
5. List five characteristics of the side of the brain identified in objective 4.
6. Describe how your personal attitude influences learning.
7. Identify if you practice a reactive or an active learning style.

DISCOVERING YOUR LEARNING STYLE

Most individuals have wondered why one classmate takes voluminous notes, while another just listens, and another equally successful student says, "I'll understand this better when I practice it." Everyone learns differently, and yet, there may be some of you that have attempted to emulate a classmate's learning style because of his or her success, or perhaps, continue to practice a learning method that has never been as successful as you would like it to be. The authors are here to say that if a learning style is not working for you, change it. After completing this chapter, you are encouraged to review what you have learned about learning style and support or change present learning styles accordingly. Before reading any further, take time to complete the self-evaluation test below.

Self Evaluation of Personal Learning Style

IDENTIFY YOUR LEARNING STYLE

Directions: Underline the answer that is most accurate for each statement.

		YES	SOMETIMES	NO
1.	Prefers to talk rather than read.	○	△	□
2.	Likes to touch, hug, shake hands.	△	□	⊙
3.	Prefers verbal directions.	○	△	□
4.	Uses finger spelling as a way of learning words.	△	□	○
5.	Likes written directions better than verbal directions.	⊠	○	△
6.	Reads to self by moving lips.	○	△	□
7.	Likes to take notes for studying.	□	○	△
8.	Remembers best by doing.	△	□	○
9.	Likes or makes charts and graphs.	□	○	△
10.	Learns from listening to lectures and tapes.	⊙	△	□
11.	Likes to work with tools.	△	□	○
12.	Might say, "I don't see what you mean."	□	○	△
13.	Good at jigsaw puzzles.	□	○	△
14.	Has good listening skills.	⊙	△	□
15.	Presses pencil down hard when writing.	△	□	○
16.	Learns theory best by reading the textbook.	□	○	△
17.	Asks to have printed directions explained.	○	△	□
18.	Chews gum or smokes almost continuously.	△	□	○

Scoring
Count all of the ○ △ □
The highest number indicates the major learning style(s).

Key: □ = visual
     ○ = auditory
     △ = tactual

Adapted from and used with the permission of Jeffrey Barsch, Ed.D. Complete copies of the test may be obtained by writing directly to Jeffrey Barsch, Ed.D., Ventura College, 4667 Telegraph Rd., Ventura, CA 93003.

Congratulations! You have taken the time to identify your major learning style(s). Now to find out what it all means.

LEARNING STYLES

Different people think differently. They think in one of three systems corresponding to one of three senses—vision, hearing, or feeling. Those who think in visions (visual learners) generate visual images, that is, they think primarily in pictures. People who think in hearing (auditory learners) talk to themselves or hear sounds. Individuals who think in touch (kinesthetic, or tactual, learners) experience feelings in regard to what is being thought about. This does not mean that a learner thinks exclusively in any one of these representational systems. What it does mean is that most people think more in one system than another, and that there are ways to enhance learning by supporting the major system. Below is an example of a response to the same statement according to the three learning styles.

INSTRUCTOR: We will meet tomorrow in the cafeteria at St. Vincent's, fourth floor, off Neurology, East wing, 0700.

VISUAL: Hmm. I can't quite picture that. Better make a note of it.

AUDITORY: No problem. I'll be there.

TACTUAL: I'll be OK after the first time. I'll go with auditory, if it's OK. (Reaches out to touch auditory.)

QUESTION: What has prompted each of the three responses? Clue: Look back at the pretest questions.

First of all, it is important not to label any of the learning styles as being better than another. Think about this. It is easy to feel connected to someone who shares a similar learning style. "We think in the same language." It is just as easy to label a peer with a different learning style as either smart or uninterested. Think also about the implication for the instructor–student relationship as the student looks away,

when the instructor asks a memory question. Resistance? Disinterest? Not necessarily. According to Bandler and Grinder (1979, p. 25) the individual is remembering images. In fact, the student, if right-handed, is probably remembering by looking up and to the left. But what has happened? If the behavior was labeled in a negative way, the instructor probably continued to talk or called on someone else. Get the picture? A learning style just is; but there are ways to increase its effectiveness. Table 6-1 suggests ideas to enhance each of the three learning styles.

QUESTION: What additional ways can you think of to enhance your learning style?

You have identified your learning style, but another important topic to be discussed involves your brain and how you use it to learn.

ONE BRAIN: TWO DIFFERENT WAYS OF THINKING

You will learn about the brain when you study the nervous system in your body structure and function class. For now, think of your brain as the control center of your body, performing more functions than the best computer you can buy today. Clench both of your fists and put them together in front of you. This is approximately the size of your brain. Now, look at two typed letters on this page. The outer surface of your brain, the cerebral cortex (the part of the brain that makes you human), is just that thick. This is the area of the brain that researchers have discovered is the seat of the mind. Personality, emotions, language, movement, sensations, thought, desires, hearing, vision, memory, and learning are some of the functions of this narrow layer. We have come a long way in brain research since Aristotle's time, when this center of mental activity was thought to be in the area of the heart and the abdomen. At least today we know that the center of mental activity is enclosed in the bony box that is our skull. Yet valentines still say, "I love you with all my

Table 6-1 How to Enhance Your Learning Style

VISUAL LEARNER	AUDITORY LEARNER	TACTUAL LEARNER
Takes notes in class	Reads aloud	Takes notes and rewrites them to condense
Writes notes in the margin of book	Reads into a tape recorder and plays it back	Learns to do sign language and does signing while reading
Looks for reference books with pictures, graphs, and charts	Discusses ideas about class content with others	
Draws illustrations of his own when studying	Requests explanations of illustrations, graphs, or diagrams	Handles visual aids provided during class
Reviews films and videotapes	Moves lips while reading	Requests to do demonstrations
Uses index cards for review or memorization	Finds a peer to study with and discusses the topic being studied	Learns best by doing
Observes a demonstration	Learns best with lectures and by using tapes	

heart," when they should say, "I love you with all my brain."

Much research on the brain has occurred since Aristotle's time and although there is a lot more we do not know about the brain, there is a lot we do know about this organ. During the late 1960s and early 1970s exciting research confirmed the fact that humans have two distinct sides of the brain that are linked by a complex network of nerve fibers called the "corpus callosum." Each side is called a "hemisphere." Although each side of the brain is generally the same in structure, each side deals with different kinds of mental activity. In other words, you have one brain, but two different ways of thinking. Before reading on, respond to the following statements as directed. Again, it is important that the answers be honest and reflect yourself.

LEARNING EXERCISE

Which Side of Your Brain Is Most Active?

You can be professionally tested for right or left brain activity. Below is a simple test designed by the authors to give you a quick clue as to which side of your brain may be more active.

In each of the following items, two different styles of learning, thinking, or acting are described. Choose the option that describes you most accurately.

1. FEELINGS AND EMOTIONS
   a. It is easy for me to express how I feel.
   b. It is hard for me to express how I feel.
2. HUMOR
   a. I am the type of person who can usually think of something funny to say.
   b. It is hard for me to think of something funny to say.
3. PROBLEM-SOLVING
   a. I usually solve problems by listing possible solutions and choosing the best one.
   b. I usually solve problems by choosing what feels right.
4. ORGANIZATION
   a. Most days my desk is very organized.
   b. Most days my desk looks like a battlefield.
5. MEMORY
   a. I'm good at remembering names.
   b. I'm good at remembering faces.
6. SENSE OF DIRECTION
   a. Sometimes I can get lost in my own house.
   b. Although I've never been there, if I had a map, I could find my way around Tibet.
7. THINKING THINGS THROUGH
   a. I am most comfortable when things are either black or white or cut and dried.
   b. I am most comfortable when things are in shades of gray.
8. LEARNING
   a. I learn a skill best by reading about it.
   b. I learn a skill best by watching someone do it.
9. VISUALIZING IMAGES
   a. When I think of an image, it is in color.
   b. When I think of an image it is in black and white.
10. MATHEMATICS (MUST CHOOSE ONE)
   a. I prefer geometry.
   b. I prefer algebra.
11. THINKING
   a. I like to look at the total picture.
   b. I like to focus on specific details.
12. Last but not least. Put down your pencil. Sit back and relax. Clasp your hands in your lap. The thumb on top is:
   a. right thumb
   b. left thumb

Use the following key to determine what your answers indicate. In the key, R means right brain and L means left brain. Add up the number of Rs and Ls. Whichever there is more of gives an indication if one side of your brain is more active.

1. a.–R	4. a.–L	7. a.–L	10. a.–R
b.–L	b.–R	b.–R	b.–L
2. a.–R	5. a.–L	8. a.–L	11. a.–R
b.–L	b.–R	b.–R	b.–L
3. a.–L	6. a.–R	9. a.–R	12. a.–R
b.–R	b.–L	b.–L	b.–L

Congratulations! Now you have identified the side of your brain that is more active. Perhaps you have found that you use both sides equally. So what does all this have to do with learning?

In most people, the left side of the brain is associated with academic activities and the right side of the brain is associated with creative intuition. One side of the brain is no more or less important than the other. You need each side to make sense out of the world. Table 6-2 compares the different functions of the right and left sides of the brain.

The two sides are designed to form a partnership and are complementary to each other. Take the activity of speech, for example. The left side of the brain, being very verbal and fluent, would wind up having us talk in computer-like patterns if the right side were not available to add tone and inflection to our voice. The right side of the brain would help us to recognize a face in the crowd quickly, even if the person had shaved off his beard, while the left side would puzzle over this missing part. At school, the left side helps us break new information down into bits and pieces so we can master it, while the right side gives us the total picture of our learning. In nursing, the right side generates new ideas to use in improving patient care and the left side verifies the safety of these new methods.

This brain partnership can be encouraged or discouraged in an individual. We have been accused of living in a left-brained world. Education in the United States has typically encouraged activity of the left side of the brain and ignored the right side. Individually, we have allowed the left side of our brain to be more active and this bad habit helps make our brain's

Table 6-2 Comparison of the Two Sides of the Brain

LEFT BRAIN	RIGHT BRAIN
Thinks in words	Thinks in images
Looks at the parts that make up the picture or entire situation	Looks at the whole picture or entire situation
Logical side	Emotional side
Breaks down the whole to individual parts and takes them one at a time, step by step (analyzer)	Combines parts to make a whole (holistic, a synthesizer)
Works like a digital computer	Works like a kaleidoscope
Speech, word center	Visual center
Slower working	Faster working
Special activities: 　Reasoning 　Numbers (mathematics) 　Expression of thoughts in words 　Verbal awareness 　Verifies ideas	Special activities: 　Music 　Rhythm 　Insight 　Imagination 　Intuition 　Nonverbal memory 　Generates ideas 　Daydreams 　Visualize in three dimensions 　Visualizes in color

partnership a lopsided one. We can learn to be aware of both sides of our brain and from the standpoint of learning it would benefit each of us to do so.

Blakeslee (1980, p. 74) states that when the full power of both sides of the brain are used together, humans can achieve great things. To overlook one side or the other in everyday life, including learning situations, is to function with only half of our potential. This has occurred throughout the history of humans by favoring one side or the other.

You have identified which side of your brain is most active. This is your strong or active side. In Chapter 7, "Learning How To Learn," you will find out how to develop the "forgotten" side so that you may learn with your personal full potential. When you do so, you can increase your learning and understanding. Remember, continue using the ways of thinking with your more active side while learning how to use newer ways of thinking with your less active side.

Wow! Chapters 4, 5, and 6 have exposed you to information that traditionally has not been shared with students. You are on your way to success.

ATTITUDES THAT AFFECT LEARNING

A perfectly good learning style can be sabotaged by the attitude of the learner. Consider some of the student attitudes listed below.

Student Nurse Sponge: This student feels inferior to the other students in class and consequently does not participate. What this student does not realize is that to risk is to learn. The student has had many life experiences that relate to what is being taught, and once the student learns how to connect new information to previously learned information, real learning will begin. This student nurse, in essence, sits on knowledge, absorbs from others, and gives nothing in return.

Student Nurse Gabby: This student feels that the class information is too simple or that it is not being presented in a desired manner. This plus a strong need for personal recognition, re-

sults in a student who dominates the class discussion and frequently intimidates other students in the process. What this student does not realize is that impatience is actually impeding reaching her desired personal goal. It would be appropriate for this student to seek out the instructor individually, express concerns in a straightforward manner, and request additional study assignments to meet personal needs.

QUESTION: Who is responsible for Student Nurse Gabby's learning?

Student Nurse I-Can't-Do-It: This student does not know just what is expected in order to meet class objectives. Consequently, requirements are seen as being overwhelming. It is this student's responsibility to ask for clarification, make special needs and problems known, and request additional help as needed. The instructor is the immediate resource. Should additional help be needed, most schools offer tutoring and counseling services.

Student Nurse Fidget: This student generally has decided that the instructor's class is boring and does not see how it applies to the clinical work. Consequently, the student has decided that each class period is a test of endurance, rather than learning. The lack of participation and constant fidgeting affect peers in a negative way. This individual needs to decide that learning is available and set a small goal prior to each class period. For example, an initial goal might be to contribute one item of information per class or to ask one question during class time. The comment or question can be developed in advance while preparing for class. In this way the comment or question is appropriate to the topic being discussed. As the student becomes increasingly comfortable, the goal can be advanced.

Student Nurse Put-It-Off: This student delays preparing for class, doing required work and projects, and studying for tests until the deadline has arrived. Enter panic and stress, and a promise not to do this again. Chances are that procrastination is a way of life for this individual. Procrastination is sometimes engaged in by people who are concerned that they may fail and consequently rationalize why it is impossible to do things on time. When a deadline arrives they are forced to do the work, but "no one can blame me if I don't do any better. I just ran out of time." Often these students are very capable, and if they desire to change this stressful pattern of learning, it is possible to do so consciously. For example, they can make a reasonable daily schedule and adhere to it, and check progress at regular intervals. There will be a tendency to go back to the previous way of functioning. When this happens, it is important to continue with the new plan rather than scrapping it and saying, "I'll start again on Monday." Remember that this pattern developed over a long period of time and will need time for change. A rule of thumb for the amount of time before you see change in any behavior, once a plan is instituted, is a minimum of two to three weeks.

Student Nurse Opportunity: This student takes the initiative in learning and sees every experience, whether positive or negative, as a learning experience. The most important lesson of all has been learned by the student—no one can make anyone else learn; the instructor's role is that of a facilitator only.

REACTIVE VERSUS ACTIVE LEARNING

The reactive, or passive, learner waits to be taught while the active, or assertive, learner takes the responsibility for learning. It is a fact that the assertive learner learns better and retains the information longer than the passive learner. According to Knowles (1988, p. 15) "the main purpose of education must now be to develop the skills of inquiry."

QUESTION: Are you a reactive or an active learner? Support your answer.

PUTTING IT TOGETHER

It is not unusual to read information and end up saying, "But of course, this doesn't apply to me." But this information does apply. You have had the opportunity to (1) identify your major learning style; (2) receive hints on how to enhance your learning style; (3) differentiate between a reactive and active learner; and (4) put the results of your self-evaluation together in practice, as you move toward your education goal.

Houle (in Knowles, 1988, p. 68) offers some principles for becoming a self directed learner.

1. Behave in a successful manner. Success will reinforce this attitude.

QUESTION: How do you act successful? Think of four ways.

2. Set realistic goals and evaluate results to see if these goals are being met. Houle cautions that it is an obstacle to learning to think that learning can take place without effort.

3. A personal point of view affects learning. Houle cautions not to let established values harden into such fixed beliefs that new ideas cannot be tolerated: at that point education ends.

4. Tie in new learning to previous learning and experiences. This gives the material meaning and makes it easier to remember.

5. Seek help when needed; sometimes studying alone is best, sometimes it is best done with others. Beginning studies, problems with studies, or the need to be with someone are reasons for seeking out others.

6. Learn beyond the point necessary for testing or performing the skill. Keep reviewing and practicing the skills.

Summary

People think in different representational systems; this determines their major learning style. Some think in pictures (visual learners), some hear sounds or talk to themselves (auditory learners), and some experience the feeling in regard to what they are thinking about and learn best by doing (tactual learners). Each learning style can be enhanced through specific techniques.

The right and left brain have separate and distinct functions. Thinking and learning are affected by the active side. Left-brain-active students tend to read and write well, solve problems logically, and enjoy learning details and facts. Right-brain active students are more creative, express their feelings freely, use an intuitive approach to problem-solving, and prefer an overview of the subject. Learning to use the less active side enhances functioning of both sides of the brain.

One's personal attitude toward learning also influences the learning process. Attitude is closely related to whether you are a reactive learner who expects to be taught or an active learner who takes charge of his own education.

REFERENCES

Bandler R, Grinder J, Stevens J, ed. *Frogs into Princes.* Moab, Utah: Real People Press, 1979.

Barsch J. *Understanding Your Learning Style.* Ventura, Calif.: Ventura College Learning Disability Clinic.

Blakeslee T. *The Right Brain: A New Understanding of the Unconscious Mind and Its Creative Powers.* New York: Berkley, 1980.

Buzan T. *Use Both Sides of Your Brain.* 3rd ed. New York: NAL-Dutton, 1991.

Garity J. Learning styles basis for creative teaching and learning. Nurse Educ 1985; March/April:12–16.

Houle C. *Continuing Your Education.* New York: McGraw-Hill, 1964.

Houle C. *Patterns of Learning.* San Francisco: Jossey-Bass, 1984.

Knowles M: *Self-Directed Learning: A Guide for Learners and Teachers.* Englewood Cliffs N.J.: Cambridge Books, 1988.

Rezler A, French R. *Personality types and learning preferences of students in six allied health profession.* J Allied Health 1975; Winter:20–26.

Williams I. *Teaching for the Two-Sided Mind.* New York: Touchstone Books, 1986.

CHAPTER 7
Learning How to Learn

Learning Objectives

Upon completion of this chapter, you will
1. Identify techniques to increase your degree of concentration when in learning situations.
2. Identify techniques to improve your listening skills when in learning situations.
3. Describe techniques to enhance understanding of information needed to be a practical nurse.
4. Evaluate personal need for help with reading skills to increase speed of reading and degree of comprehension.

Of all the reasons for not succeeding in school, lack of study skills is high on the list of causes. From our teaching experience, we have seen student failure due to lack of study skills more often than lack of time to devote to school. In fact, when failure is attributed to "I don't have the time," in reality it is many times due to lack of knowledge as to how to study and to use time to advantage. Many vocational schools and junior colleges offer courses in how to study before entering a program and have departments that offer study skill services after a student is enrolled, but not everyone who needs these services is aware of their personal need. Many adult students seem to think they will succeed because they have succeeded in high school. Adult students cannot assume they have the study skills necessary for success in the practical nursing program just because they have attended high school. The students who have developed study skills will be surprised at how much more effectively they can learn after reviewing their study habits. In addition, educators have learned much about how to learn that was not known even five years ago.

Before going on, you must be aware of two things. First, you must get yourself organized into a study habit. Some people dislike the thought of being organized. Many times this feeling arises out of habit, and can be overcome by keeping your educational goals in front of you and developing some organizational skills for studying. Second, you must realize that it is hard work to acquire the knowledge and skills needed for your chosen career. Sorry, we cannot say it will be easy. Learning is hard work and takes time and effort. Study skills are like any other skill. They are developed by practice and hard work.

GENERAL HINTS FOR LEARNERS
Concentration

Concentration is the ability to keep your mind completely on the task at hand. The major enemy of concentration is distraction. And there are many distractions in an adult's life that compete with the need to buckle down to school assignments. These distractions can be summarized as two types: Those that come from outside yourself, or external distractions, and those that come from inside yourself or internal distractions.

External Distractions

Personal study area. Your physical environment is a potential enemy of concentration. Locate one or two realistic areas for studying. The chosen areas should be associated with learning and not daydreaming or napping. The learning resource center at your school can be used between classes and after school. Another area can be one in your home or apartment. Your area could be the kitchen, a corner of your bedroom, or part of the basement. The place you choose should be away from family or roommates. The area should have a writing surface, a lamp, and a chair. Have a supply of pens, sharpened pencils, a highlighter felt marker, loose-leaf paper, scrap paper, index cards, a calendar, an English dictionary, and a medical or nursing dictionary at hand. You will save time and aggravation by not having to look for your study tools each time you sit to study. Choose a chair you feel comfortable in, but not one that you associate with snoozing.

Lighting. The light you choose for studying is almost more important than your chair. Most students have a table lamp and this is fine as long as the bulb is shaded and your writing surface is light colored to reflect light. It is important to eliminate glare; the shade and light surface will help in this matter. Try a "soft-white" light bulb to reduce glare further, but be sure that it is screwed into its socket for a tight connection in order to reduce flicker. If a ceiling light is also available, turn this on in addition to your table lamp to reduce the chance of shadows. Eyestrain can occur if lighting allows glare, shadows, or flicker to exist in your study area. If you have tried to eliminate these three unwanted lighting conditions and you experience symptoms of eyestrain, such as headaches, dizziness, tiredness, or blurred vision while reading, it is time for an eye examination to rule out the need for corrective lenses. Many students have discovered the need for glasses only after enrolling in an educational program demanding much reading, such as the practical-nursing program.

Background noise. Keep in mind that some research studies show that students can concentrate in noisy surroundings and other studies show that students have trouble concentrating in quiet surroundings. You should strive for a study environment without background noise. If this is not possible, you can discipline yourself to ignore noise and concentrate on your studying. Television, stereos, radios, and a Sony Walkman are considered background noise. Frequently, students will state that they study best with these external distractions. Some studies have shown that background music can maintain productivity when routine and manipulative tasks are involved but not when learning must occur. If these habits are a carryover from high school, try to establish new habits to help you with your more difficult subjects in the practical nursing program. High school study habits do not automatically guarantee success in educational programs beyond high school. List here any external distractions that are affecting your concentration. What can you do to eliminate these distractions?

_____
_____
_____
_____

Internal Distractions

You can have the perfect desk, lighting, chair, noise level, and equipment for studying but still not be able to keep your mind on the task at hand. The culprit may be distractions arising from inside yourself. Here are some common examples of internal distractions and suggestions for overcoming them.

Complaints of mental fatigue. Scientists have yet to prove that your billions of brain cells actually do get tired. Most students confuse boredom with fatigue. In setting up a study schedule, make sure you do not study one subject so long that you get bored with it. Keep up your physical self with proper food, sleep, and exercise. At the first sign of "getting tired," take a short break (not a snooze) and come back to

new material so that you can get your mental second wind.

Daydreaming. To daydream is to waste time. Everytime you find your mind wandering from the topic at hand to that wonderful Saturday night, next weekend, or what it will be like when you don't have to study anymore, put a check mark on a piece of paper that you keep at your side. This will remind you that you are drifting off and need to get back to work. Students who use this technique find that the number of check marks decreases dramatically as the days go on.

Thinking about things you have to do in addition to studying. "I must remember to buy milk for tomorrow." "Bobby's shirt needs to be mended." "Return that library book." These are all important, but play havoc with concentration. Write the thought down on the paper at your side that you are using for daydream check marks. Now you can get back to concentrating without fear of forgetting the item. When you are done studying or the class is finished, the reminder will be there in black and white.

Thinking about personal problems. The nature of these problems can be as numerous as there are students. Each student must devise personal strategies to deal with them. A suggestion is to write down the problem on the paper at your side. After you are finished studying, try to deal with the problem. If this does not work, seek help from friends or counselors, set up a plan of action, and follow it. Learning cannot take place when you have personal problems competing with concentration time.

List here any internal distractions that are affecting your concentration. What can you do to eliminate these distractions?

_____
_____
_____
_____

Other Techniques for Improving Concentration

The following are additional techniques that have been used successfully by students to improve concentration. Try them out to see if they can help you.

1. Look at studying as an opportunity to advance your career and not just an unpleasant task you must engage in.

2. Simple tools such as a pencil or highlighter will keep you active in your learning. Underlining or highlighting main ideas, writing in the margins, etc. will keep you active and your concentration at its peak.

Listening

The human voice takes up much of class time. Whether you are in a lecture class, a discussion, or are viewing films as part of a course, if your mind wanders, you are going to miss a lot. Listening is much more than the mechanical process of hearing. There are two kinds of listeners. Which type are you?

The **passive** listener receives sounds with little recognition or personal involvement. This "listener" may be doodling, staring out the window, or even staring at the instructor but thinking about having to change the oil in the car or deciding what to cook for dinner. The **active** listener is searching for relevant information and strives to understand it. This listener realizes that listening is a primary way of gathering information and works at developing this skill. The active listener looks for ways that the speaker's words can be put to practical use, regardless of the student's level of interest or degree of fondness for the instructor or the instructor's dress or mannerisms. Are you an active or a passive listener?

Notemaking

An important part of listening is remembering what you have listened to. Some students will tell you that taking notes will interfere with their listening skills. They are correct if they are in the business of *taking* notes. Research has shown that a student will give evidence of remembering only 50% of a 10-minute lecture when tested immediately afterward and only

25% of that lecture when tested two days later. The secret to improving those percentages to as much as 80 to 90% is to engage in **notemaking** whenever you are listening (since teachers will derive test questions from lectures, discussions, films, etc., that 80 to 90% could translate into a test score). Notemaking will help you to pay attention, concentrate, and organize your ideas, whether you are attending a lecture, watching a film, or participating in a discussion.

Hints for Notemaking

Never try to capture every word of the speaker or narrator. This is **notetaking,** and also impossible. A speaker can put out about 110 to 160 words per minute. Time yourself to find how many words you can write per minute. Have a peer time one minute and another peer read for the same time while you try to write everything down. The number will shock you. Besides not being able to get every word down, you will also not be able to capture the meaning of what was said. Strive for **notemaking,** forming condensations of what is said in a telegramlike manner. Actively listen for the main ideas and capture them in a way that is efficient for you. You are recording ideas or key concepts for later additions, corrections, and study.

Have one $8\frac{1}{2}$-by-11 loose-leaf notebook with dividers for each class. Spiral notebooks have the disadvantage of not allowing handouts to be easily included with daily notes. With the loose-leaf system, the notebook can be left at home and a supply of paper taken to school daily. Make sure your name, address, and telephone number are in the notebook, in case you misplace it when you do bring it to school.

Do not tape record classes. To do so just postpones the inevitable. You eventually have to listen to the tape so why not actively listen to the lecture and take notes? To listen to a tape after class is very time consuming, often requiring three times the length of the lecture itself. That's not good time management.

Do not take notes in shorthand. This involves having to transcribe your notes after class, another poor time-management technique. Develop your own personal symbols, abbreviations, and shorthand of sorts to help you capture the main ideas yet retain readability without having to transcribe. Use your medical abbreviations as presented in your charting classes. Make your notes in pen so that they don't smudge. When a mistake is made, cross out the error. Erasing is time consuming. Avoid typing or rewriting your class notes word-for-

word. Instead, use this time to think about what is important in the notes and condense them as you rewrite. This is especially helpful for tactual learners. At first your notes may seem to be a disaster, but remember that you are not competing for a penmanship award. With practice, things will improve. Your goal is a set of notes you can use today, next week, and even next year for review.

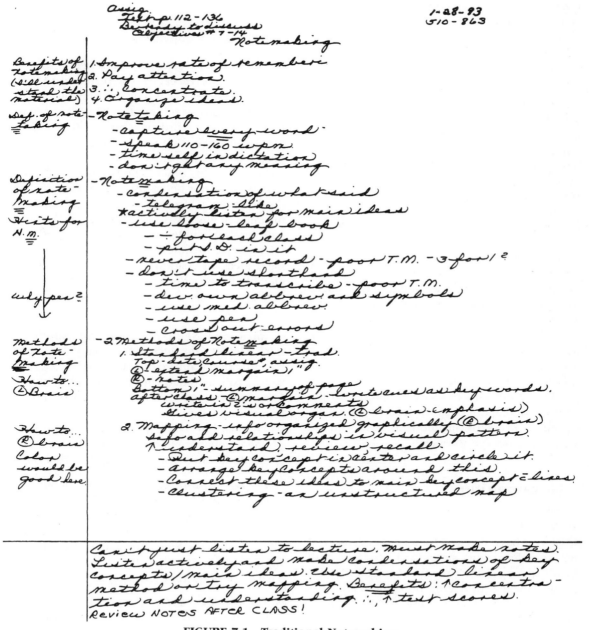

FIGURE 7-1 Traditional Notemaking

Two methods for making and reviewing notes. The first method is the *outlining method,* which has been used for ages, and involves adapting normal loose-leaf paper so that you have room to take notes, summarize content, and have a method to test yourself on your notes, thereby preparing yourself continually for testing of the material. Figure 7-1 is an example of traditional **notemaking,** used to summarize this chapter so far. Use the margin at the top of the page to write the date and course number and any assignments that are given. Extend the left margin another inch and take your notes in your personal style to the right of this line. After class, in the area at the left of the page, record key words or phrases that serve as cues for the lecture notes on the right and as a space for questions or comments. This will be useful in testing yourself. The bottom inch of each page should be left blank so that a summary of the content of lecture notes on that page can be made. This forces you to think about and come to grips with the ideas in your notes.

An alternative to the linear method of note making has been suggested by brain researchers and encourages using the right side of the brain and its emphasis on images. In *Use Both Sides of Your Brain,* Buzan (1983, p. 91) explains how information presented in a linear manner is not as easily understood as information presented by key concepts—the primary way in which the brain processes information. The brain takes these key concepts and integrates them and makes relationships. So, if the brain does not work in lines or lists, then the method of notemaking called **mapping,** in which information is organized graphically so that information and its relationships are in a visual pattern, should enhance your ability to understand, review, and recall this information. Figure 7-2 summarizes the information in this chapter so far in an unstructured mapping form called clustering.

Remembering and Forgetting

We all can recall things from the past, indicating that our brains have the ability to store informa-

tion. But how many times have you said "I forgot," or "I can't remember?" Possible causes for forgetting include a negative attitude toward the subject, interfering with motivation to remember, new knowledge interfering with the recall of old learning, and old knowledge interfering with the recall of new learning. Valid though these causes of forgetting may be, perhaps the most common reason why students cannot remember is that they had never grasped it in the first place. They really did not internalize the information and understand it to begin with. Perhaps they did not listen actively or they just read words and created a mental blur. In order to store information in your long-term memory, a neural trace or a record of the information must be laid down. Psychologists have found that it takes four to five seconds for information to move from temporary, or short-term, memory to permanent, or long-term, memory. In order to form long-term memory of information, you must strive to understand that information and in doing so, you will have given your brain the chance to lay down a neural trace. Presto! You have a memory. Short but frequent study periods will help you to understand information and store it in long-term memory.

How to Understand (Comprehend) Information

You will be exposed to much knowledge during your year in the practical nursing program. You will gain knowledge as stated in course objectives. Your real test as a practical nurse will be your ability to understand that information and apply it in the clinical area. The national licensing examination for practical nurses tests mainly at the level of understanding and application. The following will help you comprehend the meaning of *knowledge* (knowing), *understanding, and application:*

1. Knowing means the ability to repeat back information you have memorized. This is the lowest level of learning. Defining a concept *as stated in a dictionary* is an example of knowledge.

2. *Understanding* (comprehension) means to grasp the meaning of the material. This is the lowest level of understanding. Repeating information *in your own words* indicates that you understand the concept.

3. *Application* means being able to use learned material in new situations. An example of application is applying what is learned in class to your clinical work. This is a higher level of understanding, which helps you retain what

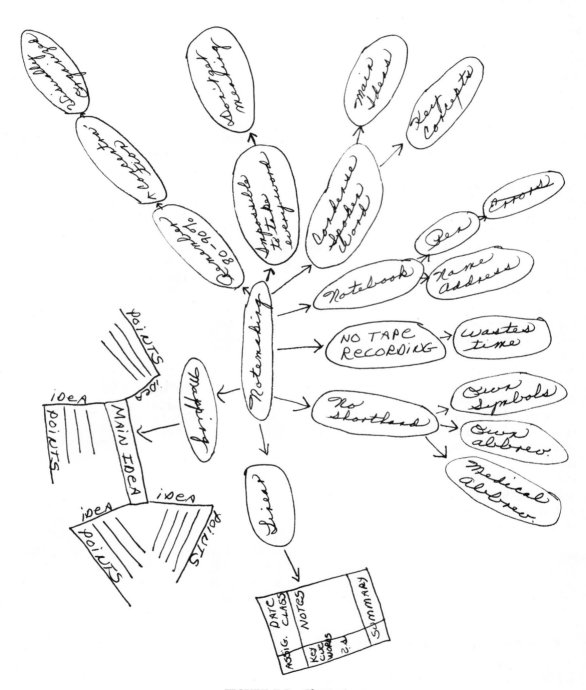

FIGURE 7-2 Clustering

you are learning. Understanding and application are what employers expect of a practical nurse on the job. Your instructors will also expect this on the clinical area.

Your scholastic world is bombarded with words, sentences, and paragraphs. One of the most beneficial techniques to understand and remember all the information you are exposed to is to balance this verbal mixture with visual strategies. Each of the following visual strategies will help you to understand and ultimately remember information better because they deal with the right side of the brain. You will be tapping a resource that perhaps you have not been using.

Draw Idea Sketches

These drawings will probably be comprehensible only to the maker. The emphasis is not on the quality of the drawing but on the process you must go through to take a verbal concept and represent it graphically, without words. To go through this process you must reach understanding of the verbal concept. You can even set it up as a cartoon. Use stick figures if you have to and verbally describe the concept. Figure 7-3 is an idea sketch used to illustrate the function of the drug lanoxin, which is used to slow and strengthen the heartbeat.

Choose a concept you are having trouble with in one of your classes; draw an idea sketch to help you increase your understanding of that concept.

Use Color in Whatever Form of Notemaking You Use

Use highlighters, crayons, colored pencils, or felt-tip pens. Avoid merely underlining the page. Use the different colors to help capture and direct your attention to information that fits in different categories. The different colors will help your brain organize and retrieve information.

Make Your Own Diagrams as You Read

If you commit ideas to memory only by using words, then you are using one half your brain's resources, those of the left side. If you also produce a sketch of that idea, you will have brought the right side of your brain into use and the use of both sides is a powerful tool to encourage the storage and retrieval of information.

Engage in Mental Imagery

This technique will really help you to remember, because it demands that you understand the information. During mental imagery, you become the idea that you are having difficulty understanding. The right side of your brain is used to generate pictures of the idea, while the left side of your brain supplies the script to explain what is going on in the pictures (and always in your own words). The following is an example of mental imagery developed by a

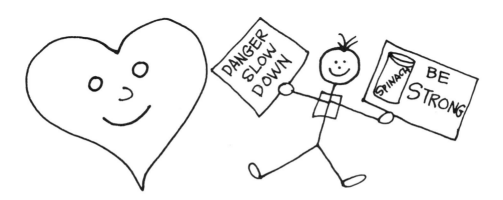

FIGURE 7-3   Idea Sketch. Action of Lanoxin (digoxin).

practical nursing student to give herself a simple understanding of the function of insulin, a hypoglycemic agent that increases glucose transport across muscle and fat-cell membranes. Notice how she used the senses of hearing and feeling and also body movement to help achieve understanding. She also uses a metaphor, equating something she knows about with something she is trying to learn. The student recites this image to herself while she closes her eyes and visualizes it. In the beginning, she had her roommate read the story while she visualized the scenario.

I am insulin—a job description. I am insulin and I am shaped like a canoe. In fact, I am a canoe, a green one. My job is to make the sugar or glucose in the blood available to most of the cells of the body for energy. I like my job. I like things that are sweet but not too sweet, so blood sugar is just my thing. Sometime after the person who owns the pancreas where I am stored in my canoe rack eats a meal, a whistle blows and I know this is a signal for me to launch myself into the bloodstream. As I ride the currents of the blood, I rock gently back and forth and the sugar in the bloodstream jumps right in to be passengers. Blood sugar likes me. I think this is because I am green, but I might be wrong. When I am pretty full, but not full enough to swamp, I pass through the blood vessels, paddle through the sea of tissue fluid (boy, it smells salty) around the cells, pass through the cell membrane, and deposit the sugar by making these molecules jump out of the canoe and into the fluid inside the cell. I feel pretty important in my job. Without me, the blood-sugar molecules would be unable to pass through the cell membranes. Because of this, I am given the official job title of hypoglycemic agent, because I lower the level of sugar in the blood. Excuse me, there goes the whistle.

Perhaps a physiologist would wince at this description. But it is nothing to be ashamed of if it helps you understand a concept. Plus, mental imagery can be fun!

Form a Neural Trace

Since positive mental attitude is a factor in allowing you to understand and remember, it is good to remind yourself that all the basic courses in which you are now enrolled are essential because they are the building blocks for all the remaining courses you will take in the practical nursing program. You have already started your career. Most of the following techniques also help increase understanding of your work by allowing neural traces to be recorded in your brain.

As you listen or read, seek out key concepts, basic principles and key ideas. Be selective and learn to sift out and reject unnecessary details. You cannot memorize everything, and if you could, you would not have an understanding of anything. The activity of being selective helps you lay down neural traces. Put your emphasis on accuracy, not speed. You want correct information to make a clear neural trace. It is difficult to unlearn wrong and to relearn correct information.

Short study periods followed by short rest periods are better than long study marathons. This type of study will reenergize you and allow neural learning to continue during rest periods. Those seemingly wasted 10 minutes between classes or standing in the cafeteria line can be used to your advantage.

Use as many body senses and as much body movement as possible when trying to learn new information. Recite the information aloud as you read, and in your own words. If you can explain it, you must understand it, and will know it. Hearing yourself say the information is an additional channel to allow neural traces to be recorded. Write down the information in your own words. Do not copy verbatim from a book. This muscle action will help you clarify ideas and improve thinking. Vary your body position while studying, lean against a wall, sit on the floor, pace. You will keep alert and awake. Using muscles by gesturing can help improve memory of information by matching a gesture to information that needs to be remembered. When the gesture and word are associated in your mind, sometimes the word can be retrieved by performing the gesture. Physical motion can jog memory and promote recall. You should see some of the motions students go through during an exam. If it works, don't knock it. These techniques of using body senses and body movement all help lay down the neural trace.

You do not have to adopt all of the suggestions we have given to help you understand the material in your classes and therefore increase your long-term memory of that information. You should, however, be working on discovering the memory tricks that work for you.

Another Memory Aid

We have not included mnemonic devices as a memory aid. You know what they are. Some examples:

- Rhymes
  Thirty days hath September . . .
  I before *e* except after *c* . . .
  In fourteen hundred and ninety-two . . .
- Acronyms
  Every good boy does fine . . . to remember the line notes of the treble clef.

Although these devices can help you remember information, they do not allow understanding of that information to occur. Use them only when necessary to remember lists of words, or facts, but do not use them as a substitute for remembering by understanding.

Reading

Since you are responsible for large amounts of reading in a practical nursing program, it is necessary for you to know how to handle this task effectively. Most of us are able to read the printed words on a page, but the reading demanded of a learner and future employee involves much more than this act. Reading to learn and understand involves a rate of speed and a degree of understanding that are effective, not just reading words on a page. You probably had a reading test as part of your pre-entrance tests for the practical nursing program. Generally, these tests are brief, and if you scored low, you were referred for help with this skill. We are concerned with those of you who scored an acceptable score on these short reading tests,

but could use some hints on how to increase your reading efficiency, that is, your rate of speed and degree of comprehension. Evaluate your reading habits by answering "yes" or "no" to the following questions.

1. Do you ever reread a sentence before you come to its end?

2. Do you ever have trouble figuring out the main point of an author?

3. Do you stop your reading every time you come across a word you cannot define and look up the word immediately?

4. Do you read novels, popular magazines, newspapers, and textbooks at the same speed?

5. Do you ever have trouble remembering what you read?

6. Do you ever have trouble understanding what you have read?

7. Do you ever think of other things while you read?

8. Do you ever read every word of a sentence individually?

If you answered "yes" to any of the above questions, you could benefit from some help with your reading efficiency. We suggest a visit to your school's skill center for assistance with reading your textbooks and technical material with more organization and efficiency.

Hints to Increase Reading Efficiency

Read in phrases, a few words at a time, rather than word by word. Although the brain can only view one word at a time, it only understands when words are in phrases. For better understanding, you should read as you speak, in phrases.

Moving your lips while reading. Although some authors feel that moving your lips or trying to hear the words while you read will slow you down, other authors feel that speaking and reading cannot be separated. Vocalization, whether out loud or to yourself, is considered to be important to the reading process, as it increases understanding. However, reading aloud word by word can decrease speed and comprehension.

Put expression into your reading. You do not speak in a monotone, so why read that way?

Be aware of your reading assignments that are technical or scientific in nature and vary your reading speed accordingly. The more recreational your reading (novel, newspaper, etc.) the faster you can read. For more technical or scientific material, you must slow down accordingly. As you get accustomed to this type of reading, you will find yourself increasing your speed.

Underline unfamiliar words as you read. When finished reading, copy the words on an index card and look them up in an appropriate dictionary. Most of the unfamiliar words you come across will be medical terms and found in your medical dictionary. At first you will think these words are Greek and you are right. Quite a few of them are derived from the Greek language. The rest are derived from Latin. Write the definition on the other side of the card.

Break the word down with vertical slashes into its prefix (the word beginning), root (core word), and suffix (word ending), so that you can begin making associations with other words with the same prefix, root, or suffix. If your medical dictionary does not include this information with each word, the information can be found in your learning resource center.

Nursing involves learning a whole new language. If possible, include your own drawing to represent the definitions of these words with the verbal definition and this can help you recall the word. Using index cards allows your language development to progress because you can take the cards with you wherever you go, to be used for learning when you have a few minutes to spare.

Underline key phrases and write in the margin. We assume you own your textbooks. This will keep you active and result in the identification of key concepts for study and review.

Summary

Learning how to learn is important, so that the theory and skills needed by a practical nurse can be stored in long-term memory and be retrieved or recalled when needed for patient care and exams. There is no easy way to learn information, but there are techniques that have been proven effective in increasing your level of concentration, improving your listening skills, and enhancing your ability to understand information. Perhaps your most important skills for success in the practical nursing program are your reading skills.

REFERENCES

Apps J. *Study Skills for Those Adults Returning to School.* 2nd ed. New York: McGraw-Hill, 1982.

Blakeslee T. *The Right Brain: A New Understanding of the Unconscious Mind and Its Creative Powers.* New York: Berkley, 1984.

Building Better Study Skills. Iowa City, Iowa: The American College Testing Service, 1989.

Buzan T. *Speed Reading.* New York: E.P. Dutton, 1983, 1991.

Buzan T. *The Brain User's Guide.* New York: E.P. Dutton, 1983.

Buzan T. *Use Both Sides of Your Brain.* 3rd ed. New York: E.P. Dutton, 1991.

Ellis D. *Test Taking Strategies* (videotape). Rapid City, S.D.: College Survival, 1990.

How Adults Can Learn More—Faster. 4th ed. Washington, D.C.: National Association for Public School Adult Education, 1969.

Make Top Scores Every Time. Del Mar, Calif.: Learning Forum, 1988.

Pauk W. *How to Study in College.* 4th ed. Boston: Houghton-Mifflin, 1988.

Pauk W. *Study Skills for Community and Junior Colleges.* Clearwater, Fla.: Reston-Stuart, 1987.

Shepherd J. *College Study Skills.* Boston: Houghton-Mifflin, 1990.

Sotiriou P. *Integrating College Study Skills.* Belmont, Calif.: Wadsworth, 1988.

Success Through Notetaking. Del Mar, Calif.: Supercomp, 1987.

What Works: Research about Teaching and Learning. Washington, D.C.: U.S. Department of Education, 1986.

Williams LV. *Teaching for the Two-Sided Mind: A Guide to Right Brain/Left Brain Education.* New York: Touchstone, 1986.

CHAPTER
8
Hints for Using Learning Resources

Learning Objectives

Upon completing this chapter, you will
1. Describe each step in the PQRST method of textbook study.
2. Discuss the value of reading assigned periodicals.
3. Locate an article related to nursing by using the *Cumulative Index to Nursing and Allied Health.*
4. Discuss six hints to be used to gain full value from lectures.
5. Discuss your responsibilities for each of the following learning methods:
    a. lecture–discussion
    b. skills lab
    c. audiovisual materials
    d. computer-aided instruction
6. Discuss the value of the following to your personal learning:
    a. librarian
    b. card catalogue
    c. computerized catalogue
    d. periodicals
    e. vertical file
    f. reserve materials
7. Discuss hints for taking multiple-choice and short-answer tests.

TEXTBOOKS

"I read the material four times and got a D. My friend read the material one time and got an A. It isn't fair." The learner speaking is correct. It takes a lot of time to read material four times for a test. Earning only a D is a poor return on your time investment. The experts in study skills have come up with a variety of study systems for using textbooks and related reading materials. These systems are basically the same in that they present a method of reading that will increase comprehension by ensuring that information is stored in long-term memory. We have chosen the PQRST method as described by Staton in *How to Study* (Staton,1982), first published in 1951 and now in its seventh edition. It is the method we used in nursing school, but do not ask which edition we used. Believe us, this method has stood the test of time.

The PQRST Method of Textbook Study

Each letter stands for a step in the study method. Studies have shown that learners who use each step of this method, regardless of the length of time available for studying, consistently scored higher on tests. But each of the five steps in the method must be used. Learners have reported that the system is easier to use than they thought it would be. Each of the five steps will be discussed by identifying the meaning and benefits of each step, how to carry out the step and why it works.

P = Preview

What it means. Preview is an overview or survey of what the material is all about. It gives you the general, big picture of what the author wants to accomplish, not the fine details.

Benefits. Previewing helps you look for and recognize important points or main ideas of the reading material.

Why it works. The Preview step makes you reflect or think about the material and increase your concentration level. These are important elements in the storage of information in long-term memory.

How to do it. When you first buy your textbooks, look at the table of contents. This will give you a general sense of the organization of the book. Read the Preface to find out the author's purpose for writing the book, the organization of the material, and suggestions for reading the book. Since authors have different ways of organizing and presenting material, preview the method of the author of each of your textbooks. Observe topic sentences and headings. With each reading assignment, instead of just plunging in and reading: (1) read each of the topics and headings, (2) read the summary, (3) read the first and last sentence of each paragraph, and (4) read the assignment, using the general hints listed for reading.

Q = Question

What it means. As you preview the reading material, ask yourself questions that may be answered when you read.

Benefits. Formulating your own questions along with using the author's will give you pointers as to what details to look for in your reading. These questions will help you prepare for exams.

Why it works. By providing you with clues, this step points out what to look for in your reading. The Question step will also make you reflect on your reading and increase your concentration level.

How to do it. Take the chapter title and each heading and turn them into questions. Some authors include questions at the end of a chapter; if so, read these before going on to the next step. Most authors include learning objectives at the beginning of each chapter. Use these to keep your mind inquisitive and to seek ends to these objectives.

R = Read

What it means. In this stage you actually read the material. You are now gathering information to be stored. Look carefully at pictures and charts, as they may contain new information or clarify what you have read.

Benefits. You will build up an intake of information and facts and hopefully be able to store it in long-term memory.

Why it works. Being an active reader by seeking answers to the questions you have formulated will keep up your level of concentration and allow you to store information in your brain.

How to do it. Review the general hints under Reading in Chapter 7 and practice them so you can remain active during this step. You are seeking the answers to the questions you formulated. Remember to underline key phrases and to write in the margin.

S = State

What it means. To state means to repeat in your own words what you have read.

Benefits. You will understand the organization of the material you are reading and the relationship of facts to each other. By increasing understanding, you will be able to apply the information in the clinical area. Rote memory fails when it comes time to apply information. Stating will help you evaluate if you did indeed store the information you read.

Why it works. Stating something out loud involves another sense (hearing) and provides an additional channel for information to be stored. Stating in your own words indicates a knowledge and understanding of the material.

How to do it. At first, at the end of each paragraph, look away from your book and ask yourself the main ideas that were covered in that paragraph. State the ideas out loud and in your own words. This is the key to the success of this step. As you become proficient in this step, you will find yourself being able to read more than one paragraph and still state the main ideas and the answers to the questions you formulated. Look at your marginal notes and try to elaborate on them.

T = Test

What it means. This final step occurs some time after your first study session and involves testing yourself on what you remember.

Benefits. Since the testing step is ongoing, it will point out weak areas and give you time before an exam to remedy them. Better grades are sure to follow.

Why it works. This stage settles once and for all whether the information is in your long-term memory. It also indicates comprehension of the material. In identifying your weak spots, you can review these areas and get them into your long-term memory. Since this step is ongoing and occurs at intervals, you will be covering the information in small doses but more frequently, the type of activity that is the best way for the brain to remember.

How to do it. This testing stage is really a review stage. Review your marginal notes. Restate the main ideas in the chapters. Review your class notes and relate them to the information in the textbook. For information you are having trouble with, place the information on index cards to carry with you so you can test yourself while on the run.

To be effective, it is suggested that about one half of your study time be devoted to Preview and Read, steps that primarily help you get the author's picture. The other half of your study time should be devoted to Question, State and Test, three steps that require reflective thinking, use of your memory, and organization of ideas through your own efforts. The strength of this system lies in the State step. The thinking in this step takes hard work, so resist the temptation to skip over State.

An important part of any textbook is the index found in the back of the book. The subject index includes a list of topics that can be found in that book, in alphabetical order, followed by page numbers where that information is discussed. This index will help you quickly locate information you need.

ARTICLES

Learners are all looking for the perfect textbook, the one that is complete and self-contained. But it does not exist! When a textbook comes off the press, it is approximately 1 to $1\frac{1}{2}$ years out of date. For this reason you will be assigned to read articles on selected subjects from professional journals and magazines. They are assigned to give you more accurate and up-to-date information to supplement the readings in your textbooks. (Magazine articles are only six months to a year out of date when published.) Use the same general reading principles and hints for reading textbooks. Copyright laws prohibit the instructor from copying an article for each of you so they will generally be available on a reserve basis. You can make notes from these articles or photocopy the article itself for your use and underline, highlight, and write in the margins. Remember, the instructor knows you are busy. Articles are not busy work but are a necessary part of any career education.

LECTURES

Many of your teachers were taught using the "bucket theory" of education. This implies that knowledge is transmitted from a teacher's mind to the consciousness of the student through the lecture method (Erickson and Curl, 1972, p. 6). This teaching method evolved from the time of Aristotle. The teacher was considered to be the source of information and the vehicle of transmission of that information. Of course, the printing press had yet to be invented! Traditional lectures can be valuable as a means of enhancing your assigned readings. They are passive learning experiences that do not actively involve you in the learning process. Research has shown that "most students learn best from methods other than lecture" (Jerit and Taylor, 1991). A lecture situation should enhance your reading assignment, never replace it. A lecture should reflect the fact that the teacher spent time searching, reading, selecting, and organizing information for your benefit. The instructor has done all the work and has become smarter in the process. You need to remain especially alert during the lecture to be able to benefit from this method of teaching.

What goes on in the classroom is just as important as what goes on in a reading assignment. There is, however, one great difference between the two. You can repeat a reading assignment but you can never repeat a missed class. Here are some hints to help you learn from a lecture.

1. Never skip a lecture unless you have an emergency. Some students skip lectures to get another hour's sleep, use the time to prepare for another class or an exam, or to get in their legal number of cuts. When an emergency does make it necessary for you to miss class, photocopying notes is not the answer to catch up on what you missed, because every student develops a personal note-making system. Instead, ask a peer to go over his notes and tell you about the class. Then take your own notes as he talks.

2. Come to class prepared. By having the assignment completed, key terms and concepts will be familiar to you and you will not embarrass yourself by asking questions that are answered easily by the readings. Come to class in time to get a seat close to the lecturer and blackboard. Heading for the last row is heading for distractions and lower grades. Have a pen and paper ready to go.

3. Listen for verbal cues that will inform you of key points. Some examples can be found in Table 8-1. Keep vigilant for nonverbal cues that will also inform you of key ideas. Examples are raising the hands, a long dramatic pause, raising or lowering the voice, and leaning toward the class. Be sure to copy everything that is written on the blackboard.

4. Although the lecturer speaks at about 110 to 160 words per minute, you are capable of thinking at 650 to 700 words per minute

Table 8-1 Verbal Cues for Key Ideas in Lectures

"The most important difference is. . . ."

"The major principle in this situation is. . . ."

"To sum up. . . ."

"The main point is. . . ."

"Finally. . . ."

"In conclusion. . . ."

"Moreover. . . ."

"To repeat. . . ."

(Lenier and Maker, 1980, p. 244). The fact that you can think faster than the lecturer can speak allows you to relate this new information to information you have learned in the past and formulate questions when you do not understand. Ask these questions in class or seek out the instructor after class. Do not be afraid to question.

5. *Look over your notes as soon after class as possible.* It should take no longer than 10 minutes to correct, add details, write key concepts and questions in the left-hand margin, and summarize at the bottom of the page. Review these notes weekly until test time or daily if the tests come up more often.

6. *Never doodle, knit, or listen to music by earphones while in class.* If you question why, read the section on Concentration.

LECTURE–DISCUSSION

In this teaching method, the instructor will share several ideas with the class and then stop so that the class may discuss the ideas. Sometimes, the instructor may say that the next class will be nothing but discussion of the assignment. The instructor then will act as a discussion leader. Here are some hints for participating in discussions.

1. Be prepared to discuss by completing your assignment.

2. Be sure to have gathered a list of questions about the assignment. Discussions are the perfect time to clear up questions.

3. While other learners are speaking, listen to what they have to say. Some learners make the mistake of using other learners' speaking time to formulate their next comment.

4. You may disagree with others during a discussion. Do so assertively and firmly, but avoid yelling matches at all costs.

COURSE OUTLINES

Some schools of nursing use outlines for each course the learner takes. These outlines are a

great help to an adult learner, because they contain unit-by-unit course objectives, which indicate exactly what the learner must know. Each objective will begin with a verb. Watch the verb carefully and you will know the level of understanding you must achieve to meet the objective. If an objective states you must *list* something, that task is quite different from having to *compare* and *contrast* the same information. Instructors will develop their test questions from the objectives. The course outline may also include a list of resources indicating where the information to answer the objectives may be found. Also, supplementary material in the form of worksheets, charts, and activities may be included to round out your learning.

AUDIOVISUAL MATERIALS

In addition to lectures, textbooks, and articles, the instructor may have included films and videotapes as part of your assignment. Audiovisual (AV) materials are no longer considered extra or additional; they are a significant part of all areas of learning. These learning resources give credence to the saying that "one picture is worth a thousand words" and provide an additional sensory channel for learning compared to reading. In some nursing courses, especially autotutorial skills courses, the AV medium is the course, and the student progresses independently, seeking out the instructor when questions arise and attending periodic lecture–discussion classes. Approach the AV material as you do a lecture, but realize that you have the benefit of repeating all or part of the presentation when you do not understand. Do not forget television as a source of information on nursing and related topics.

COMPUTER-AIDED INSTRUCTION (CAI)

The development of the computer has been accompanied by much technical jargon and supposed complexity. Perhaps no segment of society has been left untouched by the computer, and education in general and nursing education in particular have benefitted from the use of this technology. CAI is an increasingly used teaching method in nursing education, with the following benefits:

- CAI allows learners to be actively involved in their learning.
- CAI encourages problem solving in the learner, a needed skill for practical nurses.
- CAI provides immediate feedback to the learner by quickly evaluating answers and decision-making strategies.
- CAI provides the opportunity for learners to develop their ability to follow directions.

Learning by CAI is enhanced for students who are right-hemisphere–dominant learners. CAI can also be used effectively by any student to master new material. It simplifies concepts and reinforces skills previously presented.

If CAI is used in your practical-nursing program, you will be taught the skills necessary to use the computer. You will be surprised how simple the process is even if you do not have any computer experience. Many of you will also be using the computer in the clinical area to store and retrieve patient information.

Computer Simulation

Computer simulation is a learning activity that uses an imaginary patient situation. The student is required to gather data, set priorities, plan, and evaluate care as in an actual clinical situation.

The computer patient simulation continually changes, as it would in the clinical area. This requires the student to evaluate the situation and plan new nursing interventions. Computer simulations are used when the patient census is inadequate for patient assignments, when a desired patient situation is unavailable, or to enhance learning of specific concepts. A review of software reveals few computer simulations specifically for practical nursing students. Your instructors can modify existing simulations for your use or may design their own.

LEARNING RESOURCE CENTER

If you are over 30, you know this resource as the library. Its new name, often abbreviated LRC, merely reflects the increased scope of the library in the 1990s. It is a lot more than books. How do you feel when you find out you must use the LRC? If you have some negative feelings, perhaps it is due to the fact that you are unfamiliar with the sources of information this resource contains and their location. Investigate your school library and you will find that it contains a wealth of services that will help make your time in the practical-nursing program much easier. Ask the librarian for a tour. Some libraries have self-guided tours on audiotape. An hour spent touring can save you many wasted hours later on. Ask for a library brochure so that you have an idea of the library's general hours of operation and its layout. Identify the special study areas available to you and groups of learners. Since the library is a learning area, you should help keep it a quiet environment.

Librarian

This is perhaps the best resource in the whole building. This person is a college-educated specialist on what the library has to offer in the area of information and where that information can be found. Look at the librarian as a professional educator about information for learning and as a person who is always ready to assist you. When you do go for assistance, be sure to watch the process that the librarian goes through to obtain the information you need. Next time, you will be able to help yourself.

Card Catalog

Although the following discussion will concentrate on the traditional card catalog, the student should be aware that more and more libraries are converting their card catalogs to an on-line (computerized) catalog. The information to be derived from the computer screen is similar in many respects to what is found in the card catalog. However, the search techniques will, of course, be different, and in general, more points of access will be available. If the library you use is on-line, it behooves you to become familiar with these new techniques as quickly as possible, by taking advantage of instructional sessions offered by the library and soliciting personal help from the librarian when necessary.

There is a lot of information you can obtain in a library by yourself once you understand the card catalog. This catalog is an alphabetical index or listing of the books and materials that are contained in the library, with a description of each and where each can be found. This information is placed on index cards and stored in drawers in file cases. This system makes the total resources of the library easily accessible to the user.

There are three types of cards: the author or main entry card, the title card, and the subject card. Sometimes you have an author's name but not the title of the book you need. You would look up the author's name in the author card file and the title would be listed underneath it. If you have the title but not the author, look up the title and the author's name will be underneath it. Look up the subject you are interested in and authors and titles relating to that topic will be listed. Figure 8-1 gives you an example of an author or main entry card and the information this card gives you. The title card has the identical information, but the title is typed in black above the author's name. The subject card differs from the other two cards in that the subject is typed at the top of the card in red letters or in black capital letters. The remainder of the subject card is similar to the author card.

Now to locate a book. Libraries may choose to use either of two systems to classify materials so they are easy to locate: The Dewey Decimal System and the Library of Congress Classification system. Regardless of the system your library uses, the call number on the author, title, or subject card will be the same number as on the spine of the book. Get in the habit of copying, in order, all the letters and the numbers in the call number.

The Stacks

Armed with the call number, you can proceed to the stacks—the collection of the majority of materials that can be checked out. When you do find the book you are looking for, note that since books covering the same subject are shelved in the same area, you can find additional useful books on the same shelf.

Reference Material

Reference materials include dictionaries—including medical and nursing dictionaries—encyclopedias, almanacs, yearbooks, atlases, handbooks, and many other categories. You will find up-to-date information on any subject in this area. Reference material generally does not circulate; that is, it cannot be checked out. Some libraries allow certain reference books to circulate for brief periods.

Periodicals

Since magazines are published weekly, monthly, and quarterly, that is, periodically, they are often called periodicals. They are also referred to as journals—publications that contain news or material of current interest in a particular field. Professional journals contain articles including the most recent material on a specific subject and subjects that are too new to be included in books. This is why periodicals are very important resources to a learner in a field changing as quickly as nursing. The titles and authors of various articles cannot possibly be included in the card catalog and are found instead in bound books called periodical indexes. Entries are listed by author, title, and subject. There are two periodical indexes of special value to practical-nursing students.

Reader's Guide to Periodical Literature

This comprehensive index to more than 160 popular American nontechnical magazines in-

```
                        2
                        |
   LB                  Pauk, Walter
   2395              3—How to Study in College, 2nd ed.—4
1  P3               5— Boston, Houghton Mifflin, 1974,—7
                                              |
                                              6
   1974              8—274 p. illus.
                                |
                                9
                    10—Includes bibliographical references.
                    11—1. Study, Method of
```

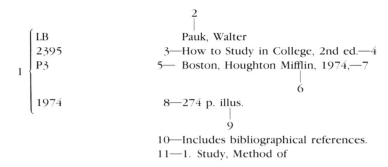

Key: 1. Call number, 2. Author's name, 3. Title of book, 4. Edition number, 5. Place of publication, 6. Publisher, 7. Date of publication, 8. Number of pages, 9. Illustrated, 10. Special features, 11. Subject heading (the subject that is fully treated in the book). If you look up this subject in the subject file, you will find a list of authors and titles covering this subject.

FIGURE 8-1 Author or Main Entry Card

cludes articles published between the dates printed on its cover. This guide is useful for recreational reading on specific topics, such as raising petunias, color analysis of pets, and tattooing the painless way. The *Reader's Guide,* or green book, can keep you up to date on nursing topics presented to the consumer of health care.

Cumulative Index to Nursing and Allied Health (CINAH)

This comprehensive and authoritative periodical index contains current listings for nursing and allied health professionals and others interested in health care issues. Three hundred nursing, allied health, and related journals are reviewed, indexed, and included in five bimonthly issues and cumulative bound volumes of past issues.

Figure 8-2 illustrates the information found in a typical entry in a periodical index. Near the indexes will be a listing of magazines and dates of the issues that are found in your library. If the article you want is in a magazine not found in your library, see the librarian, and he or she will track down the article in another library and arrange for you to receive a photocopy. If your library has the date and issue you want, go to the section of the library that contains the periodicals. If the issue you want is not there, it may be on microform. To conserve space, back is-

FIGURE 8-2 An Entry from the *Cumulative Index of Nursing and Allied Health*

```
1—GERONTOLOGIC CARE
  2—see also GERONTOLOGIC NURSING
  3—Home health care and the elderly in
       the
     4—1980s (Jackson BN) AJOT 1984 Nov;
        38(11): 717–20 (17 ref)
        |          |       |   |    |
        7          8       5   6    9
```

Key: 1. Subject, 2. Topic under which to look for additional material on the subject, 3. Title of the article, 4. Author of the article, 5. Article has a bibliography, 6. Journal in which the article appears. The periodical index will have a list of periodical abbreviations in front of the book and the full name of the magazine for which those abbreviations stand. 7. Volume number, 8. Pages of the article, 9. Date of publication

sues of magazines are microphotographically produced. Two commonly used microforms are microfilm and microfiche (mī-crō-feesh).

1. Microfilm—this is the most popular form for reproducing information to save space. A whole year's issues of magazines can be reproduced on 16-mm or 35-mm film that threads on a wheel about $3\frac{1}{2}$ inches in diameter, with room to spare.

2. Microfiche—this form involves a four-by-six-inch film card that carries reduced images that are placed on the card in rows. One microfiche can contain up to 98 pages of text.

Both of these microforms must be read with a device that enlarges the very small image. Many libraries have reader–printers that will print the image seen on the screen on a sheet of paper you can take with you. See the librarian for help with microforms.

Vertical File

This file contains pamphlets of various subjects arranged in alphabetical order by topics.

Circulation Desk

This is the area to check out and return library materials. Materials that your instructor reserves will probably be found here and checked out, along with audiovisual equipment to use with the material, if needed. Materials on reserve can be checked out for short periods.

LEARNING EXERCISE

How well do you understand the information found in a periodical index entry? Use the CINAH entry below to test yourself by answering the questions found underneath it.

> Day Gynecologic Chemotherapy Unit: an innovative approach to changing health care systems (Torosian LC, et al.) CANCER NURS 1985 Aug; 8(4): 221-7 (8 ref)

Author _____

Title _____

Volume number of magazine _____

Name of magazine _____

Date _____

Pages _____

SKILLS LAB

This resource will allow you to practice and develop your physical bedside skills and is to be used throughout your program of study. This lab contains the physical items to help make the practice area as similar to the hospital or nursing home as possible. Skills must be practiced. Reading about them, watching a film, and watching other students practice do not allow you to develop a physical skill. Practice until you are proficient in each skill, so that you will feel comfortable performing these tasks in the clinical area. Remember that you recall 10% of what you hear, 20% of what you see, 50% of what you read, and 90% of what you do, so *do* all you can.

NURSING ORGANIZATIONS

Nursing organizations frequently organize speakers, seminars, and workshops on nursing and related topics and make them available to students. Nursing organizations will be discussed in Chapter 17.

COMMUNITY RESOURCES

The city library and museums sometimes sponsor programs and exhibits on topics of interest and use to practical nursing students. Health care facilities such as hospitals and clinics offer lecture series.

TEST TAKING

Does the thought of having to take a test leave you feeling numb? Welcome to the club. Some anxiety about test taking is normal and can work to your benefit. Without it, you would probably watch television instead of studying. Once again, research results are on your side. Even when learners complain of fear and anxiety in test-taking situations, researchers (Culler and Holahan 1980, p. 19; Moshe et al., 1981, p. 823) have found that if you do not do well on tests, odds are that one or more of the following variables apply to you: less intelligence, poor study habits, or weak test-taking skills. The first reason does not apply in your situation, otherwise you would not have been admitted to the practical-nursing program in the first place. Chapter 7 dealt with overcoming poor study habits, and the remainder of this chapter will deal with weak test-taking skills.

In our experience, lack of preparation of subject matter and poor test-taking skills have been observed as the most common reasons for low test scores. Occasionally a learner will have fear and anxiety about test taking that interferes with what was studied and will require knowledge of relaxation techniques, even drugs, but this is the exception, not the rule.

Hints for Successful Test Taking

Focus on remaining an active learner. Anticipate the types of questions that will be asked.

Set a goal to *understand* the information you are learning with an eye to *application* of that learning. NCLEX-PN will be testing you at the level of understanding and application, with very few straight knowledge questions.

Test-taking skills are divided into two general areas: preparing for the test and actually taking the test. The following list will address these areas.

Preparation for the Test

Preparation for Test Taking Begins the First Day of Class. This includes (1) your system of notemaking for class and assignments and (2) your goal of *understanding* information as a preparation for tests and for clinical performance.

Clarify Content to Be Covered on the Test and the Form of the Test. Hints for actually taking different forms of tests begin on page 99.

Periodically Review the Material You Have Already Studied. This will result in 80% retention of material (Pauk, 1988, p. 210). Utilize the Test step of the PQRST method frequently and the audible recitation suggested. Make index cards of the material you are having difficulty understanding. Cramming—last-minute studying of new material for a test—sometimes results in short-term memory of material that might help you pass a test. But since you did not engage in repetitions spaced over days, storage in long-term memory will not occur and application of the material will be impossible. Cramming for an exam is like packing your suitcase at the last minute for a vacation. You will wind up with a suitcase filled with things you do not need and a whole list of things you forgot to bring.

Use Time-Management Techniques to Help You Organize Your Time before the Test. Make a schedule to help identify study times to do a grand review for each test. Do not reread the textbook. Since you have studied the material periodically since the last test and used study-skill techniques, all you must do at this point is focus on your summaries, margin writings, underlinings, and index cards to check your retention. The night before the test, do not be tempted to watch television or go to a movie. These activities will interfere with remembering. Instead, do your grand review as described above and get a good night's sleep.

Taking the Test

Arrive at the classroom in plenty of time to get your favorite seat and arrange your pencils, etc. Beware of peers who may get you nervous by saying "You didn't study that did you?" or "You mean you didn't study that?" Keep a positive mental attitude. You organized your time and systematically reviewed for this test after clarifying the content of the exam. Silently rehearse your facts to keep out distractions. Take slow deep breaths to reduce tension. It is almost test time and you are ready.

Would you believe that some people who have organized their notes and their time, systematically reviewed, and understood the material have nevertheless done poorly in tests? The main reason for this is that they did not follow the directions on the test. How well do you follow directions? Take out a blank sheet of paper and test yourself on the following directions.

*L*EARNING EXERCISE

How Well Do You Follow Directions?

Directions: Read the following directions carefully. You will have one minute to do the exercise after reading the directions. Be sure to write legibly. When you have finished, check your answers against the directions before handing in the paper. *Be sure to read the exercise before beginning.*

1. On a sheet of paper, print your name in the upper left-hand corner, last name first.
2. Under your name, write your Social Security number.
3. In the upper right-hand corner, write the name and number of the course for which you are taking this exercise.
4. In the lower left-hand corner of the paper, write today's date.
5. In the lower right-hand corner, write your instructor's name, last name first.
6. Fold your paper in half lengthwise.
7. Number the left half of your paper 1 to 6, skipping three lines between each number.
8. Number the right half of your paper 7 to 12, skipping three lines between each number.
9. Now that you have read all of the exercise, do only number one of the exercise and hand your paper to the instructor.

How did you do? If you did not follow the directions, do you feel tricked? You were not. The directions were clear and you simply did not follow them. Meticulously listen to oral directions and read the written directions completely before each test. To those of you who did follow the directions for this exercise: keep up the good work! If directions are ever unclear, ask the instructor before proceeding. Clarify the time limit of the exam. Now you are ready to begin.

Quickly skim the entire exam to set up an overall picture of the types of questions on the test so you will be able to figure out the amount of time you can devote to each section. Then answer the questions you know well. This will boost your confidence level. Do not spend large amounts of time on difficult questions and do not get upset about them. Both of these activities waste time and do not earn points. Go on to the next question and return to the skipped item later. Watch for absolutes such as always, never, all, and only.

Take the full time for the test. If you finish early, try to answer the questions you skipped. This brings up the point of guessing at answers.

If you are not penalized for guessing, answer all the questions. But if the test will be graded by subtracting the number of wrong answers from the number of right, generally speaking, do not guess. Make sure you have not missed an item or group of items. Make sure your answers match up to the proper answer slot. The instructor cannot possibly know you put the answer to number 37 in the slot for number 36. Should you change an answer? Although research has shown that test scores are generally improved by changing answers, we have seen many learners decrease their test scores by the same action. If you have given the item further thought and feel the item should be changed, change it. Test by test, keep tabs on your test scores to see if changing answers is helping your final score and modify your behavior accordingly. If you are using a separate answer sheet that will be machine corrected, then be sure you erase your first answer completely. Chapter 4 discussed tests as a learning tool. When the exam is corrected and returned to you, do the following:

1. Read the items you missed. Why are they wrong? Did you make a careless mistake? Did you know the material? Can you correct the item without looking in your textbook or notes? If not, look up the answer.

2. Read the items you answered correctly. What did you do right to get credit for these items?

3. Decide which of your study skills and test-taking techniques are and are not working to

your benefit. Modify your strategies accordingly.

Hints for Specific Tests

The types of tests you will be taking in the practical-nursing program, including the NCLEX-PN, are achievement tests, because they measure how much you have learned. Achievement tests are of two types—objective and subjective. Objective achievement tests include multiple-choice questions. In objective achievement tests, the answer is generally included in the test item and you must pick it out. The format of NCLEX-PN is multiple-choice items. Subjective achievement tests include short-answer questions. In subjective tests, you must answer the question by formulating the answer. We will use samples of these two test forms to help you understand them and provide hints for taking each of them.

Multiple-Choice Items

Before taking the short multiple-choice test that follows, here are some hints for taking this type of test. Read over all the options given before making any decision. Eliminate options you know are definitely wrong. When a number answer is involved, choose the number in the mid-range. Remember the course subject matter for which you are being tested, and eliminate options that are not related to the subject matter.

*L*EARNING EXERCISE

Choose the appropriate option for the following multiple-choice items. There is only one answer to each multiple-choice item.

1. Multiple-choice items are examples of
  A. items for which one-word answers are required.
  B. incomplete statements with four options for answers.
  C. two vertical columns that must be matched item by item.
  D. items that require a sentence to be written on the answer sheet.
2. When answering multiple-choice items, it is not necessary to
  A. read the directions.
  B. match lists of items

C. read each of the options.

D. watch out for negative words.

Answers

1. B. The beginning of a sentence is given with four options. Usually only one option is correct and the rest of the options are distractors, that is, options that are there to see if you really have learned the material. Option A describes fill-in-the-blank items, option C describes matching tests, and option D describes short-answer items.

2. B. This multiple-choice item contains a negative word in the stem that can complicate things. To sort out your answer, read the stem without the negative word to get some meaning out of it and read the options. One option should not fit in with the others. Now reread the original stem with the negative word and see if the option you have already isolated fits in. Even though the test begins with directions, there may be additional directions before multiple-choice items. These directions may ask you to select one best answer or select all of the correct answers. Remember, do not stop reading when you think you have the correct answer. There may be a better option yet to come. Incidentally, options A, C, and D are true.

Multiple-choice items are not multiple guess. Think thoroughly through each response before choosing your answer. Should you ever guess? To be able to make a decision regarding guessing, you must know if you will be penalized for wrong answers. Even if you are, figure out the odds. If you can eliminate one distractor for certain, you have a better chance of answering correctly. Can you eliminate two out of four distractors? Your chances are now even better. You make the decision.

Short-Answer Items

1. Describe a short-answer item.

2. List five hints that the test taker should use

in answering short-answer items to receive full credit for those items.

Answers

1. A short-answer item is one in which you are given a simple command to carry out.

2. Five hints for answering short-answer items:

a. Be sure to give the information that the item asks for. Watch the verbs in these items, and do what they ask you to do.

b. Give objective answers.

c. Write in complete sentences.

d. Concentrate on packing information into your answer.

e. Think before you write.

Summary

The hints for learning resources found in this chapter will help you obtain the information you need to be a practical nurse and get better grades on tests. The PQRST method of reading a textbook is an effective technique to store information in your long-term memory so that it is available for recall for tests and application in the clinical area. Specific learning resources that most probably will be used by the practical nursing student, in addition to textbooks include lectures, lecture–discussion, articles from periodicals, computer-aided instruction, the Learning Resource Center, and the skills lab. After learning the information you need to be a practical nurse, you must demonstrate that learning has taken place in a variety of ways: performance in the clinical area, multiple-choice tests and short-answer tests. Testing helps instructor and student discover areas that are not understood and need further study. Knowledge and application of test-taking techniques will help to decrease test anxiety.

REFERENCES

Assisting students with exams. Nurse Educ 1985; 10(6):24–25.

Benedict S, Coffield K. The effect of brain hemisphere dominance on learning by computer assisted instruction and the traditional lecture method. Computers in Nursing, July/August 1989; 7(4):152–156.

Building Better Study Skills. Iowa City, Iowa: The American College Testing Service, 1989.

Culler R, Holahan C. Test anxiety and academic performance: the effects of study-related behavior. Educ Psychol 1980; 72(1):16–20.

Ellis D. *Test Taking Strategies* (videotape). Rapid City, S.D.: College Survival, 1990.

Erickson C, Curl D. *Fundamentals of Teaching with Audiovisual Technology.* New York: Macmillan, 1972.

Gates J. *Guide to the Use of Books and Libraries.* 5th ed. New York: McGraw-Hill, 1983.

Jerit L, Taylor B. *Towards a Definition of Critical Literacy.* (Unpublished paper for Critical Literacy Project of Oakton Community College, Des Plaines, Ill.), 1991.

Lenier M, Maker J. *Keys to College Success.* Englewood Cliffs, N.J.: Prentice-Hall, 1980.

Make Top Scores Every Time. Del Mar, Calif.: Learning Forum, 1988.

Moshe B, McKeachie Y, Holinger D. Test anxiety: deficits in information processing. J Educ Psychol 1981; 73(6):816–824.

Pauk W. *How to Study in College.* 4th ed. Boston: Houghton-Mifflin, 1988.

Shepherd J. *College Study Skills.* Boston: Houghton-Mifflin, 1990.

Sotiriou P. *Integrating College Study Skills.* Belmont, Calif.: Wadsworth, 1988.

Staton T. *How to Study.* 7th ed., 1982. Distributed by HTS, P.O. Box 40273, Nashville, TN 37204.

Success Through Notetaking. Del Mar, Calif.: Supercomp, 1987.

part III
KNOW YOURSELF

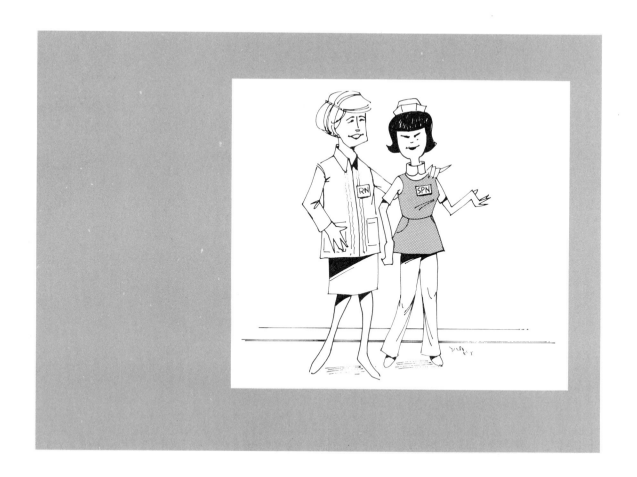

CHAPTER
9
Personality Development

Learning Objectives

Upon completing this chapter you will
1. Describe how the subconscious records real and imagined images.
2. Discuss how the body acts out what the mind imagines.
3. Discuss four characteristics needed for a positive attitude.
4. Monitor personal "self-talk."
5. Explain how positive affirmations and images can be used to develop a positive attitude.
6. Describe "getting along" as a major issue in the workplace.

When reading the title of this chapter, you may have assumed that you are going to receive information on personality development theories. Not so. This entire textbook is dedicated to your personal advancement: as a current student and as a future nurse. This chapter provides an opportunity for you to take a look at your own personality development: present and future. On what kind of information are you functioning? How did it get there? Is it real? Can it be changed? How do you feel about yourself? Do you see yourself as being successful? What are your personal goals? Most important, do you have choices, and how can you exercise those choices? These and many other questions will be dealt with. However, before going any further, take the brief test that follows. It will help to personalize the information for you. Once again, answer the questions as honestly as possible, as they relate to you at this point in your life.

*L*EARNING EXERCISE

Test

Read the following statements and determine if they are true or false in regard to how you feel right now. Check the appropriate column.

	TRUE	FALSE
1. I have personal written goals.	_____	_____
2. I can usually find alternatives to a problem.	_____	_____
3. I say "thank you" to a compliment.	_____	_____
4. I work well with groups.	_____	_____
5. It is my responsibility to learn.	_____	_____
6. I evaluate my own work.	_____	_____
7. My parents did the best they could.	_____	_____
8. I believe that I can excel.	_____	_____
9. I can change how I feel about myself.	_____	_____
10. Self-talk determines my behavior.	_____	_____
11. I treat me like a best friend.	_____	_____
12. I find something good in everyone.	_____	_____
13. I can learn anything I want to.	_____	_____
14. I express myself with "I"-centered statements.	_____	_____
15. I rarely explain my behavior.	_____	_____

KEY: (count the number of True items)
    10–15 Trues = Positive Attitude
    0–9 Trues = Need an attitude adjustment

Look closely at the result of the test now, and then again at the end of the chapter, at which time you are encouraged to write some realistic, time-limited goals for yourself in a special way.

*A*TTITUDE AS IT AFFECTS SUCCESS

Here is that word again—attitude. But what does it have to do with success? A lot, according to a five-year study supported by the Carnegie Foundation. The research showed that only 15% of a person's ability to get a job, keep a job, and move ahead in that job is due to his or her knowledge: the other 85% is attitude. Furthermore, it has been shown that people like to be around positive people and that positive people are more productive on the job because they have more energy and motivation. In essence, knowledge is the key that unlocks a career door: Once inside, attitude is the key to success.

The characteristics of optimism, motivation, discipline and confidence that result in a positive attitude will be considered separately. Suggestions for changing a characteristic, as needed, will be included. All the characteristics are intimately related to getting along with others.

Optimism

Life is an adventure, and as pointed out in Isaiah 14:24, "Surely as I think so it shall come to pass." Immediately, it sounds as though you are responsible for what happens to you. Can this be? Yes, definitely, for you set the tone for each day of your life. For example, think about what you say to yourself when you first awaken. Is it a positive message? Do you anticipate new opportunities for learning and experience that will prepare you for your career? Do you expect it to be a good day? Do you see the problems that you face as challenges that have solutions? Or do you wake up feeling resentful that you must get up? Do you anticipate problems with class content and tests? Do you just know this will be a bad day because you spilled your juice—"A sign, you know"? Do you personalize the behavior of someone immediate, who is cross or ill—"I just can't win"?

Let's take a look at what happens during those first few minutes of your day. All of us are constantly involved in self-talk. That talk and the images it evokes are being recorded by the subconscious, the part of our mind below our immediate awareness or conscious mind. Interestingly, it does not matter to our subconscious mind if our perceptions are accurate or inaccurate. It records the messages and images as being the truth and the conscious mind operates on this "truth." In other words, you become what you fear or you become what you expect to be. Life is a self-fulfilling prophecy. With that in mind, go back to what happens when the alarm clock goes off.

SCENE 1: "Terrific, it's Monday. I'm going to ace the test. I know the material."
SCENE 2: "Ugh. Monday already? I studied a lot, but I never do well on Monday."

You already know which self-talk is most likely to result in passing the test. Chances are that if the nurse in Scene 2 does pass the test, it will be dismissed as "just luck."

Optimism has far-reaching effects not only for schoolwork, but for overall health and personal relationships as well. Certainly, hereditary and environmental factors are significant. But consider the fact that your conscious mind is trying to follow the messages you provide it, for recording in your subconscious: the body acts out what the mind holds. So, if you provide self-talk messages of "I can't take this much longer," "I'm getting run down," "I usually get a cold when I'm overworked," "I get a strep infection every year at this time," your body will try to follow directions for what it believes to be the truth. The same is true in regard to personal relationships: Negative self-talk begets negative results. For example: "With my luck, this relationship is bound to fail." "What can you expect? Teenage is a disease to be endured." "That kid cries just to annoy me." "My childhood was so rotten. I don't have a chance." What do you think the outcome will be?

Hopefully, you have had a lifetime of self-talk that is optimistic. For those of you who continue to practice negative self-talk leading to pessimism, there is hope. You can *choose* to become optimistic by changing your self-talk.

The negative self-talk recorded in your subconscious cannot be erased, but you can provide and practice an entirely new script of optimistic self-talk. The subconscious will accept what you give it and the conscious mind will begin to function based on this new information. You will not experience a difference in feelings right away. Just continue to practice the new self-talk and your feelings will eventually catch up. After all, your old feelings have been a part of you for quite some time. Maintaining the new scripts with relatively few slip-ups will take a minimum of two to three weeks. You will note that as new challenges (formerly called problems) arise, there will be the tendency to return to the old self-talk, that is, "I knew this wouldn't work—not in my life. It's different." Just remind yourself, firmly, that it will work, and continue practicing the new self-talk. It may initially feel as though you are acting. That's fine. Fake it until you make it. This feeling that you are only acting will go away as your optimism begins to grow and becomes a part of you.

How to Change Your Outlook

Decide on your own positive self-talk. Write it down. For example: "I did a good job today. I will do even better tomorrow." "I will be a terrific nurse." "I can cope with this new challenge." "I'm pleased to have this opportunity to go to school."

Begin your positive self-talk before going to sleep. For example: "I'm capable and smart." "I'm going to have a great sleep." "I'm lucky to have a teenager who is practicing independence." "We'll make it. There's bound to be a solution." "I grow from every challenge."

Plan what you want to wake up to and take a few minutes for preparation the night before—a favorite tape, record, radio station, TV channel, chilled juice, an inspirational saying—whatever is special for you and starts you in a positive way upon awakening.

Greet yourself in the morning with more positive self-talk. For example, "It's going to be a good day for me." "I'm glad to be alive."

Deliberately look for something good in anything that doesn't go just right during the day. It may be necessary, especially at first, to write down daily what you see as problems and then rewrite these statements of problem as challenges—an opportunity to grow and gain inner strength. For example, *Problem:* car stalled. *Challenge:* I proved to myself that I can find a solution to a challenge, and I feel stronger because of it.

Treat yourself as you would your best friend. Certainly you would treat him or her with empathy, respect, encouragement, and reassurance that there are alternatives for dealing with the current situation.

Avoid negative people. Those who are involved in criticizing and complaining tend to pull you down, especially when you are attempting to change a pessimistic outlook to an optimistic outlook. Right now, you need your energy for you. If you do get hooked into complaining, move away from the person or group as soon as you recognize what is happening.

Look for a positive person to be with and/or to model yourself after, even if being with that person is not possible.

Plan for positive visual and auditory experiences. Play tapes, records, and radio music—inspirational messages that say "I can." When

you really listen to many of today's lyrics, they say, "I can't. It won't work, and if it doesn't I'll probably drink, cheat, or kill myself." Meanwhile, your subconscious records all as you sing along. Consider the same in regard to television and movies, especially prior to going to bed. Negative sensory experiences will support more negative recording into the subconscious as you sleep.

QUESTION: Did you ever have a weird, scary dream after watching a violent TV show and awaken feeling fearful or anxious?

Look for something good in everyone you meet. This is initially difficult since it is easier to think of people as all good or all bad.

QUESTION: What is a more realistic way to view every individual that you contact?

Optimism is closely related to your state of health. Be aware of the messages to yourself and to others when they ask how you are feeling. Furthermore, you can also influence others' health through your statements to them. Consider the following:

SCENE 1: "You're looking good. Looks like you've found positive ways of dealing with your studies."
Nurse: "Thank you. You're right. I'm proud of being able to juggle my life successfully."

SCENE 2: "You don't look so good today. Are you getting ill?"
Nurse: "Well, I thought I was OK, but maybe you're right. I have been putting in long hours."

QUESTION: What do you think will happen to each of the nurses in Scenes 1 and 2?

Motivation

According to Viktor Frankl, what a person really needs in life is struggling for a goal that is worthy of him. Each man knows in his heart what his assignment in life is. Aim at what your conscience wants you to do and success will follow you (Frankl Workshop, 1984). That seems to coincide with findings that motivation is one of the major characteristics common to individuals who are outstanding successes in their fields. Interestingly, these individuals have developed personal goals similar to those of major corporations. Far off? Maybe, but it works.

QUESTION: Do you have stated goals for your life or is life just a happening?

Where does motivation come from? Perhaps you have always looked for someone or something to motivate you from the outside, like a "good" teacher, friend, parent, deadlines, or crisis. It is true that all these people and factors can get you going, but let's face it, that kind of motivation lasts only as long as the teacher is with you, until the deadline is met, or until the crisis is over—and then it is back to the old habits again.

Motivation means that you are moved from inside of you, because you have decided that you want to attain certain goals. You will go on to do what needs to be done happily and to the best of your ability because you want to. As Frankl puts it, "The struggling for a goal is worthy of you."

As you consider this characteristic, you may be aware of some internal resistance to change. This resistance to change is named fear, another powerful force in our lives. After all, changing the ending of a story also shakes up your present security. Have you ever noticed how much easier it is to share a story about a crisis with someone when it is a thing of the past and you know the whole story, and how much more difficult it is to talk about a present, unresolved situation? There is a sense of security in knowing how the situation in the past ended. So it is with holding on to negative characteristics. You know what the end of the story is. The thought of making a change arouses fear—fear that this new way of behaving will not work out. Your self-talk is a powerful factor in motivation, because you do, in fact, do what you think about most.

"Wait a minute," you are saying, "that is quite a sales pitch. I'm paying my teachers to teach me and to tell me what to learn and to tell me if I am doing well." Read that statement again. It sounds like you are creating your own bondage. The instructor, at best, is a facilitator only, who sets an example of personal motivation by researching the class content in order to set up the best course possible. In nursing, this generally means a course outline, references, visual aids, clinical guidelines, and student evaluation. The instructor must trust that you will do your part in the instructor–student relationship. It is at this point that internal motivation is a significant factor that lets you take control of your learning. A clue: most courses continue to be based on minimal expectations, that is, what is the least you can get by on to pass the course. The word minimal tells you that there is a great deal more that you can learn from the course if you are motivated and choose to do so.

QUESTION: Economically speaking, how do you get your money's worth from a course?

QUESTION: Futuristically speaking, how will you become best prepared to meet the needs of your patients?

Consider the following suggestions and look for applications that will increase personal motivation for you.

1. High achievers have identified goals. Write down three things you want in the near future and how you expect to benefit from attaining each one of them. Place the list where you can read it first thing in the morning and last thing at night.

2. Do the following exercise: Read a single direction and complete it before reading the next direction, and so on.

   a. Take a piece of paper and write "I can't" on the top. Make a list of all the things you think you cannot do.

   b. Cross out "I can't" and replace it with the word "won't." Read your list again. Notice that almost every item on the list, unless related to severe mental or physical disability, is actually a choice on your part.

   c. Cross out the word "won't" and replace it with "want." Read the list again.

d. Cross out "want" and replace it with "can." Circle the one item from the list that you desire to accomplish within the next six months.

e. Write your choice as a positive "I will" statement on an index card that you can carry with you. For example: "I will say no without feeling responsible for other's feelings." "I will speak with a lower, warm, authoritative voice." "I will exercise vigorously for 20 minutes three times per week." "I will weigh 136 pounds." "I will practice rapid relaxation techniques as needed daily."

3. Practice saying the "I will" statement daily, for example, in the shower, in the car, upon arising, before going to sleep, when exercising. What a great idea for a video.

Have you noticed how much of the choice in this chapter is yours? You truly have a choice. The instructor need never know if you have chosen to follow suggestions made to you or if you have chosen to complete minimum requirements in life. It is indeed, a very personal, private, internal decision.

Discipline

Think for a moment how you view discipline. Do you view it as something internal that helps you accomplish your personal goals or do you view it as something external, imposed by another, that forces you to comply? There is a significant difference between the two. Internal (self) discipline permits you to be in charge of your own life. For example, "I am finally going to have an opportunity to learn about other religions." "I like the idea of learning about home health, but would like to visit an agency, instead of using the pamphlets as my resource." External discipline, usually referred to as punishment, means that you are dependent on others to make you do what you should and should not do. It also helps to set up a pattern of manipulation between you and the system or person involved. For example: "If she does not ask for a return demonstration, that's one more skill I don't have to worry about." "This instructor

does not care if we come in late or leave early: good deal." "I'll just change the charting: no one will know I did not give the medicine." "I'll read the chapters before the test: she never calls on me in class anyway."

Far-fetched examples? Not really. There continues to be the tendency, as there was in childhood, to do only what you absolutely have to, and to get away with whatever you can, until such time as personal discipline becomes internal reality, and therefore, a way of life for you. Self-discipline is saying, "I have decided that I am going to do whatever is necessary in order to gain the knowledge, skills, and experience available during school to prepare me for nursing. I am doing it because I choose to do it."

QUESTION: Is discipline related to personal health and interpersonal relationships? Support your answer with an example.

The following suggestions are offered to support you as you make an internal decision to excel through personal discipline.

1. Check your vocabulary: What kind of self-talk are you involved in? For example: What do you say to yourself when you are given an assignment or look at a course outline for the first time? Do you say, "Looks like I cannot get out of doing this." Or do you say, "I want to learn about this topic." It does make a difference, because the subconscious continues to record, and the message it receives will make a difference in how you act and feel. The power of the choice is yours, so pick your self-talk carefully. Avoid phrases like: "I cannot get out of this, I should, I should not, I cannot, I have to, They made me, I have no choice." And consciously change your self-talk to "I want to, I choose to, I have decided to, I would like to, I am going to, I am doing it for me."

2. Use imagery to support the change you desire to make, whether it relates to study habits, health, or interpersonal relationships. Feelings and thoughts are pulled toward one's mental images and you most often become what you imagine you will become. The nervous system operates on imagery and your personal images serve as a self-fulfilling prophecy. Images go directly to the nervous system. Images are used for or against yourself, and when tired, the negative images seem to make the maximum impression. To counteract this process, create positive images for yourself. Visualize successfully completing the task you have to do. Take time to include enough detail for it to be real to you—smells, sights, sounds. Visualize feeling happy about having completed the task success-fully and on time. See yourself being praised for choosing to do the task completely and on time.

3. Take any size note card. Divide it into three columns. In column 1, list the following words: choose, want, decided. In column 2, list three tasks or projects that have been put off. In column 3, list a completion date specific to each task or project. Look at the sample below.

1	2	3
Choose	Study Chapter 3	Tonight
Want	Nutrition Assessment	Monday morning
Decided	Talk to George	Sunday afternoon

Read across. You have created three personal guidelines for discipline.

4. **Practice, Practice, Practice.** Old habits will want to creep back before new ones are well established. Do not worry about it. Just re-instate the new behavior, immediately, where you left off.

Confidence

Confidence is made up of many factors. Most important among those factors is how you see yourself and your ability to respect what you see. "It is not what you are that holds you back, it is what you think you are not" (Waitley, 1983, tape 3). Traditionally, parents and circumstances in childhood have been held responsible for how the individual views himself as an adult. Consider the following opposite views. "I always felt self-conscious because my parents were so poor." And "I grew up in the shadow of successful parents and can't measure up to them." In each example the individual rationalizes his present internal state by blaming the parents' state of being. It is worth noting that parenting, at best, is an inexact science and that parents can only give emotionally what they have attained up to their present state of growth. This, in turn, is influenced by your interpretation of events. Parents are, like you, involved in the adventure of living and continual growth. The positive aspect of all this is that you can be in charge of the rest of your life—

usually from age 18 on—and change (not erase) any of the scripts you do not like. Continuing with current personal scripts that are negative and/or you do not like simply provides an excuse for lack of success.

QUESTION: What do you think are the components of developing confidence?

Number one is knowledge. In this case, you do not fake it. Knowledge belongs in the realm of thinking and it is imperative to have a strong knowledge base on which to make observations and think through decisions based on those observations. Overlearning has already been suggested as a way to learn classroom content. If you are lacking in reading and writing skills, ask the counselor or instructor how to get help in these areas. Interestingly, in many schools, you have already paid for these services through the fees charged at the time that you pay the tuition. Many schools have learning labs set up just waiting to serve you.

A close second to knowledge skills is clinical practice. Once again the principles of over-learning apply, since it is not always possible to have every experience desired during a clinical assignment. Seek the needed experiences through clinical simulation in the lab and by viewing teaching films. It is your responsibility to be actively involved in the learning process. Personal discipline provides the push for developing this aspect of confidence.

Third, deal with negative scripts and feelings that are getting in the way of absorbing the knowledge available to you. The counseling service in your school is also probably already paid for through the fee system, so use it to your advantage. The counselors are prepared to deal with you on "here-and-now" issues and to look at alternatives that will fit your life style.

Fourth, learn to deal with criticism. In this case, the best defense is a good offense. Decide now to critique your daily work in as objective a manner as possible. It is sometimes said that human objectivity is a myth; but this should in no way prevent you from striving for it. In order to critique yourself objectively, it is necessary to (1) look at what you did well and give yourself credit for it, and (2) look at areas that need improvement and make an immediate plan for change. This process needs to be devoid of emotion in that you are simply looking on a daily basis at strengths and areas that need improvement. This is also an excellent prelude to evaluation by the instructor or floor personnel. It is helpful to have the "head set" that you and the others are critiquing your work in order for you to be the best possible nurse. If you are accustomed to critiquing yourself, you will be able to be more objective with regard to the comments offered to you by the instructor and others. The following ideas will help you with this process.

Remind yourself that this is not an attack on you as a person. Evaluation is meant to look at performance and how to improve it.

Consider the information unemotionally, as though it applies to someone else. Evaluate whether it is a valid criticism, and if so, ask for suggestions for improvement and/or offer suggestions of your own.

If the information is based on miscommunication, offer a brief statement of explanation, being careful not to get on an emotional roller coaster. If the error is yours, avoid "over-apology." This simply makes it more difficult for all involved to cope. The important issue is the plan of action. Take the blame and go on to other things. Feeling guilty takes energy away from the solution and creates a new problem.

And finally, if the criticism is unwarranted and continual, there are avenues available to you—through your coordinator, counselor, student senate, etc. Your student handbook is usually a good resource with regard to student rights.

There is an interesting phenomenon that is still a factor in criticism. In our society, more males continue to be involved in team sports and have been conditioned to having behaviors corrected by the team's coach. With this upbringing, many males have learned early to separate their personal selves from their actions—a preparation for criticism on the job—listen, make an adjustment, go on. Many females, on the other hand, have continued to focus on being liked by others and often get feedback on their external selves: looks, clothes, etc., and equate criticism with "You do not like me" (the person) as opposed to "You do not like what I did" (the action).

Fifth is the issue of compliments. Do you accept a compliment by saying "thank you" and allowing yourself to believe it or do you quickly neutralize the compliment by pointing out your shortcomings. Did it even occur to you that you are insulting the person offering the compliment by not accepting it? You are, as a matter of fact, telling that individual that he is "dumb" in regard to the observation he has made.

Sixth, deal directly with what you fear. The usual outcome is that the issue is not as great as you imagined it to be. Even if the result is not ideal, give yourself ample credit for having dealt with your fear directly. If, for example, you have decided to confront someone directly, remember to use "I"-centered statements denoting that you take responsibility for what you are saying. Take responsibility for your side of the conversation only.

CORRECT: I feel angry when you criticize me in front of the other students.

INCORRECT: You make me angry when you criticize me in front of other students (gives responsibility and power for personal feelings to the other person). Maybe you were not aware of doing this (offers an excuse for the other person's behavior and takes responsibility for both parties involved).

It is also sometimes helpful to imagine the worst possible thing that could happen, in an exaggerated sense, prior to taking action. For example: "If I tell the instructor I am angry, she might hit me. Then I will have to press charges.

She will go to jail, there will be no one to complete the rotation, so I will flunk it and the other students will be angry with me and picket my house . . . ," etc.

Seventh, learn from someone who is confident and whom you admire. Look at how this person deals with situations. Listen to the tone of voice and observe the body language. Practice techniques that have already been shown to be successful. Approach the individual and ask for tips on how to develop confidence. You have just paid him or her a sincere compliment, and most individuals will be willing to offer information to you. Pick and choose what will work for you.

Finally, monitor your self-talk. Imagine succeeding in advance; learn from errors and do not dwell on them—save the energy for solutions.

Getting Along

A 1986 survey reported on the national news revealed that executives spend more of their time—equivalent to a full month per year—on the problems of employees not getting along with each other. Consider the losses in productivity, money, and of course, personal satisfaction and happiness in the workplace.

The four characteristics that influence personal attitude are the essential ingredients for getting along with others. Optimism permits you to see the positive side of yourself and others. The optimistic individual knows that there are alternatives for dealing with current challenges and uses his or her energy to solve problems. This individual spends little or no time and energy at the complaint counter.

Motivation provides the impetus for commitment to worthwhile goals. The motivated person puts out his or her best effort daily, both to do his or her own work and to work with oth-

ers: common, worthwhile goals—the bottom line in nursing being excellence in patient care. He or she is willing to learn new tasks and is not imprisoned by his or her own fears.

Discipline provides the internal control to do whatever is necessary to function effectively and to stay current within the field. It also provides the push to deal with issues that arise in the work setting, knowing that unresolved personal issues with peers limit effectiveness and cooperation with others. Discipline also provides the strength to change personal negative self-talk into positive affirmations. How you feel about yourself is reflected in the way you treat others.

Confidence reduces anxiety in those around you—whether at a peer level or as the one in charge. It says, "I am in charge of me. I do my best at all times. I learn from my errors and go on even stronger on the inside than before." The confident person is not defensive and is capable of listening to those he or she works with. He or she accepts critiquing from others and feels the responsibility to provide feedback to others regarding their patient care. Patient care becomes, collectively, "Our business." The confident individual is willing to compromise on issues that do not affect the quality of care. She treats others in the manner in which she wishes to be treated. It is well to remember that confidence is earned, not learned.

GETTING ALONG

CHARACTERISTICS	HOW DO I RATE?
1. Optimism	
2. Motivation	
3. Discipline	
4. Confidence	

Summary

The individual becomes the most powerful force in the continuing development of the personality. Self-talk must be constantly monitored, for you become what you imagine you are. Old images cannot be erased, but they can be replaced by new images through positive affirmations. Knowledge is the key that unlocks a career door, and attitude is the key to success. Characteristics that result in a positive attitude are optimism, motivation, discipline, and confidence. These in turn provide the total package for getting along with others, considered a major problem in the workplace.

REFERENCES

Bandler R. Using your brain—for a change. Moab, Utah: Real People Press, 1985.

Bauer B, Hill S. *Essentials of mental health care: planning and interventions.* Philadelphia: W.B. Saunders, 1986.

Frankl V. An evening with Victor Frankl workshop. Milwaukee: Mount Mary College, March 1984.

McCaffrey M. Focus: how to use the power of self-image psychology (audiotape). Chicago: The Human Resources Company, 1983.

Rutkowski BL. Six steps to building your confidence. Nurs Times 1986; 6(1):26–29.

Waitley D. The psychology of winning: ten qualities of a total winner (audiotape). Chicago: The Human Resources Company, 1983.

CHAPTER
10
Wellness and Personal Care

Learning Objectives

Upon completing this chapter, you will
1. Evaluate your own level of wellness and personal care in regard to
   a. The image you project,
   b. Present choices regarding wellness,
   c. Preventing muscle injury,
   d. Nutrition,
   e. Stress management,
   f. Negative influences.
2. Modify present wellness and personal care practices in order to make the most of what you are and can be.

As a nurse you will model wellness and personal care for your patient. The image that you project gives a far more powerful message than anything that you attempt to teach verbally. In nursing it is not sufficient to admonish the patient "Do not do as I do; Do as I tell you to."

QUESTION: Is there a relation between the nurse's level of wellness and personal care and the patient's willingness to follow postdischarge care directions?

Consider how you, as a patient, would react to being taken care of by the following nurses.

- A nurse who refuses to follow dress code: looks like she was put together by a committee.
- A nurse who smells of last night's gastronomical adventure: garlic bread, etc.
- A nurse with stained hands that smell of tobacco, as does her breath.
- An overweight nurse that comes in to give directions for a weight-reduction diet.
- A "high-strung" nurse who cannot cope with the demands of the job.
- A nurse who helps the patient in the next bed, but does not wash her hands before continuing with your care.

QUESTION: What are some other examples of incongruous nursing behavior?

THE IMAGE YOU PROJECT

A recent college graduate began her new job, which entailed intense involvement with young children, other staff, and parents. Since it was winter, she frequently wore a sweater to work. It did not take long for the children, staff, and parents to identify and complain of an unpleasant odor about her. It was soon apparent that it was body odor plus something they could not identify.

The supervisor called her aside and talked to her about the need to bathe daily and to use an adequate deodorant. The employee was quite upset and announced that she did indeed bathe daily. Furthermore, she did not see how the complaint could be true since she was careful, every night, to spray her sweaters and blouses, especially in the axillary area, with Lysol spray.

Good intentions, but a misinterpretation of the use of a product advertised as a deodorant. Her nose had adjusted to the odor, as all good noses will. It is with this in mind that we will deal with basic issues affecting personal image.

A daily bath and shampoo have a twofold purpose: to minimize transfer of "souvenir illnesses" to yourself and those you live with and to wash away body odors accumulated during the work day. Ideally, bathing takes place shortly after you arrive home: this is not possible for some of you. At the very least, change shoes and get into "home" clothes, put the uniform into the wash and wash your hands thoroughly before tackling home responsibilities.

QUESTION: 1. Why are your shoes a source of concern?
2. Why do some workplaces provide a place for you to leave your shoes and shoe polish?
3. Should you change into a fresh uniform and pair of shoes if you are going from your clinical position to a job at another agency?

Underarm deodorants and antiperspirants are not the same. Deodorants neutralize odors: antiperspirants prevent sweating. The choice should be based on your needs and skin sensitivity. If you have difficulty finding an effective deodorant or antiperspirant, talk directly with a pharmacist: he may have to make up a special substance just for you.

Some of you may experience unpleasant, although normal, all-over body odor, even though you bathe daily. Talk with your physician, since there are chlorophyll-based tablets that can be prescribed for this. Most of you do not have to seek these additional solutions, but those who do need to know that alternatives to embarrassment do exist. Remember, also, that sometimes the offender is an article of clothing that you are wearing, that is, the material retains body odor even though it is washed, and releases the odor when the article becomes warm and moist when worn. This is generally limited to a synthetic fabric that does not have a soil-release component built in. In this case, when special soaps have not solved the problem, you may have to plan a proper burial for the uniform. However, before burial, try investing in dress shields. These are hard to find, but do exist (e.g., at The Vermont Country Store, P.O. Box 3000, Manchester Ctr., VT 05255-3000). Dress shields also prevent yellow stains. Also, try spraying the armpit area of clothes with prewash before each laundry. Spray shields also.

Brushing the teeth after meals solves part of the problem of bad breath. Once a day, teeth must be flossed as taught by a dental hygienist, bridges and partial bridges cleaned, and the tongue, roof of the mouth, and insides of cheeks gently, yet thoroughly brushed with a clean, soft brush and water. Never mind the gagging when doing the tongue: the white coating that accumulates when you do not brush the tongue becomes a hidden source of halitosis. Unfortunately, mouthwash, mints, and gum are frequently used to mask the odor: a temporary solution at best. Daily brushing and flossing will also help you prevent future gum disease.

Under the fingernails and tiny scratches in the nailpolish are remarkable ways of transporting germs to your sandwich, your mouth, your eyes, your mate, your children, and your dinner salad. Actually, this list should start with the first patient, the next patient, and so on throughout the day. This is the real reason instructors discourage use of any nail polish, expect short nails, and are such terrors on proper handwashing: running water, soap, and friction. In some nursing programs, students have the opportunity to culture their nails and are surprised at the variety of "colonies" that grow from their "clean nails." Examples of cultured organisms include *Staphylococcus aureus, Staphylococcus epidermidis, Escherichia coli,* and *Clostridium perfringens.* Organisms involved depend on what you have touched in the course of the day.

Much to the annoyance of some nurses, who desire to make a statement with their hairstyles, they are told to wear it up and off the face if long, or off the face and above the collar in length. This, of course, provides a neat appear-ance desired by patients and management, but there is a hygienic reason for having clean, well-behaved hair. Visualize leaning over a portion of the patient's anatomy to change a dressing, insert a catheter, irrigate a wound. As you lean over, so does your hair. It is like shaking a rug lightly: whatever is on it falls off, providing another source of contamination for the patient. Furthermore, if you reach up to push your hair back with your hand or do the "whiplash special," you have further increased the chance for contamination.

What about the uniform itself? Some agencies no longer require a totally white uniform plus cap. They all, however, have a dress code. Adhere to it. A nurse of many years recently noted that she continues to wear her entire uniform, including the cap, and rarely has a patient refuse any medication, treatment, or direction. "It's a trick, I suppose. So easy. So pleasant. I am greeted with, 'Oh, here comes the nurse,' and a smile." Whatever your dress code, keep in mind as you dress for the day, that a patient—vulnerable, worried, and often in pain—has to look at you and view you as being believable and in charge. The "put-together-by-a-committee" look does not provide that comforting image for the patient.

Clingy, skimpy, suggestive garments may provide a topic of conversation and an impetus for inappropriate acting out on the part of the patient. This brings to mind the nurse who often wore minidresses with fruit prints to work and complained angrily when a confused patient kept trying to "pick the apples" off her "tree." Think easy care and a professional look. When shopping for the items, bend over, stretch, kneel, crush the fabric in your hand: go through the motions the garment will be subjected to. For convenience, a blend of natural and synthetic fibers is often desirable. For example, a blend of cotton and polyester will provide the comfort of cotton, because it breathes, and the ease of washing and little or no ironing because of the polyester.

Although undergarments are not meant to be seen, they sometimes are, because of the choice of color and style. Patients and other staff often discover, but will not tell, when they have seen "that itsy-bitsy, teeny-weeny, yellow polka dot bikini" when you bend at the knees to pick up an item from the floor. Interestingly, beige, not white, is the choice of color for undergarments beneath a white dress, skirt, or trousers for light-skinned individuals. Many dark-skinned individuals choose black or brown underwear beneath a white dress, skirt, or trousers.

Shoes are the most important investment of all. "American women have five times as many foot problems as men. That's because they're wearing trash on their feet" (Molloy, 1977, p. 79). Invest in a well-fitted pair of leather walking shoes. Your back, legs, feet, and whole body will thank you. If your feet perspire readily, have the shoemaker punch a hole in the instep area: an old trick, good for the shoes and the feet. Perhaps you have already noticed an interesting phenomenon for some nurses of both sexes, from the knees or ankles on down. They look sharp, and then you notice the rumpled socks, odd-colored hose, or booties with pom-poms in dirty, rundown shoes. The whole effect is destroyed for the patient. A nursing student with older, yet supple, white leather shoes offered information on how to keep the leather from cracking and the color fresh: "I use mink oil periodically to keep the leather soft and polish them at least every other work day. I also bought an extra pair of shoelaces right away: one to wash and one to wear."

Molloy, in his book *The Woman's Dress for Success Book* (1977, pp. 86–88), continues to offer on-target advice for the modern nurse:

- Regarding makeup—Light, and applied with good taste.

- Regarding perfume or aftershave lotion— If another can smell your perfume, it is too much. (Incidentally, some of the exotic oils are especially overpowering. Furthermore, no aftershave lotion and no perfume is the rule in surgery, recovery room, and short-stay areas.)

- Regarding jewelry—Simple gold posts for earrings. For rings, a plain band only— again to avoid a source of contamination.

QUESTION: Where do your "fingers do the walking"? Track the movements of your fingers for one day.

WELLNESS AS A CHOICE AND A RESPONSIBILITY

A cartoon once showed two people jogging. One asked the other, "How is your health?" The other jogger responded, "I don't know; I'll have to ask my doctor." This not-so-funny cartoon depicts an all-too-common attitude regarding wellness: that it is something out there, out of one's personal control and the responsibility of someone else. The "designated someone else" usually is a physician who is looked to as a magical "pill fairy" when something goes wrong. Please note that most visits to the doctor are focused on illness, rather than wellness. The topic is wellness, and this is where personal responsibility and choice come in.

Consider for a moment how you care for a prized possession: Very Carefully! For some of you, this is a car, and if you care for it lovingly, you are involved in a continual maintenance program in order to have it operate at peak performance. This also helps to avoid costly repair bills. It should not be any different with your self. Once you decide that wellness (continual maintenance) is a responsibility and a choice, you can design a lifestyle that will help you maintain your highest potential for personal health. Wellness does not mean a lack of imperfection, physical handicap, or a chronic condition. What it does mean is making the most of what you have and can be.

Preventing Muscle Injury: Planned Moving

Applaud yourself if aerobic exercise such as jogging, walking, or swimming is a regular part of your personal maintenance. Such exercise, which increases the cardiac and respiratory rate for a period of time, increases oxygenation and blood circulation to all parts of the body. If this already is an established part of your life, stay with it. If you are interested in beginning regular aerobic exercise and cannot decide which one, choose walking. If you have a chronic disease or orthopedic condition, call your doctor to see if there are any reasons to be cautious. Chances are that since you passed your preadmission physical, you can enjoy the healthful, yet inexpensive benefits provided by walking.

Walking is suited for people who consider themselves unathletic and out of shape, but is also effective in improving and maintaining fitness in well-conditioned people. Pain is not considered a gain. Exertion needs to be based on increasing your heartbeat to its target rate for a sustained period of time. The target heart rate is calculated by using the following formula: $220 -$ Age $\times 70\%$. Periodically check your rate by counting your heart rate for 6 seconds and adding a zero. If you do not have a watch along you know if you are close to the correct target heart rate if you can continue to converse and break into a light sweat. Walk 12 miles a week. Gradually build up to 16- to 17-minute miles. Three miles per day four times per week or approximately 45 minutes of brisk walking four times per week, excluding warm up and cool down, is recommended for cardiovascular benefit. Warm up includes 5 to 10 minutes of lighter-paced walking to gradually increase your heart rate and body temperature. Cool down follows your brisk walking. A lighter pace for 5 to 10 minutes decreases your heart rate and prevents blood from pooling in your legs.

The major investment is a good pair of walking shoes. Remember, too, that cold muscles are subject to injury. You can either begin a bit more slowly and gradually work up to the speed needed for the pulse rate or do gentle stretching exercises, both at the beginning and the end of the walk. Stretching exercises at the end are a must, since muscles, ligaments, and tendons along the back of the legs tighten up during walking.

The key is to be gentle and easy—no bouncing. Plan how to fit walking into your day so that it does not become "just one more thing to do." Some of you will be able to have this become your mode of transportation to work, errands, spending special time with a significant other, reviewing class information, or a way to relieve tension after school. Consider your needs.

A major concern in nursing is the frequency of muscle injuries, especially back injuries. Interestingly, the issue is that of flexibility, not strength. Think of people whom you consider strong who have received injuries due to twisting, bending, or any other movement common in nursing. Keeping your muscles flexible is another nursing (and personal) responsibility for you. There is a tendency to skip this responsibility because it is not as obvious, initially, as is your external image. Because it is part of the internal conditioning (and image), there is also the tendency to relate it to such words as "willpower" or "character." It is, in reality, an issue of keeping your "equipment" ready to use. Consider, also, that almost everything you do in life, you do because you have to. The things you do spontaneously and without "have to's" attached, are usually related to the one you love.

Stretching begins at the beginning of your day, may be necessary periodically throughout the day, and is often the last thing to do before going to sleep. When you awaken, think cat: think about the leisurely stretching that a cat involves itself in upon awakening. "When you wake up in the morning, have you ever lain in bed for an extra five minutes after the alarm rings? Spend those minutes stretching your sleepy muscles and getting them ready for the day" (Prudden and Sussman, 1981, p. 9). Since nursing provides an additional strain on the back, include some back stretches. Be reasonable in deciding which stretches to do and the number of repetitions. If you make your initial effort excessive, chances are you will skip all stretching on the days you feel rushed. Think in terms of a lifetime, manageable routine. And do be gentle. Listen to your body. Pain is not gain. Increase repetitions gradually to the number that leaves the muscles feeling alive and ready to face the day.

If showering is a part of your day, think of stretching, both while in the shower and when toweling yourself. For example, in basic nursing you are learning body mechanics; practice the moves in the shower.

The bathtub is a wonderful way to relax, especially with sufficient warm water and time. Do take advantage of the time for stretching the ankles, toes, wrists, and fingers. Make up your own gentle movements. Remember, your feet have held you up all day and obeyed your commands. Gently massage each foot lovingly and thoroughly. Be aware of any areas that need special care.

What about time spent sitting in the classroom? It takes up a major part of some of your days. Here are some ideas:

- Parking lot jaunt—Disappointed not to find a parking place close by? Do not be. In fact, plan to give yourself five extra minutes and deliberately park further away. Enjoy a walk to the building.

- Stairway caper—Unless there is a medical reason not to, choose the stairs over the elevator, or a combination at first, if many flights are involved. Remember to come prepared with walking shoes.

If there is some television time during the day, remember that it is a good time for stretches of your choice. Young children like to be included and it models self-care for them.

QUESTION: Which stretching exercises are needed and possible as a part of your day? Make out a plan that you will begin today.

GOOD NUTRITION: FUEL FOR YOUR MACHINE

An interesting dilemma: nurses receive specific instruction on nutritional needs and yet often have incredibly poor personal eating habits. To which of the following can you relate?

- Coffee and a cigarette for breakfast (or break or lunch, etc.).
- Over-the-counter diet pills for quick weight loss.
- Soda and chips for lunch.
- Sweetroll and coffee for breakfast.
- Coffee at the desk and when passing medications.

If you have become a nutritional dropout, get back into good eating patterns by using your head. This (like your daily stretching) is important enough to follow through without anyone else's prompting. Continuing a balanced nutritional pattern of eating is more a matter of structure and routine than a test of your character. Pull out a nutrition textbook and look at it from a personal perspective. Recommended food servings have been modified. Changes focus on foods that are (1) lower in fat, especially saturated fat, (2) lower in cholesterol, and (3) higher in fiber. In addition, it is suggested that the amount of complex carbohydrates be increased. Table 10-1 provides a down to earth look at current recommendations.

This may sound like a lifetime of boredom with meals, but what it actually suggests is moderation: putting more emphasis on some foods than others, with no reason totally to give up foods that you especially like. Moderation suggests control of the amount you consume and "trade-offs," depending on your choices throughout the day. Varying the foods decreases boredom and may open the door to some adventures in eating. In this way you combine current foods and introduce new foods gradually. Incidentally, do not be fooled by the word "natural"; read labels to find the actual composition of a product.

By now you may be saying, "Just give me some basics to begin with and forget the hype. I am so busy with school and the rest of my life." No problem.

Breakfast literally means to "break the fast" of your night and is without a doubt the most vital meal of the day. Although breakfast is traditionally thought of as the morning meal, it is in reality your first meal when you awaken. Depending on the shift you are working, someone else's dinnertime may be your breakfast. Plan accordingly. The trendy thing in recent years has been to skip breakfast and settle for a cup of coffee. A vitamin/mineral packed substitute in easy to manage containers is fresh fruit. Eat it right out of its natural package, cut up a variety of fruits into a bowl or for a change of pace, blend into a fresh fruit sauce or "smoothie." The following basic blender recipe can be varied by changing the fruit, juice or spices that are used. Blend until desired texture is obtained. Ripe fruits are the most flavorful.

Basic	Sample
2 large fresh fruit	2 large apples
$\frac{1}{2}$ cup juice (or water)	$\frac{1}{2}$ cup apple juice
$\frac{1}{4}$–$\frac{1}{2}$ teaspoon spice(s)	$\frac{1}{2}$ teaspoon cinnamon
1 or more complementary fruit	1 banana or other fruit

Table 10-1 Eat Wisely—Live Well!

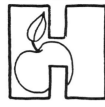 **elp** yourself to 5 servings of fresh fruits and vegetables daily. (Include at least one dark yellow or dark green vegetable and one citrus fruit.)

> **Portions: 1 Cup Leafy Vegetables**
> **1/2 Cup Cooked Fruit or Vegetables**
> **1 Medium Fruit**
> **1/4 Cup Dried Fruit**

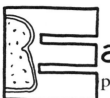 **at** at least 6 servings of whole grain breads, cereals, rice, pasta, potatoes, dried peas or beans daily.

> **Portions: 1 Slice Whole Grain Bread, Muffin, Roll, Tortilla**
> **1/2 English Muffin, Bagel**
> **1/2 Cup Cooked Cereal, Rice, Pasta, Potato, Dried Peas or Beans**
> **1 Ounce Dry Cereal**

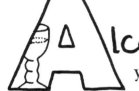 **lcohol** provides empty calories. So, if you drink, limit yourself to 2 servings daily.

> **Portions: 3 Ounces Wine**
> **6 Ounces Beer**
> **1 Ounce Hard Liquor**

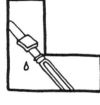 **imit** yourself to 2–3 tablespoons of fat or oil, such as butter, margarine, salad dressing, mayonnaise or cooking oil daily.

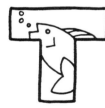 **rim** fat by choosing up to 6 ounces of fish or poultry (without skin) or well-trimmed beef or pork daily. (3 ounces is about the size of a deck of cards.)

> **Portions: 2–3 Ounces Fish, Poultry (without skin) or Well-trimmed Beef or Pork**

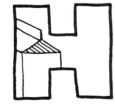 **elp** yourself to 2–3 servings of low-fat dairy products daily. Include skim or 1% milk, low-fat yogurt, ice milk, low-fat frozen yogurt and low-fat cheeses.

> **Portions: 1 Cup Skim or 1% Milk, Low Fat Buttermilk, Low Fat Yogurt**
> **1/2 Cup Ice Milk, Low Fat Frozen Yogurt, Low Fat Cottage Cheese**
> **1 Ounce Low Fat Cheese**

Note: Children under two years should not eat a low-fat diet. It may be harmful to their development. Pregnant or breastfeeding women and people with a medical condition should see their health professional for diet information.

Source: Our Nutrition Position. Two Harbors, MN: Lake County HealthWise Coalition, 1990. (Used with permission.)

Take along additional fresh fruit to enjoy during breaktime. During lunch and dinner you will be able to enjoy heavier fare that includes vegetables, starches and proteins. If you are trying to maintain your weight as opposed to gaining weight, plan to stop eating after eight p.m. (or your shift equivalent). This will give your digestive system time to do its assigned task in an uninterrupted fashion. Chances are that you will sleep better. If you still need your coffee, drink it at a nonmeal time.

The current push nutritionally is to increase daily fruit consumption. The push began in California with its "five a day" campaign. Making fruit a breakfast habit for you and your family is an easy way to meet the daily requirement.

HOW TO STAY ALIVE IN NURSING: STRESS MANAGEMENT

Without a doubt, patient care can be stressful for the nurse. Patients can be demanding and press for answers that you do not have. All patients experience some degree of regression in their behavior during their illness. Some patients are able to express their needs directly, while others express their needs indirectly, through irritability or criticism of your performance. There are, of course, patients who do not respond to treatment and continue to deteriorate.

Frequently, life and death issues are at stake. Lack of cooperation by the patient and his family may cause you to feel angry and frustrated. You in turn may be tempted to blame the patient for making you feel helpless and for the patient's lack of improvement. Patients may challenge the care they are receiving and the knowledge base of involved staff members. Family members may call and visit continuously because of concern, lack of understanding, and feelings of helplessness.

Differentiating between feelings of sympathy and empathy in regard to the patient is a major consideration in preventing burnout. Empathy is a respectful detached concern; you understand what the client is experiencing, but do not experience the emotion with him. Sympa-

thy, on the other hand, leaves you vulnerable to identifying with the patient and experiencing the emotion along with the patient. Consequently, you are no longer in control of the situation and have limited value to the patient; thus, a long-term sympathetic response is very stressful. What started out as a caring relationship becomes detrimental to the patient and to you because of overinvolvement.

You, as a nurse, function as a member of an interdisciplinary team; communication and cooperation are needed to accomplish the very best care for each patient. Remember that focus: it must be what is best for the patient. If energy is focused primarily on self, there is a limited amount left for the patient. If you find yourself saying, "I am shy, I am bashful, I have an inferiority complex," you need to be reminded that this is not synonymous with humility: it is synonymous with conceit. Do something about it.

Mutual trust of a coworker begins with you. This does not mean that you will not be hurt occasionally by those who violate this trust. However, honesty and a willingness to deal with difficult people in an assertive way pays off. Bramson (1984, pp. 46–47) offers some additional basic rules for dealing with those who attack you: (1) Stand up for yourself—otherwise you will be ignored. (2) Do not worry about being rude—when the other person is interrupting, tell him or her, then keep on talking. (3) Get the difficult person to sit down; most people are less aggressive when sitting down. (4) Speak from your point of view: use I-centered statements. (5) Avoid an all-out fight. Your purpose is to function more effectively. (6) Be ready to be friendly. Once you have stood up to a difficult person, the offer is usually genuine.

It is interesting to note that it is our reaction to a situation, rather than the situation itself, that causes stress. Everything that happens to you—either pleasant or unpleasant—creates stress. Interpretation of stress as distress or negative stress depends on personal problem-solving skills and the intensity and duration of the situations involved. Ironically, a time of boredom and understimulation is accompanied by high adrenaline levels in the body, as is a time of high stress. In other words, individuals seem to do best with a moderate amount of stress in their lives. What is defined as moderate stress varies from person to person.

While work is necessarily commendable and personally satisfying, it is, of necessity, only one part of your life. Recreation is also important and must be a part of your plan for living. Otherwise, it is too easy to brush it aside "because I have too much work to do." The ultimate choice in recreation may not be available to you consistently, but short-term recreation is available.

QUESTION: What kinds of recreation do you enjoy? List two that consume a longer time to accomplish and four recreational activities that can be accomplished in a short amount of time or on a continuing basis.

As you look at the answer to the above question, remember that some forms of recreation may be high-stress activities for you. Recreation is not the same as relaxation. Rethink your list and choose one or two short-term recreational activities that you will be able to involve yourself with on an ongoing basis without causing distress in your life. There will be times to treat yourself to longer-term recreational activities if you think it through—maybe 9 holes of golf instead of 18; read your favorite author's work during breaks, while waiting for appointments, at stoplights, on trains, in the bathtub—use your imagination.

Relaxation training is one way to manage stress. During a relaxed state, the pulse and respiratory rates decrease, the metabolic rate and blood pressure are lowered and muscular tension is decreased. Along with the positive physical changes experienced by all except about 3% of the population, you also experience a sense of well-being. If you are part of that 3%, there is nothing wrong with you. It just is, so think about what does bring about the physical changes described above for you. For example, a student shared that relaxation exercises made her "ready to climb the walls," whereas rock-and-roll music had a calming effect on her. In fact, knowing this, she insisted on listening to rock-and-roll during the birth of her child.

Many relaxation methods are available and need to be tailored to your lifestyle. Decide on a regular practice time. Some of you will want to start your day with a relaxation exercise. Some of you will want to end your day this way. Overall, relaxation is accomplished most readily before meals or at least two hours after a meal, because of the stimulant effect of food on the body. Caffeine-containing drinks, such as regular coffee and some soft drinks, are best avoided prior to the training session.

*L*EARNING EXERCISE

Meditation (Based on Benson's The Relaxation Response *1976, pp. 159–161):*

INGREDIENTS:

A quiet environment
A mental device (a word, sound, phrase, or gazing at an object)
A passive attitude
A comfortable position

DIRECTIONS:

Sit quietly in a comfortable position with your eyes closed (or open, if gazing). Let your muscles relax, beginning at your feet and progressing up to your face. Breathe through your nose as you breathe out. Repeat the mental device (or continue to gaze at an object).

For example: Breathe in . . . out . . . (mental device). Eyes may be opened as desired to check the time; simply close your eyes when satisfied, and return to repeating the mental device. Do not worry about being successful. Let distractive thoughts pass through. Simply return to repeating the mental device. In . . . out . . . (mental device). In . . . out . . . (mental device).

A quiet environment helps eliminate distractions and permits you to concentrate on a mental device of your choosing. A mental device is any sound, word, or phrase that evokes a sense of calm. You repeat the device silently or out loud with your eyes closed. If you prefer to keep your eyes open, you can fix your gaze upon an object. Either way, your mind is focusing on one thing. Concentrating on your normal breathing pattern also enhances your repetition of the mental device. A passive attitude is considered most significant for eliciting a successful relaxation response. Distracting thoughts may occur: simply let them pass through, and return to repetition of the mental device. Trying hard usually creates tension. A comfortable position prevents added muscular tension. Sit with good posture, loose-fitting clothes, shoes off, and feet on the floor. Lying down is not encouraged because you tend to fall asleep.

Imagery is another way of relaxing yourself. This kind of imagery is not the guided imagery that is used in psychotherapy and that requires a trained psychotherapist to deal with symbolic material that may emerge. Some of you are better at imagining than others. Some may see only shadowy figures, while another sees vivid, technicolor images. Images need not be particularly vivid to be effective. Mental pictures do seem to come more easily when you are relaxed and free of distraction. Begin with a relaxation exercise (some brief relaxation techniques follow later in the chapter). If you are very tense, progressive relaxation will be helpful.

Once relaxed, follow with the imagery. Two or three deep breaths are helpful prior to the imagery. In practicing the imagery, it is important to take sufficient time to include enough detail so that you can "get into" the imagery. When ready to conclude the imagery, count from 1 to 10, sit for a while with your eyes closed, open your eyes, then stretch.

It is worthwhile to remember that if you experience anxiety anytime during the imagery, you need only to open your eyes, look around, reorient yourself to your surroundings, and when satisfied, close your eyes and continue with the imagery. Some of you will be comfortable with your eyes open during the entire process and do not seem to have any problems visualizing. Imagery, like other techniques, takes self-discipline; therefore, daily practice sessions are suggested.

Imagery is an excellent way of learning to relax and once learned can be done in less-structured settings, such as during break time. It is also a way of protecting yourself against situations that you may face in the future, by visualizing the situation and how you will move through it successfully. It is also creative and fun. You already do it; you did so before embarking on your present career. What you will learn now is a more controlled way of using imagery.

LEARNING EXERCISE

Imagery: Relieving Anxiety

Design your own favorite place: whatever is your idea of complete peace, harmony, and joy. See yourself, appropriately dressed in the setting you have created. Take time to look around and visualize your surroundings with great detail. Use all of your senses to experience the sight, sound, smell, touch, and taste available in your special hideaway. See yourself staying there and feeling peaceful and calm. Remember that it is a safe place, and that you can return there to rest daily. When you are ready to leave, take one look back, knowing that you can return any time. You will continue to feel relaxed and happy as you return to your daily activities.

Progressive relaxation is a method of tensing and relaxing all of the muscle groups in order, resulting in deep relaxation. The order—from head to toes or from toes to head—is a personal choice; either is effective. If the intent is to fall asleep, then lying down is the position of choice. Otherwise, the general rules for all relaxation can be followed. Sometimes progressive relaxation is enhanced by taped (or natural) sound such as the wind or seashore sounds or by music that is close to body rhythm, such as certain Bach selections, Pachelbel's Canon in D or Steve Halpern's Zodiac Suite. Some experimentation with sound will help you discover if it enhances or distracts.

Brief relaxation techniques are useful throughout the day and can be practiced without special effects.

ᴸEARNING EXERCISE

Brief Relaxation (Based on Roon's Applied Relaxation [Roon, 1961])

TECHNIQUES	DIRECTIONS	PLACE
Brief relaxation. This exercise prevents the rush of thought. It can be used to induce on-the-spot relaxation in a public place or to promote sleep.	Part your lips slightly. Place the tip of the tongue behind the lower teeth. Keep it there without pressure for awhile. Continue with normal breathing.	Walking down the hall, in the bathroom, in class, in a meeting (not in front of the boss or instructor), during break, while studying.
Yawning. This is a one-minute tension-release exercise. The lungs expand; the back, jaw, mouth, and tongue relax. More oxygen comes into the system. Nice to do near an open window.	Drop your jaw gently until it feels large enough to take in a whole fruit. As you begin to yawn, it feels as though it will never end. As you yawn, you are taking in a deep breath. When the yawn ends you feel relaxed, clear down into your stomach. Your lungs have expanded, and your back begins to release its tension. Bauer and Hill (1986, p. 162).	

QUESTION: 1. Where can you use the above techniques? List at least two places at home, at school, and in the clinical area.
2. What method of relaxation has been successful for you in the past?
3. How can you enhance your current relaxation method?

All the methods of dealing with personal stress can be sabotaged unless you develop a regular pattern of sleep. Be aware that you can create your own insomnia by taking your worries to bed. Tell yourself firmly that you have done your best for the day and will not think about the issues until you awaken. Any of the techniques can be used to relax before bedtime if needed. Roon's "Brief Relaxation" (Roon, 1961) is excellent for inducing sleep. Continue focusing on the technique until you fall asleep.

Research on sleep has shown that most people have 90- to 100-minute sleep cycles. In order to make use of this information, do the following:

1. Go to bed at the same time: listen to what your body is telling you. Extra early or later than usual is no favor to the body.

2. Most important, when you naturally awaken, get out of bed. Better yet, do the stretching exercises and then get out of bed.

No doubt, you have at some point decided to treat yourself to a few more minutes of sleep and then ended up feeling tired much of the day. Research seems to show that the body is set on a 25-hour clock and when you get up at a different time, the body tries to "reset" the clock throughout the day. No wonder the "treat" you offered yourself did not work.

NEGATIVE INFLUENCES

The focus of nursing is wellness; yet, all too often nurses focus on wellness in others and ignore their own needs.

QUESTION: Did you practice smoking until you learned to smoke with ease and now find it a craving?

Years ago smoking was glamorized. After all, did not the hero light up the heroine's cigarette? Then, as they spoke romantically, they blew smoke into each other's face. Time to re-think that scenario; there is plenty of scientific information regarding the effect of smoking on the body to help you make an informed decision on whether to continue smoking. Our heroes and heroines of long ago did not have the data that is available to you.

So it is with alcohol and other drugs. There are many "impaired" nurses, the current term for addicted nurses. Some of you will be among the number who are looking for a painless way to relax at the end of the day, to blot out the human suffering that is a part of your new world, to sleep. Know now that there is no easy out, because if, for example, drinking is a nightly routine, you will find yourself increasing the amount that numbs you as much as the lesser amount did some weeks ago. It is an insidious process and you will not be aware when moderation ends and addiction begins. Since alcohol also affects every system in the body physically, there are multiple problems. Once again, an informed decision, in advance, is the wise decision regarding the use of alcohol and other drugs.

QUESTIONS: 1. What current behaviors in your life style support lifelong wellness?
2. Which behaviors undermine wellness?
3. What is your personal plan for change?

Summary

A nursing responsibility is to model wellness and personal care for the patient. Therefore, it is imperative for the nurse to make informed decisions about the direction of her personal life early in nursing:

1. The image you project sets the tone for the patient's level of confidence, willingness to believe, and cooperation.
2. Health care practices, especially handwashing, decrease the risk of contamination for patients, self, and family members.
3. Wellness is a personal issue under your direction and control. Planning needs to be realistic and based on your lifestyle. It begins today and is maintained for a lifetime.

REFERENCES

Bauer R, Hill S. *Essentials of mental health care: planning and interventions.* Philadelphia: W.B. Saunders, 1986.

Benson H. *The relaxation response.* New York: Avon, 1976.

Bramson R. Assertive techniques for handling difficult people. Nurs Life 1984; July/August:46–49.

Brody J. *Good food book: living the high carbohydrate way.* New York: W.W. Norton, 1985.

Idem. Jane Brody's nutrition book. New York: Bantam, 1988.

Idem. Jane Brody's The New York Times Guide to Personal Health. New York: Avon, 1982.

Davis M, McKay M, Eshelman E. *The relaxation and stress reduction workbook.* Richmond, Calif.: New Harbinger, 1981.

Lazarus A. *In the mind's eye.* New York: Rawson, 1984.

Molloy J. *The woman's dress for success book.* New York: Warner, 1977.

Our nutrition position. Two Harbors, MN: Lake County HealthWise Coalition, 1990.

Prudden S, Sussman J. *Suzy Prudden's I can exercise anywhere book.* New York: Workman, 1981.

Roon K. *Karin Roon's new way to relax.* New York: Greystone, 1961.

Ryan R, Travis J. *Wellness workbook.* Berkely, Calif.: Ten Speed Press, 1981.

CHAPTER
11

Assertiveness as a Nursing Responsibility

Learning Objectives

Upon completing this chapter, you will
1. Explain why assertiveness is a nursing responsibility.
2. Differentiate between assertive, aggressive, and passive behavior.
3. Describe three negative interactions in which nurses can get involved.
4. Maintain a daily journal that reflects personal interactions and responses.
5. Develop a personal plan for change toward assertive behavior.

Assertiveness is an expectation in nursing—a responsibility for you as the patient advocate.

Once again you are requested to do a brief exercise before going on with your reading.

LEARNING EXERCISE

Directions: Imagine for the next few minutes that the nurse/patient roles are reversed and that you are the patient.

QUESTION: What are your expectations of the nurse assigned to you? List the rationale for each expectation that you identify.

EXPECTATION

1.

2.

RATIONALE

Doing the above exercise has already begun to give you insight into the need for the nurse to be assertive. At the end of this chapter you are encouraged to do this exercise again. Evaluate any change in expectations.

Now let's take a look at three major behaviors: passive (nonassertive), aggressive, and assertive. We will also look at negative interactions specific to nursing, and at how to move toward truly assertive behavior.

PASSIVE BEHAVIOR

Passive (nonassertive) behavior is an emotionally dishonest, self-defeating behavior. The passive nurse attempts to look the other way, to avoid conflict, and to take what seems to be the easiest way out—he or she is never fully a participant on the nursing team. The passive individual does not express feelings, needs, and ideas when her rights are infringed on, deliberately or accidentally. This personal pattern of behavior is reflected in her nursing as well; consequently, she is unable to recognize and meet the patient's needs. A number of examples of passive behavior are given below. With each, the type of behavior is given in parentheses.

- Tells another nurse how "stupid" the doctor is for ordering a treatment. (Indirect)
- Limits contact with the patient she is uncomfortable with to required care only. (Indirect)

- Routinely tells the patient who questions her for an explanation about the illness, tests, medications, and treatments to "ask the doctor" or "ask the R.N." While this answer is advisable some of the time, it certainly is a "brushoff," since part of nursing responsibility is to seek the answer for the patient. (Takes the easy way out)
- Experiences inability to continue with a necessary, uncomfortable treatment ordered for the patient. (Interprets patient's expression of discomfort personally ["He will not like me if I make him do this."])
- May assume, without checking, that the patient wants to skip his daily personal care when a visitor drops in. (Avoid conflict)
- Experiences a feeling of being "devastated" when a patient, doctor, nurse, or other staff person criticizes her work. (Interprets criticism of work as criticism of self)
- Responds to patient's questions regarding her personal life and that of other staff. (Afraid of not being liked)
- Patient asks her to pick up some personal items on the way home. She frowns, but agrees to do so. (Communicates the real message indirectly)
- She is angry with the team leader and drops hints to others about her feelings. (Communicates real message indirectly)

- Another nurse asks her to take on the care of her patients. She is already too busy, but responds by saying "Well, uh, I guess I could." (Hesitance, repressing her own wishes)
- Needs help with her assignment, but says nothing. (Refrains from expressing needs)
- After making an error, overexplains and overapologizes (Unaware of the right to make a mistake. Should take responsibility for it, learn from the error, and go on.)
- Plans on finding a new job because she is afraid of approaching the supervisor to tell her side of what has happened. (Avoid conflict)
- The doctor "chews out" the nurse in front of the patient. She is angry, but says nothing. (Refrain from expressing your opinion)

QUESTION: What are some other examples of passive behavior?

By not taking the risk and not being honest, the nonassertive nurse typically feels hurt, misunderstood, anxious, and disappointed and often angry and resentful later. Since you do not allow your needs to be known, you are the loser.

AGGRESSIVE BEHAVIOR

Outspoken people are often automatically considered assertive when, in reality, their lack of consideration for others may characterize aggressive behavior. Aggressive behavior violates the rights of others. It is an attack on the person rather than on the person's behavior. The purpose of aggressive behavior is to dominate or put the other person down. This behavior, while expressive, is self-defeating as it quickly distances you from other staff and patients (Bauer and Hill, 1986, pp. 102–103).

The following examples are some of the ways that aggressive behavior can be recognized. An explanation is included in parentheses.

1. You have asked to go to a workshop and the supervisor tells you, "Why should you get to go? Everyone has worked here longer than you have?" (Attempt to make you feel guilty for making a request)

2. Another nurse points out your error in front of the other staff and adds, "Where did you say you graduated from?" (Attempt to humiliate as a way of controlling)

3. A peer approaches you with a problem. You don't want to listen and say "If it isn't one thing it's another for you. Why don't you get your act together?" (Disregard others' feelings)

4. A new rule is instituted without requesting input from or informing those whom it will involve. You protest and are told "That's tough, this is the way it is going to be from now on." (Disregard for others' feelings and rights)

5. The patient has had his call light on frequently throughout the morning. You walk in and say, "I have had it. You have had your light on continuously for nothing, all morning. Do not put your light on again unless you are dying or I will take it away." (Hostile overreaction out of proportion to the issue at hand)

6. You attempted to express your feelings to a peer about her behavior toward you. Today she greets you with an "icy" stare when you say "Hello." (Hostile)

7. The patient tells you "I thought this was a pretty good hospital but none of you seem to know what you are doing." (Sarcastic—Hostile)

8. You push yourself in front of others in the cafeteria line. (Rudeness)

9. Another employee greets you with "I hear you are a real whiz kid. Show us your stuff." (Put-down)

QUESTION: What other examples of aggressive behavior have you experienced?

Aggressive behavior certainly is a way of saying what you mean at the moment, and it often does produce temporary relief from anxiety. However, the feeling does not last and very often the aggressive person is left with residual angry feelings that simmer until the next situation and/or person comes along. It is interesting to note that sometimes this aggressive person was once passive and made a decision that "no one will step on me again." However, instead of practicing assertiveness, this individual practiced and became involved in another destructive, self-defeating behavior. The aggressive nurse, like the passive nurse, is unable to function as a true advocate for the patient since she is too busy taking care of what she perceives to be her personal needs.

ASSERTIVENESS

Assertiveness is a current name for honesty, that is, to live the truth from your innermost being and to express this truth in thought, word, and deed. The concept seems simple enough, but actually to practice being truthful all the time is difficult. Assertiveness, according to Webster's dictionary, is characterized by taking a positive stand, being confident in your statement, or being positive in a persistent way. You, the nurse, work in a setting that requires speaking frankly and openly to others in such a way that their rights are not violated. While it is not the nurse's right to hurt others deliberately, it is unrealistic to be inhibited to the point of never hurting anyone. Some people are hurt because they are unreasonably sensitive, and some use their sensitivity to manipulate others. The nurse has the right to express thoughts and feelings. To do otherwise would be insincere and would deny patients and other staff the opportunity to learn to deal with their feelings. Assertiveness, then, is a way of expressing oneself without insulting another person. It communicates respect for the other person although not necessarily for the other person's behavior (Bauer and Hill, 1986, p. 103). Being assertive does not guarantee that you will get your way. What it does guarantee is that you will experience a sense of being in control of your emotions and your responses and that, win or lose, you gave it your best shot. The real bonus is freedom from residual feelings of anger.

The following examples, with rationale in parentheses, are expressions of assertive behavior.

- The doctor orders a medication or treatment that seems inappropriate. You request to talk with him privately, ask about expected outcomes, and then present any new information you have that may potentially affect the decision to continue with the order. (Direct statement of information)

- The patient has been giving you a bad time. Pulling up a chair and sitting down, you say, "Mr. Smith, I would be interested in knowing what is going on with you. I have noticed that whatever I do, you are critical of my work." Then listen attentively and with understanding; respond nondefensively. (Direct statement of feelings, does not interpret patient's criticism as a personal attack)

- When the patient requests information you are unfamiliar with regarding his illness and treatment, you say, "I do not know but I will find out for you," and follow through by checking with appropriate staff and determining who is to inform the patient. (Respects the patients right to know)

- The patient has an order to be walked 10 minutes of each hour. She complains that it hurts and asks you not to make her walk. You respond by saying, "I know it is uncomfortable, but I will walk along beside you. We can stop briefly any time you like. I will also teach you how to do a brief relaxation technique that you can use while you are walking." If pain medication is available, you will also be sure that this is given prior to walking and in enough time for the medication to take effect. (Respects patient's feelings, but supports need to carry out doctor's order)

- Unexpected visitors arrive when it is time for you to help the patient with his personal care. Go in and ask the patient directly if he wishes to have his care done now or to postpone it briefly. State the time that you will be available to assist with care. (Respect the patient's right to choose, as long as it does not compromise his care)

- You have just been criticized for your work; you respond by saying, "Please clarify. I want to be sure I understand." If the error is yours, ask for suggestions to correct it and/or offer alternatives of your own. (Separates criticism of performance from criticism of self)

- The patient asks for personal information about you (or another staff member). You respond by saying "That information is personal and I do not choose to discuss it." (Stand up for rights without violating rights of others)

- Your patient asks you to pick up some personal items for him. Since this would mean doing it on your own time, which is already very full, you say, "I will not be able to do the errand for you." (Direct statement without excuses)

- The team leader has been "on your case" constantly and, you think, unfairly. You approach him or her and say, "I want to speak with you privately today before 3 P.M. What time is convenient for you?" (Direct statement of wishes)

- You are being pressed by other staff members to help with their assignments. You are too busy to do so and say "No, I do not have the time to do so today. Try me again on some other day." (Direct refusal without feeling guilty. Leaves the door open to help at a future date)

- Overwhelming day. You approach your team leader "I know you want all of this done today, but there is no way to get it all done. What are your priorities?" (Direct information and request for clarification)

- The doctor has "chewed you out" in front of the patient. You feel embarrassed and angry. You approach the doctor and tell him you want to speak to him privately. Using I-centered statements, you begin by saying "I feel both embarrassed and angry because you criticized me in front of the patient. Next time, ask to talk to me privately and I will listen to what you have to say." (Stand up for your rights without violating the rights of others)

- You are ready to leave work when a peer approaches you about a personal problem. You respond by saying, "I have to leave now, but I'll be glad to listen to you during lunch-time tomorrow." (Compromise)

- Another staff person gets in the cafeteria line ahead of you with a nod and a smile. You are in a hurry too, and feel put-upon. You say firmly, "I do not like it when you get in line ahead of me. Please go back to the end of the line." (Stand up for rights)

QUESTION: What are additional examples of assertiveness with which you are familiar?

Three rules of thumb are helpful overall in being assertive (Bauer and Hill, 1986, p. 102)

1. Own your feelings: That is, do not blame others for the way you feel.

2. Make your feelings known by being direct and by beginning your statements with "I."

3. Be sure that your nonverbal communication matches your verbal message.

NEGATIVE INTERACTIONS

With the availability of so many types of preparation for nurses and lack of differentiation in the roles based on preparation, nurses sometimes experience insecurity in their role and the worth of the role as they understand it. This negative interaction involves use of the coping/mental mechanism of *projection,* whereby an individual attributes his own weaknesses to others. The interaction can be characterized as "My education is better than yours" or "I'm more competent than you are" or "You're only a _____ nurse," etc. Unfortunately this negative, aggressive interaction uses up energy that could be used to provide the patient care that is being alluded to. In work areas where nurses are confident and assertive, excellent examples of working together to enhance each other's knowledge base and legal responsibility can be witnessed, and the patient benefits.

Another negative interaction is based on a previous unresolved incident between the patient and the nurse(s). The nurse uses the coping/mental mechanism of *rationalization* in which she offers a logical, but untrue reason as an excuse for her behavior. The nurse quickly informs others that this patient is a "troublemaker" or "manipulater" or "uncooperative," as the case may be: a passive, indirect behavior on the part of the nurse. Obviously, if other nurses incorporate this information into their transactions with the patient, the patient will never be seen as his or her self and anything that he or she does can be interpreted in the context of the label given by the nurses. A vicious circle can ensue: if the patient's needs are not met due to this obstacle, this increases his or her frustration and threat to self, resulting in anxiety. Depending on the patient's personal strength at this time, it can lead to problem solving or use of coping mental mechanisms, and/or symptom formation. See Figure 11-1.

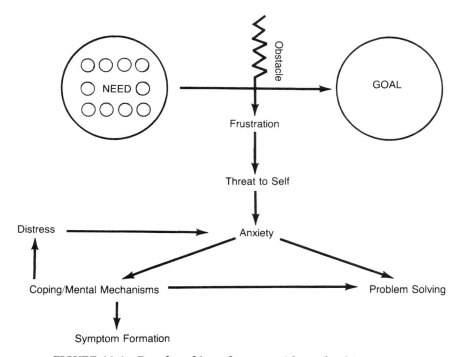

FIGURE 11-1   Results of interference with goal achievement.

Source: Bauer B, Hill, S. *Essentials of Mental Health Care: Planning and Interventions.* Philadelphia: W.B. Saunders, 1986.

An honest, assertive response on the part of the original nurse involved would lead to dealing with the patient directly in regard to the previous situation and not involve other nurses as allies to "get this patient." An example of how extreme this seemingly innocent rationalization can be happened at a nursing home. A young man who was paralyzed from the waist down as a result of a car accident was being transferred from one nursing home to another. A transfer form arrived before he did. The information on the form created immediate anxiety for the nurses involved—before they had even met the man. The form labeled the man as "manipulative" and explained that "he will be pleasant and polite at first, but watch out because it is a trick, and when he has won you over, you will see his 'real colors.'" The nurses discussed the prospective admission and expressed gratitude to have been warned by their colleagues in the other nursing home. After all, "what are colleagues for." And now "forewarned is forearmed."

When the patient arrived and attempted to get acquainted, he was dealt with coldly and abruptly and made to wait: "we will show him he cannot manipulate us." As his frustration and his discomfort increased, he began to demand that his treatments be done on time and shouted angry comments at the nurses when they finally arrived to assume his care. The nurses called him "demanding" and "hostile" and the original title of manipulative was supported when the patient had his roommate put on the call light to get help to take him to the bathroom. Each day seemed worse than the day before. The showdown finally came when a longtime nurse employee left, saying she would not come back until the patient was transferred to another facility and she would even volunteer to do the transfer note.

Other nursing staff threatened to follow suit. Finally the administrator gave in—the patient was transferred and the nurses congratulated each other for having worked together!

QUESTION: 1. What factors contributed to the patient's behavior?
2. What factors contributed to the nurses' response to the patient?
3. How could this have been handled differently?
4. Was the behavior of the nurses passive, aggressive, or assertive? Explain your answer.

Another negative transaction involves patient rights and can be known by many titles, depending on the issue. It can, for example, be called "no guts" or "I have got a secret" or "It is not my responsibility" or "She will be upset" or "She is too weak to know." Responsibility to inform the patient about his condition or transfer plans is not carried out so that present staff does not have to deal with the full impact of the patient's reaction to the information. The coping/mental mechanism used by the nurses is *denial,* whereby the nurse refuses to recognize the existence and significance of the patient's personal concern. The nurse further uses denial as a way of excusing her responsibility: "The doctor should tell him" or "It's the team leader's responsibility." Although the decision may not be entirely yours, it is clearly your responsibility to check out what portion of the information is yours to give, and who is going to present the information and when.

QUESTION: Is the nurse's refusal to take responsibility to seek out the information the patient needs to know a passive, aggressive, or assertive transaction?

Although there are many possible negative interactions, certainly the passive and/or aggressive game of "gossip" or "Did I tell you" or "I just found out" is a destructive interaction, with potential for ruining reputations, of both patients and personnel. The nurse involved in this interaction generally experiences low self-esteem and tries to increase it by being "in the know." The coping/mental mechanism is *compensation,* whereby the nurse is covering for real or imagined inadequacy in her work by developing what she considers desirable traits: observation, listening, and reporting. Unfortunately the energy is misguided, since reputations are at stake and time spent socializing while at work is time away from quality patient care. Listeners can squelch this game by assertively saying, "I will work on a relationship with you and me, but I do not wish to have you talk to me about others." Instead, too often, the listener, while calling the other nurse "a gossip," listens with interest, thus supporting continuation of this behavior.

QUESTION: 1. What other negative interaction between staff or between patients and staff are you familiar with?
2. How is the continuation of this interaction supported by others?

GUIDELINES FOR MOVING TOWARD ASSERTIVENESS

The following poem by an anonymous author captures the reason for working toward assertiveness: Being able to feel good about yourself as you continue to grow as a person.

Myself

I have to live with myself and so,
I want to be fit for myself to know.
I don't want to stand with the setting sun,

And hate myself for the things I've done.
I want to go out with head erect.
I want to deserve all man's respect,
But here in this struggle for fame and self,
I want to be able to like myself.
I don't want to look at myself and know,
That I'm bluster and bluff and empty show.
I never can fool myself, and so
Whatever happens, I want to grow
More able to be more proud of me,
Self-respecting and conscience free.

—Author Unknown—

"Making the decision to change may be the toughest part of all. Change is not easy. It cannot be imposed on anyone by logic, or rhetoric, or a persuasive assertive training leader. The decision to change can come only from ourselves" (Bloom et al., 1980, p. 67).

The problem-solving process is a conscious growth-producing method of dealing with this challenge in your life. It is important to note that problem solving is an active process and is more than simply developing an intellectual awareness of the challenge at hand.

Step 1—Define the Problem

Ironically, sometimes what is perceived as the problem is not the problem at all. Furthermore, before making a commitment for change, it is important to look objectively at the gains and losses associated with the present behavior. After all, your present way of responding to others developed as a response to anxiety-producing situations in life and usually has its roots in childhood.

Another important consideration is that when you change the way you act toward others, you change the way they will act toward you. What has been a predictable reaction will no longer be there. Initially the "others" will test you and increase their behavior as a way of getting you to give up the new behavior. However, if you persist with your new way of dealing with and responding to situations, their behavior toward you will also change. This is actually the only way to influence change in any one's behavior. No amount of "telling" or "scolding" makes a difference as long as they can count on you to behave in a predictable way.

Therefore, defining the problem depends on gathering data for two or three days and then writing your problem statement based on this information.

Gathering data needs to be done in an objective manner—as though you were observing someone else. Keeping a daily journal helps to pinpoint specific situations. Bloom (1980, p. 99) suggests a chart form as follows:

SITUATION AND DATE	PHYSICAL SYMPTOMS, BODY CUES, AND BEHAVIOR PATTERNS	MY BEHAVIOR	HOW I FELT	WHAT I WOULD LIKE TO HAVE DONE	WHY I DIDN'T DO WHAT I WANTED TO DO

Reviewing the data you have gathered will give you insight into the pros and cons of your present behavior. The problem statement you develop will have to be personal and specific.

SAMPLE: I am afraid to say what I mean for fear that others will get angry with me.

This is characterized by

Saying "yes" to babysitting when I need the time for homework.

Not asking for help with household chores even though I am a full-time student plus homemaker.

Saying "yes" to added requests at school that I must complete on my own time.

Feeling tired and resentful much of the time and eventually "blowing up" over something insignificant.

Step 2—Decide on a Goal

At this point you review the problem statement and say "So what?" In other words, what do you want to do differently? This can be stated as a single goal, but often it is more useful to break the goal down into a long-term goal and several short-term goals (sometimes called objectives) —the steps to attaining the desired long-term goal. All goals must be realistic, measurable, and time limited. At this time, write a goal for yourself.

SAMPLE	LONG-TERM GOAL	SHORT-TERM GOAL
	I will say what I mean without fear of others being angry with me, within 6 months (Give actual date).	a. I will say "no" to "babysitting" requests when I need the time for homework, within 2 weeks (Give actual date).

As you read each of the goals you have written, ask yourself if they are realistic, that is, reasonable to attain. Next, review each goal and ask if it is measurable, that is, so specific that you can use the senses to detect the change. Also note that each goal begins with "I will," that is, a personal commitment to work on the goal. Finally, note that the goals are to be attained within a designated amount of time; that is, they are time limited. This is also the only way to give that personal push to get started.

Obviously, all the changes are not going to occur exactly at the projected date and you will have to revise the goal dates from time to time. But most important, they provide target dates to strive for. As you accomplish each short-term goal, cross it out and go on to the next one. Do not be alarmed if you find yourself working on more than one goal at a time. This is possible and even desirable when the opportunity presents itself. Meanwhile, it is important to continue recording in the journal that was begun initially to obtain data. Its value now is in keeping a record of the process you are going through and in seeing the changes taking place. Unless you do this, you may not fully appreciate your work and its progress. Many changes will be subtle and not accompanied by bells and claps of thunder.

Step 3—Choose Alternatives

Alternatives are the approaches that you will be using to attain each of the established goals. When beginning to make a list of alternatives (in your journal) let your imagination run wild. Consider all the possible solutions—from serious to humorous—that you may have already considered at some time. This may even provide some comic relief to a serious challenge with which you are dealing. Remember to include "Do nothing" in the list of alternatives, since to "do nothing" is a choice and, therefore, an alternative. Look at each of the goals and think of specific things you can do or say to help support the goal.

SAMPLE: Approach: Practice in front of a mirror. In an even tone of voice say, "No, I will not be able to babysit tonight, but try again another time." If she persists, say "No, I do not have the time tonight." Repeat as needed until heard. Compliment yourself for not giving in.

Do you see how the approach (alternative) corresponds specifically to the short-term goal?

Step 4—Try out the Alternatives

The initial plan has been made and it is time to put the plan into action. For many of you the paperwork is far easier than taking the first step to make the "paper trip" become a reality. You may have also discovered that it has been far easier to offer ideas to peers, than to take the first step into action with your own plan.

QUESTION: What are you gaining from staying nonassertive? What are you losing from staying nonassertive?

The answer belongs in your journal. Whether you are writing or tape recording a journal depends on your learning style. Regardless of the journal method, it has by now become an important part of the process. At this point you may wish to change the headings as follows:

SITUATION AND DATE	PHYSICAL SYMPTOMS, BODY CUES, AND BEHAVIOR PATTERNS	MY BEHAVIOR	HOW I FELT	ALTERNATIVE USED	RESPONSE TO THE USES OF THE ALTERNATIVE

It is also a good idea to build in an incentive to continue using the new assertive approaches. Promise yourself something that is worthy of you (a worthy goal). You will note as you go along that sometimes you will slip back into old, familiar ways of behaving. Do not be dismayed; this is normal. Simply reinstitute the newly planned approaches immediately and continue. The more you practice the new approaches, the more they will become a part of you and ultimately a replacement for old passive or aggressive behaviors.

Step 5—Evaluate the Effectiveness

The evaluation mechanism is built into the overall plan for change by making the goals time limited. This tells you that each goal, along with the alternatives that you have chosen, will be evaluated as indicated. Remember not to change a goal or approach too quickly—give it at least two to three weeks. There are two reasons for this: (1) The negative behaviors of other individuals toward you will increase initially as they attempt to resist change created by the change in you. (2) It takes a minimum of two to three weeks for the new behavior to become a part of you. As a part of the evaluation, review your entire journal. It is an excellent source of information for what happened, how you dealt with it, and if the present course is effective.

Step 6—Repeat the Process if the Solution Is Not Effective

Going through Step 5 gives you information as to whether or not to pursue the established course. If changes are needed, go back to Step 3 and identify additional alternatives or perhaps choose alternatives that you originally identified but did not use. Then go through the rest of the steps as before.

As you pursue an assertive way of behaving, remember to monitor your nonverbal messages. The nonverbal communication you provide is even more powerful than your verbalization. It is possible to have the words just right, only to have them sabotaged by hesitancy, a look of sarcasm, or emphasis on certain words. Practice in front of a mirror. Busy schedule? Try bath time. Listen to the way you sound. A tape is helpful or even speaking into an empty corner and hearing your words bounce back. Try lowering your tone of voice and being sure that the last word of a sentence is no higher than the one before. Listen for this in others. It makes a statement sound like a question. Posture plays an important role—sit up straight, walk with shoulders back and with a confident stride. Provide eye contact when speaking. If this is new and difficult for you, look at the area between the eyes of the person you are addressing—it provides an illusion of eye contact. Periodically look away so that it does not look as though you are staring. Avoid annoying characteristics such as nail biting, finger or foot tapping and jiggling, playing with your hair, chewing on a pencil or glasses, and artificial laughter. And finally, when someone asks you what you think of an issue or what you would like to do, answer them instead of saying "I really do not know" or "Whatever you like; it does not matter." Life is an adventure, and all of it, including your ideas, count.

CULTURAL DIFFERENCES

It is not safe to assume that all cultures are focused on moving toward assertive behavior. In some cultures, for example, what is thought of as manipulation in the mainstream culture of the United States is an accepted norm. Skillful manipulation is especially applauded.

It is easy to jump to the conclusion that the person is trying to "trick" you because you do not share the same cultural background. Make time to talk. The differences will be interesting and revealing for both of you.

Summary

Passive (nonassertive) behavior is an attempt to look the other way, avoid conflict, and take what seems to be the easiest route; in short, never truly being a participant in life. The end result is often one of resentment and anger. Aggressiveness, at the other extreme, is an uncontrollable response to fear, anger, and anxiety and holds others responsible for the inability to deal with life's challenges in a tranquil, honest way. Assertiveness is a synonym for honesty, that is, to live the truth from your innermost being and to express this truth in thought, word, and deed. To always be truthful is difficult, but as the patient advocate, this becomes a major goal toward which to strive.

Undesirable behaviors and interactions can be changed through using the steps of the problem-solving process. Both verbal and nonverbal interactions must be dealt with during this change.

REFERENCES

Alberti RE. *Your perfect right: a guide to assertive behavior.* 6th ed. Broomfield, CO: Impact Publishers, 1990.

Bauer B, Hill S. *Essentials of mental health care: planning and interventions.* Philadelphia: W.B. Saunders, 1986.

Bloom L, Coburn K, Pearlman J. *The new assertive woman.* New York: Dell, 1980.

Levin P, Berne E. Games nurses play. Am J Nurs 1972; 72(3):483–487.

Smith M. *When I say no, I feel guilty.* New York: Bantam, 1985.

CHAPTER 12
Pitfalls to Success in Practical Nursing

Learning Objectives

Upon completing this chapter you will
1. Discuss two ways to prevent burnout in nursing.
2. Describe abuse of alcohol and/or other drugs as a path to becoming labeled "Impaired Nurse."
3. Explain the effect of smoking tobacco by the nurse on the nurse and the patient.
4. Identify the need for personal weight management as a health issue for the nurse.
5. Describe fears of occupational risk such as AIDS, tuberculosis, and hepatitis.
   a. Myths/facts about AIDS
   b. Tuberculosis and AIDS connection
   c. Hepatitis: What are the risks?
   d. Universal precautions as a way of life in nursing.
6. Discuss codependent behavior as an obstacle to success.
7. Determine specific pitfalls, if any, that may prevent your success in practical nursing.

As a nurse you must learn to take care of your-self. In turn, you can be more effective in meeting your patient's nursing needs. In taking care of yourself positively, you serve as a positive role model for both your coworkers and patients. There is stress involved in patient care. However, it is not the event, it is how you view the event that determines the amount and kind of stress that you experience. Sage advice from Frankl (1984) gives you the control: "Change your attitude if you cannot change the situation."

QUESTION:
1. What current situation in your life is creating negative stress?
2. In what way can you view the event in a more positive way?

BURNOUT

Burnout is like looking at your career world through black glasses. The positive attitude you held about nursing, working with clients, and self-care begins to change.

Symptoms include gradually losing a sense of caring about clients; talking about emotional exhaustion; losing positive feelings, sympathy and respect for clients; seeing clients cynically; blaming clients for their illness; increasing the use of alcohol and other drugs; talking negatively about oneself and having conflicts at home (Haack, 1987, p. 240).

Differentiating between feelings of empathy and sympathy in regard to your patient is a major consideration in preventing burnout. Empathy is a respectful, detached concern. As a nurse, you understand what your patient is experiencing, but do not experience the emotion with him. A sympathetic reaction leaves you vulnerable to both identifying with and experiencing the emotion along with the patient. This means that you no longer are in control of the situation. Consequently, you have limited long-range value to the patient. A long-term sympathetic response is very stressful. What starts out as a caring relationship can become detrimental to you and your patient because of overinvolvement.

Another significant step in preventing burnout is to develop a detached way of evaluating your daily personal performance. Waiting for a patient, doctor, or nurse manager to notice your performance is rarely helpful or rewarding. Perhaps they notice only what is missing. However, a detached, daily evaluation of your performance leaves you free to credit yourself for what you have done well. Furthermore, it alerts you to areas in which you need more study, assistance, and/or practice. *You are your most effective boss!*

Time management is another important factor in dealing with both the personal and the professional areas of your life. Because of its significance, Chapter 5 is devoted to the topic.

QUESTION: What change have you made using information from the chapter on Time Management? If you said "none," read the chapter again. Repetition reinforces learning.

Humor—do not forget humor. No matter how seriously you take yourself, you are never going to get out of this life alive. So lighten up. There are many things that happen in a nursing situation that can be lightened up through humor. Case in point: The nursing instructor walked into the room to see how the student nurse was doing with her patient. As she approached the patient, she extended her hand and greeted the patient by name. As he opened his mouth to speak, he simultaneously expelled flatus—a thunderous clap! The patient's eyes opened wide—momentary silence—the student looked shocked—and then the instructor chuckled! "It happens," she said with a shrug. Soon all three were laughing; the embarrassment was gone. The real issue of the patient's condition and nursing care was again the priority.

Maintaining nursing skills is essential. Even if you are in a situation that requires less hands-on care, make time to perform nursing procedures. Also, learn to do new procedures as they are introduced to your facility. This helps to feed your self-esteem, an issue closely related to preventing burnout. Otherwise you may develop a secret fear of being put on the spot and perhaps, will lie your way out of requests to demonstrate or assist.

Finally, remember that there is life after patients. Separate your personal and your professional life. Otherwise you will find that you are never completely in either place.

QUESTION: 1. Do you find yourself frequently focusing on home issues when at work?
2. Are you talking often about work when you are with your friends and family?
3. Name one change that you will begin to work on starting now.

*I*MPAIRED NURSE

Impaired and nurse sound like contradictory terms. There are, however, nurses that become chemically dependent on alcohol and/or other drugs. You may be one of them.

Early intervention is essential. Not only is your health and life at stake, but so is that of your patients. It will help you to take the first step for yourself or another nurse if you remember that chemical dependency is a disease, not a character flaw (Abbott, 1987, p. 1105). It is also interesting to note that "alcoholics have the same psychological and emotional problems as everyone else before they start drinking. These problems are aggravated, however, by their addiction to alcohol. Alcoholism undermines and weakens the alcoholic's ability to cope with the normal problems of living. Furthermore, the alcoholic's emotions become inflamed both when he drinks excessively and when he stops drinking. Thus, when he is drinking and when he is abstinent, he will feel angry, fearful, and depressed in exaggerated degrees" (Milam & Ketcham, 1983, pp. 12–13).

The most telling sign of chemical dependency is a gradual decline in performance usually noticeable in three to six months. Behaviors that need to be checked out include

1. Complaints by staff and patients;
2. Accidents, errors in documentation, a greater number of injuries caused while moving patients or equipment, errors in practice;
3. Increased visits to employee health department or emergency room;
4. Increased volunteering to take call for others;
5. Arriving early or staying late to assist in the narcotic count;
6. Frequent absenteeism after days off and for personal emergencies;
7. Irritability and mood swings'
8. Performing only the minimum work required; and
9. Inability to perform psychomotor skills due to intoxication or tremors (Abbott, 1987, p. 1108).

Two emotional characteristics of chemical dependency make it difficult to begin treatment. The denial system is very strong, and the person is usually a skilled manipulator. A recovering alcoholic who is a commercial photographer explained, "I was always drinking with the finest professionals. My companions included a judge, a lawyer, the town's top surgeon and the police chief. Obviously *they* weren't alcoholics and anyway there was always someone in a more advanced stage than I was. As my alcoholism continued to progress I would point to someone in a more advanced stage and say—'look at them. I'm not doing that. I'm not an alcoholic.—and then one day I almost died after I fell down a flight of stairs. I finally heard when the doctor said, 'Either you quit drinking or you will die'" (Michael L., 1990). Unlike Michael L., it is not necessary to hit bottom to intervene.

QUESTION: 1. Do I turn to alcohol and/or other chemicals for relief from pain or stress on a regular basis?
2. If the answer to 1 is yes, whom will you seek out for intervention?
3. List names of facilities and persons in your area who assist with chemical dependency issues.
4. If you realize that a coworker is drinking and impaired while on duty, what is your responsibility to the patient?

You can seek help from counselors, treatment centers, Alcoholics Anonymous, Narcotics Anonymous, and other local resources. The yellow pages in your phone book list "Alcohol Abuse Information and Treatment" and "Drug

Abuse Information and Treatment" resource numbers. You can also look in the white pages under "Business and Professional Listings" for alcohol or drug abuse services, helpline and hotline numbers. Risk making a phone call for information on your own or a friend's behalf.

SMOKING

Nurses and smoking—another set of contradictory terms. "None of the habits that can damage the health of human beings has been as clearly documented, or as widely publicized, as smoking. There is simply no room for debate: Smoking promotes heart disease and cancer and is the major cause of premature, preventable deaths in the United States. Smoking can make you sick if you're healthy, and make it harder to recover if you do get sick" (University of California, Berkeley, 1991, p. 53).

As a nurse you will be asked to encourage your patients to decrease or discontinue their use of tobacco. Visualize the contradiction if you, too, are a smoker. Your breath, hair, skin, clothes, and hands quickly make your words unconvincing.

It is interesting to note that the rate of smoking by men has continued to decrease. The rate of smoking for women has increased. Approximately half of American smokers who have ever smoked have quit. Most heavy smokers continue to smoke even after a life-threatening illness. It is thought that many of those smokers are physically addicted to the nicotine in tobacco. Meanwhile approximately three thousand young people begin to smoke each day. If you are a smoker take the following test.

Why Do You Smoke?

True of False: I smoke . . .

1. because I light up automatically and don't know I'm doing it.

2. because it's relaxing.

3. because I like handling cigarettes, matches, and lighters.

4. to help deal with anger.

5. to keep from slowing down.

6. because it's unbearable not to.

7. because I enjoy watching the smoke as I exhale it.

8. to take my mind off my troubles.

9. because I really enjoy it.

10. because I feel uncomfortable without a cigarette in my hand.

11. to give myself a lift.

12. without planning to—it's just part of my routine.

Results: "True" answers to 5 and 11 indicate that you smoke for stimulation; to 3 and 7, that the pleasure of handling is important; to 2 and 9, that you seek relaxation; to 4 and 8, that you need a tension-reducing crutch; to 6 and 10, that you have a physiologic addiction; to 1 and 12, that you smoke from habit. No doubt you smoke for a combination of these reasons (*Source:* U.S. Department of Health and Human Services).

Because there is no safe way to smoke, it is important that you quit—for your sake and for your patients' sakes. "Nothing you do for your health—not even dieting and exercise—pays as many dividends so quickly as giving up smoking" (University of California, Berkeley, 1991). Benefits to the heart show up so quickly that in 2 years much of your risk of heart disease has disappeared. In 5 to 10 years your risk will be as though you had never smoked. The risk of lung cancer and other malignancies begin to decrease steadily when you quit smoking. After 10 years your risk is almost as low as that of a nonsmoker. If you have bronchitis or emphysema you can expect improvement with breathing almost at once. Plus, nonsmokers have stronger bones and less chance of getting osteoporosis (University of California, Berkeley, 1991, p. 55).

Whether you are helping your patient to quit or doing it for yourself, the method used must meet individual needs. Ask your instructor to help you identify resources, or contact your local Cancer Society or Lung Association.

WEIGHT MANAGEMENT

Too little or too much weight? Either have possible implications for energy, strength and personal health.

Dietary Guidelines for Americans, 1990 (U.S. Department of Agriculture).

HEIGHT WITHOUT SHOES	WEIGHT WITHOUT CLOTHES	
	Age 19 To 34*	35 And Up*
5'0"	97–128	108–138
5'1"	101–132	111–143
5'2"	104–137	115–148
5'3"	107–141	119–152
5'4"	111–146	122–157
5'5"	114–150	126–162
5'6"	118–155	130–167
5'7"	121–160	134–172
5'8"	125–164	138–178
5'9"	129–169	142–183
5'10"	132–174	146–188
5'11"	136–179	151–194
6'0"	140–184	155–199
6'2"	148–195	164–210
6'3"	152–200	168–216

*Women or men.

QUESTIONS:
1. At what weight do you feel most healthy?
2. At what weight do you experience the greatest amount of strength and energy?
3. Do you have any illnesses or injuries that may be related to overweight or underweight?
4. Are you able to do the nursing work assigned to you without excessive tiredness and/or soreness? Too much weight, meaning 20% over your desirable weight is a health risk.

Studies are showing relationships between obesity and hypertension, high blood cholesterol, heart disease, heart attacks, and possibly diabetes. Also connected are certain cancers—colon and prostate for men and uterus and breast for women. There is also a direct relationship between too much and too little weight and back and joint injuries.

You may have heard reference to pear-shaped versus apple-shaped bodies. *Pear-shaped* refers to fat primarily in the hips, buttocks, and thighs. This fat is stored primarily under the skin. *Apple-shaped* refers to fat primarily in the abdominal area. The apple shape, abdominal fat, is stored deeper inside the body. It is theorized that more fatty acids are released into the system of the apple-shaped person, who becomes more susceptible to the aforementioned illnesses.

In Chapter 10, "Wellness and Personal Care" you learned a common-sense approach to combining good nutrition and exercise. One fuels the body; the other strengthens and aids with flexibility. As a nurse you promote or do not promote health, just by being. So take time to review how you manage your weight and if necessary, set some reasonable, reachable goals. No personal badgering allowed.

OCCUPATIONAL RISK

You come into nursing knowing that you will be expected to provide nursing care for patients with infectious or contagious disorders. In fact there are times when a patient is admitted and the diagnosis is unknown until a series of tests are completed. In order to protect yourself and your patients, you need to perfect your technique for following universal precautions and/or sterile technique when needed. Basic nursing instructors traditionally will not pass you on either of these skills unless you demonstrate perfection. Once out of the classroom, it is up to you to maintain technique.

Although human immunodeficiency virus (HIV) is a fragile virus, a great deal of misinformation continues to instill fear in nurses. It seems prudent to review facts as we know them today. Casual contact is not a risk. You will not be infected by touching or being near a patient or coworker. There is no evidence that HIV is spread by sharing facilities or equipment. This includes sharing phones, computers, pencils, cups, and bathrooms. Neither is it passed through the air by coughing and sneezing. Furthermore, you will not pick up HIV infection through casual social contact. Nor will you get it from a food handler or a waitress. You will not get it from eating utensils, drinking fountains, or swimming pools. Sitting next to someone in a bus, car, or plane does not put you at risk. There is no evidence that a child will be infected by sitting near or playing with a child infected with HIV or the acquired immunodeficiency syndrome (AIDS).

To understand more completely the progression of HIV infection it is helpful to think in terms of three steps:

Step 1: HIV enters the body. HIV is transmitted from one person to another through blood and body fluid. The most common way is during sexual intercourse or by sharing needles during intravenous drug use. During sexual intercourse HIV in the semen, vaginal fluid, or blood of the infected person travels to the bloodstream of another through the tissue lining the rectum, vagina, penis, or mouth. In intravenous drug use, HIV enters the bloodstream through a puncture made by a needle contaminated with infected blood. Less common means of transmission include an infected woman to her child during pregnancy or birth, breastfeeding by an infected woman (rare), blood transfusions. The current risk of transmission through blood transfusion is small because donated blood is tested. You cannot be infected with

HIV by donating blood. All equipment is sterile and used only once.

Step 2a: HIV attacks the immune system. When HIV enters the bloodstream, the immune system tries to fight off the virus by developing antibodies to destroy it. But HIV enters a special immune cell, the T cell, where it can hide from antibodies. The virus may remain dormant for an indefinite time—the *asymptomatic* period. The only sign of HIV infection may be a positive blood test for antibodies to the virus. This first appears approximately six weeks to six months after the initial infection.

Step 2b: HIV weakens the immune system. After the virus reproduces itself, the new viruses burst from the T cell and infect other immune cells. As more and more immune cells are destroyed, the body becomes less able to fight other germs. The person with HIV becomes more susceptible to other infections. Each new infection weakens the person and the immune system. During this *symptomatic* period, persistent symptoms may develop in the infected person. These may include swollen lymph glands, night sweats, fever, cough, diarrhea, and/or weight loss. The symptoms are often mild at first and become progressively worse.

Step 3: The body cannot fight back. Eventually, the virus destroys almost all the disease-fighting cells. This gives a number of uncommon infections the opportunity to overwhelm the body. When these opportunistic infections appear, the person is considered to have AIDS. The most frequent opportunistic diseases are *Pneumocystis carinii* (a severe lung infection) and Kaposi's sarcoma (a rare cancer). The infected person may also experience severe weight loss (wasting) and neurologic problems. Eventually, the person will die from these diseases.

Are there risks for you as a nurse? Perhaps. But not in the way you think. Rarely is the patient with HIV infection or AIDS a source of transmission unless there has been a serious break in technique. Do not try to second guess if a person has an infectious disease by how they look or who they are. Resolve to follow universal precautions and bloodborne pathogen standards with every patient contact.

Some clues as to who may be at risk is to think back to the 1970s. This is when HIV first started spreading in the United States. Those at risk include persons who have been sexually active, who have not been in a mutually monogamous relationship since then, who themselves or their partners have shared intravenous drugs, or who have received a blood transfusion or blood product prior to 1978. If anyone has been living differently they may have been exposed. Confidential free testing is now available in most parts of the country. Encourage at-risk persons to be tested.

The connection: TB and HIV

Tuberculosis (TB) is occurring in persons infected with HIV. When the disease is not recognized or treated, it provides a potential hazard to nurses and other health care workers.

TB is spread from person to person through tiny airborne droplets that contain the tubercle bacilli. The person with active pulmonary TB coughs up these particles. By being in the same airspace for a prolonged time a susceptible individual inhales the bacilli. The organisms travel to the lungs. If they reach the air sacs and multiply, TB begins.

Most individuals who become infected with TB do not develop active TB. A healthy immune system can often keep it in check. However, even a healthy immune system cannot kill all of the TB organisms. Therefore, infected individuals remain at risk of developing active TB at a time when the body's immune system is weakened. Since HIV weakens the body's immune system it is far more likely for active tuberculosis to develop in an individual with TB infection.

Incomplete treatment of persons with TB has resulted in drug resistant TB—a new concern for nurses. Homelessness is thought to be a contributing factor to noncompliance and the inability to track persons with TB to complete treatment. The medications developed in the 50s and 60s are ineffective in treating drug resistant TB.

The most common site for TB is in the lungs, that is, pulmonary TB; however, it can occur in any site in the body. TB of the lymph nodes and miliary (disseminated) TB are also commonly seen in the patient with HIV. Characteristic

symptoms for active pulmonary TB include cough, fever, night sweats, weight loss, and fatigue. Symptoms for extrapulmonary TB (other body sites) depend on the site that is affected.

In 1989, the Centers for Disease Control, Atlanta, Georgia recommended that all persons who are HIV seropositive should be given a Mantoux tuberculin skin test. Similarly, persons with high-risk behaviors, such as intravenous drug users, should also be tested for TB.

Some persons with both HIV and TB may show falsely positive skin tests. Chest x-ray and other studies may be needed to confirm the diagnosis. Meanwhile, it is important for the nurse to practice infection-control techniques for preventing spread of airborne infections. Basic nursing is dress rehearsal for real life on the clinical unit. Remember too, to teach your patient to cover the mouth and nose when coughing, sneezing, or expectorating. Dispose of tissues properly—just the way you learned in basic nursing. Adequate ventilation helps to keep the TB organism count down. Check with your instructor for direction.

*H*EPATITIS

The greatest bloodborne risk that health workers face is hepatitis B virus (HBV). According to Assistant Labor Secretary Gerald Scannell, occupational exposures alone account for 5900 to 7400 cases of HB infection a year (Scannell, 1992, p. 82).

During 1985, the Center for Disease Control (CDC) first recommended universal precautions. However, their guidelines were not legally binding. Consequently during December 1991, the Occupational Safety and Health Administration (OSHA) developed a standard on bloodborne pathogens (HIV, HBV, and others). The standard makes universal precautions mandatory in all health care settings. The new rules also order employers to offer hepatitis B vaccine free of charge to every employee who can be "reasonably anticipated" to have "skin, eye, mucous membrane or parenteral contact" with blood or other potentially infectious materials. Besides being free, vaccine must be offered "at a reasonable time and place" and "within 10 working days of initial assignment." OSHA is able to back up their standards with fines up to $10,000 for "serious or willful" violations (Scannell, 1992).

The term *hepatitis* means inflammation of the liver. Its numerous causes include bacteria, drugs, alcohol, and other toxins. Of serious concern is hepatitis caused by hepatitis viruses that infect the liver. There are at least five types of hepatitis caused by different hepatitis viruses. They are currently known as hepatitis A through E. Study Table 12-1. Focus especially on hepatitis viruses B, C, and D.

Table 12-1 Hepatitis

HEPATITIS	A	B	C	D	E
Former Name	Infectious hepatitis	Serum hepatitis	Non-A, non-B hepatitis	Delta hepatitis	Epidemic or waterborne non-A, non-B hepatitis
Mode of transmission	Excretion in feces. Unwashed hands. Passed on to food and other items that go into mouth. Contaminated drinking water or food, including raw or steamed clams, oysters, and mussels	Found in all body fluids in infected people, including blood, semen, saliva, and urine. Spread by intimate contact with infected people and exposure to body fluids. Spread by piercing of skin by contaminated instruments: tattooing, ear piercing, acupuncture, dental, or medical procedures. Spread by intravenous drug use sexual intercourse. Spread to babies at birth by infected mothers	Transfused blood. Intimate contact	Must have hepatitis B before being infected; Combination of two diseases is more severe than hepatitis B alone. Transmission same as HBV. In United States, occurs primarily in those receiving blood products, i.e., through dialysis, by hemophiliacs, through IV intravenous drug use	Ingestion of contaminated water or food

HEPATITIS	A	B	C	D	E
At risk	Persons exposed to unsanitary conditions, i.e., who consume virus contaminated food or water Common in day care centers or nurseries Infected children transmit disease quickly to others	Health care workers Patient and staff on units where blood is handled Staff of institutions for mentally handicapped Certain military personnel Those who have personal contact with infected persons Morticians and embalmers Blood bank workers Anyone with risk taking sexual behaviors Intravenous drug users People of Asian African, Eastern European, Caribbean, Pacific Island, American Indian, Native Alaskan, or South American descent	Anyone who receives transfused blood or blood products.	Anyone who already has hepatitis B	Same as hepatitis A
Prevention	If exposed: gamma globulin	HBV vaccine If exposed and not vaccinated: HBIG (hepatitis B immune globulin)	—	HBV vaccine	—

Table continued on the following page.

HEPATITIS	A	B	C	D	E
Diagnosis	Blood test	Blood test	Blood test	Blood test	—
Outcome	Usually resolves without long-term effects	Complete recovery Death (less than 1%) Chronic liver disease that may progress to liver cancer in 5 to 10%	50 to 60% chance of lifelong liver disease	Generally progresses to chronic active disease or death due to severe hepatitis	In developing countries, leading cause of acute viral hepatitis Mortality rate in infected pregnant women nearly 20%

CODEPENDENCY

Before you read any further, answer the following questions:

1. What is your reason for making nursing your career choice?

2. Who supplies the most important critique of your day's work?

3. How do you feel if the patient does not tell you that you did a good job?

There is increasing speculation that as many as 90% of nurses may be codependent. What this means in nursing is that "the codependent nurse has a pathological need to be needed" (Cavello, 1991, p. 132). Codependent nurses relate to their patients and to their coworkers in unhealthy ways. For some a painful childhood that included sexual abuse, violence, or chemical abuse may have paved the way to codependency. Some characteristics of the codependent nurse follow.

Using denial and manipulation to gain satisfaction in unhealthy ways has usually been practiced for many years. It takes special courage to really look and see if any of these behaviors are present. Both self-help groups and books are available. How about codependency as a topic of discussion during class in relation to personal life and/or relationship with classmates? Replace the words "patient," "coworkers," and "staff member" with "others" in the preceding characterization. Determine your codependency traits outside of nursing.

Codependent Nurse	Possible Behavior
1. Says "yes"—really means "no."	Agrees to help another staff member and then complains to someone else about being taken advantage of.
2. Feels the fate of nursing care rests on her shoulders.	Takes on nonnursing duties that belong to other departments.
3. Feels responsible to solve other's problems.	Sympathetic, rather than empathetic response to patients and other staff.
4. Competes for attention rather than supporting coworkers.	Engages in one-upmanship and intershift rivalries over patient care.
5. Often feels angry, unappreciated, and used.	Comes in early and works late. Works extra shifts to "help" coworkers.
6. Does not support patients need for autonomy and return to self-sufficiency.	Does for the patient what he needs to do in order to regain optimal health and self-confidence.
7. Makes excuses and conceals negative practices rather than working for change.	Feels powerless. Takes on extra duties because of chronic understaffing.
8. Shows feelings of anger indirectly.	Pouts, procrastinates, forgets, gets sick, or is late.
9. Perfectionistic: gossips and judges.	Unrealistic expectations of others.
10. Avoids conflict.	Too nice, loving, and forgiving. Smiles when having negative feelings.

Summary

Major pitfalls to success in practical nursing are most often personal rather than work-related. As a nurse it is essential to take care of yourself. By doing so, you give permission for others to take care of themselves. "Should" and "ought" type of messages need to be replaced with "I choose to" or "I choose not to" messages. Maintaining and practicing nursing skills such as universal precautions are an expected part of nursing.

How you see your patient gives you important clues about your needs. If you are able to separate your personal and professional life, develop an empathetic approach to patient care, and be your own best friend and boss, chances are nursing will continue to excite you.

Behaviors that impair nurses are harmful not only to the nurse but are potentially dangerous to the patient as well. Codependent behaviors encourage patients to become dependent rather than to regain control of their lives. Neither you nor your patient is satisfied. Nursing is a wonderful vocation. Take time to evaluate your behaviors at this time. If changes need to be made, reach out. You will find there is someone out there ready to reach out to you.

REFERENCES

Abbott C. The impaired nurse. AORN J 1987; 46:1104–1108.

Bauer B, Hill S. *Essentials of Mental Health Care*. Chapter 12. Philadelphia: WB Saunders, 1986.

Beattie M. *Codependent No More*. New York: Harper & Row, 1987.

Bradshaw J. *The Family*. Deerfield Beach, FL: Health Communications, Inc., 1988.

Cavello B. Codependency paints nursing's goals. RN 1991; 54:132.

Czarnecki G. Presented at The Hurt and the Healing, A Workshop on Codependency, at University of Wisconsin–Green Bay, Green Bay, WI, October, 1991.

Flaskerud J, Ungvarski P. *HIV/AIDS: A Guide to Nursing Care*. 2nd ed. Philadelphia: WB Saunders, 1992.

Frankl, Viktor. An Evening with Viktor Frankl, Workshop at Mount Mary College, Milwaukee, 1984.

Franklin F. Hooked. Health 1990; November/December:39–52.

Haack M. Alcohol use and burnout among student nurses. Nurs Health Care 1987; April:239–242.

Long P. Great weight debate. Health 1992; February/March:42–47.

Milam J, Ketcham K. *Under the Influence*. New York: Bantam Books, 1983.

Morrow L. A nation of finger pointers. Time 1991; August 12:14–23.

Hepatitis: Everything from A to E. Abbott Park, IL: Abbott Laboratories (pamphlet).

Regs put new legal force behind universal precautions. Am J Nurs 1992; January:82–84.

Scannell G. "OSHA" stiffens bloodborne rules, decrees free hepatitis B vaccine. Am J Nurs 1992; January:82.

Simons SB. Willpower workout. Ladies Home Journal 1989; March:64–70.

Snow C, and Willard D. *I'm Dying to Take Care of You: Nurses and Codependence Breaking the Cycles.* Redmond, WA: Professional Counselor Books, 1989.

University of California, Berkeley. *The Wellness Encyclopedia.* Boston: Houghton-Mifflin Company, 1991; 53–59.

Does alcohol really prevent heart disease? University of California at Berkeley Wellness Letter, 1991; November: 1.

York P, York D, Wachel T. *Toughlove.* New York: Bantam Books, 1983.

York P, York D, Wachel T. *Toughlove Solutions.* New York: Bantam Books, 1984.

part IV
KNOW YOUR PATIENT

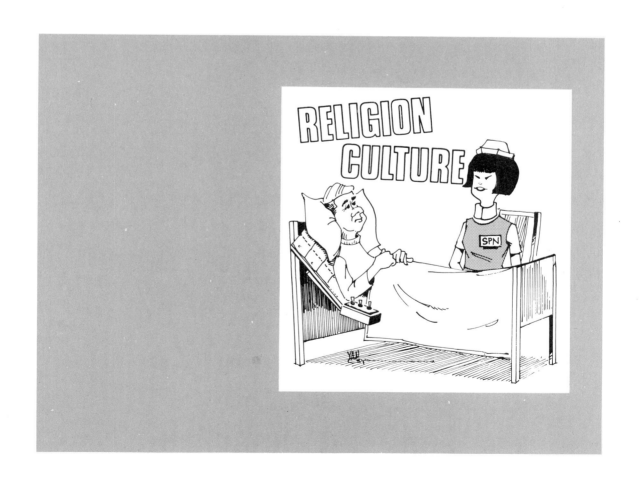

CHAPTER 13
Job-Related Communication

Judith A. Mix, R.N., M.S.N., Ed.D.

Learning Objectives

Upon completing this chapter, you will
1. Explain the significance of effective communication skills (verbal and nonverbal) in health care.
2. Describe the communication process and its components.
3. Describe the purposes of communication in nursing.
4. Contrast verbal and nonverbal communication.
5. List seven examples of nonverbal communication.
6. Develop verbal communication skills: speaking, reading, and writing.
7. Discuss factors that influence the communication process.
8. Develop beginning listening skills.
9. Utilize and explain the rationale for each therapeutic communication.
10. Identify and explain the effect of the blocks to therapeutic communication.
11. Describe the significance of effective communication with colleagues and the benefit of transactional analysis in this interaction.
12. Describe techniques that may be useful for communicating with children and with the elderly.
13. Explain why it is essential for nurses to have an understanding of computer use in health care, that is, to be computer literate.

SIGNIFICANCE OF COMMUNICATION

Imagine that suddenly you find yourself in an environment or on a planet where all human communication has ceased. There is no verbal or written language, and the humans in this environment do not respond even nonverbally, using no gestures or facial expressions. There are no newspapers, books, radios, television sets, computers, or videocassette recorders. What problems would result from the absence of communication? Fortunately, it is highly unlikely that an environment totally lacking communication exists anywhere, because communication is necessary for physical as well as emotional and social survival.

Our waking day is almost totally consumed in some form of communication. Communication activities link us to our environment, to people in our environment, and to people outside our immediate environment. These activities include reading, speaking, writing, listening, watching television and other forms of audiovisual media, satellite communications, computer use, word processing, and nonverbal methods such as body movement and facial gestures (body language). Our expressions of love and acceptance, or dislike and nonacceptance, are communicated mainly by nonverbal means. Touch is a powerful communicator of how we feel about another human.

Communication (verbal and nonverbal) is essential to formal and informal learning. We learned how to function as humans by utilizing all of the communication activities available to us, as well as by listening to others and mimicking their behaviors. Communication enables you and others to work and play together and to establish harmonious and productive relationships. Poor communication leads to problems in human relationships and consequently to social problems. Effective communication skills are essential tools for the nurse.

The forerunner of effective communication is establishing a rapport. Patients will confide in you only after a trusting relationship has been developed. How do you establish a rapport or a trusting relationship with another person? Effective relationships with coworkers are essential to teamwork and the attainment of the team's or the institution's goals. Effective communication skills assist us in our interactions with others by helping us to present ideas clearly and by helping us to understand another person's message.

This chapter includes a discussion of what communication is and is not, the components of communication, types of communication (verbal and nonverbal), barriers to communication, techniques of therapeutic communication, blocks to effective communication, listening techniques, transactional analysis, and computer communication in health care.

COMMUNICATION: WHAT IT IS AND WHAT IT IS NOT

Communication is a dynamic, changing, never-ending process. You communicate through the senses of sight, sound, taste, smell, and touch. How well you communicate with another human depends on mutual understanding of verbal and nonverbal signs and symbols. When I say to you it looks reddened, feels soft, sounds like a doorbell, tastes sweet, smells like a rose, you need to have the same image as I do for effective communication to occur. We express what we have sensed in a verbal or nonverbal manner. When you feel something hot, such as the vinyl seat covers in your car on a hot summer day, you respond by sitting down slowly or by jumping off the seat. A small child communicates fear and pain by crying. We recognize and understand the signal. When the signal is not understood, communication has not occurred.

Communication is conveying a thought or idea from a sender to a receiver. It means making something known to another person or asking for information from another person. It can be done verbally (spoken or written) or nonverbally (through the expression of feelings, attitudes, or thoughts). Communication requires two people or more who interact for some reason. Communication usually does not occur between two people who are in a casual relationship, such as riding the same bus or patronizing the same restaurant or supermarket.

People who communicate also interact, and by doing so, respond to messages they receive.

COMPONENTS OF COMMUNICATION: A MODEL

The essential components of communication are the sender (person conveying an idea or asking a question), the message (idea or question), and the receiver (person or group for whom the message is intended). Communication is an active process and requires a vehicle or channel to transmit the idea or question. The sender uses the senses to convey messages verbally (spoken or written) or nonverbally through body language. The receiver receives and interprets the message. The receiver frequently gives the sender feedback regarding understanding of the message. When you are the sender, you can ask for understanding of the message from the receiver should the receiver not give you feedback or if you are uncertain as to the understanding of your message. When you are the receiver you can ensure your understanding of the message by saying to the sender, "Is this what you are asking?" Figure 13-1 illustrates the communication process.

Exchanging messages requires knowledge. The sender must have knowledge about the topic in order to send the message, and the receiver must have basically the same knowledge to understand the message. Use language and terminology that your receiver will understand, and check for understanding. Past experiences of the sender and the receiver influence messages sent and received. If you have not experienced an event such as a loss, childbirth, or hospitalization, it is difficult to understand the intimacies of those experiences. Unless the sender and the receiver have similar past experiences and knowledge, communication is difficult (Wolff et al., 1983, p. 226).

Communication is influenced by feelings and values. That is, if you think a topic is important or not important you will communicate that feeling or value to the receiver. For example, it would be extremely difficult to effectively encourage another person to stop smoking if you yourself are a smoker.

PURPOSES OF COMMUNICATION

The intent of communication is usually one of the following: social, relationship development, receiving information, giving information, clarifying and validating information, and conveying feelings. As the nurse, you need to have a sense of purpose before communicating with patients,

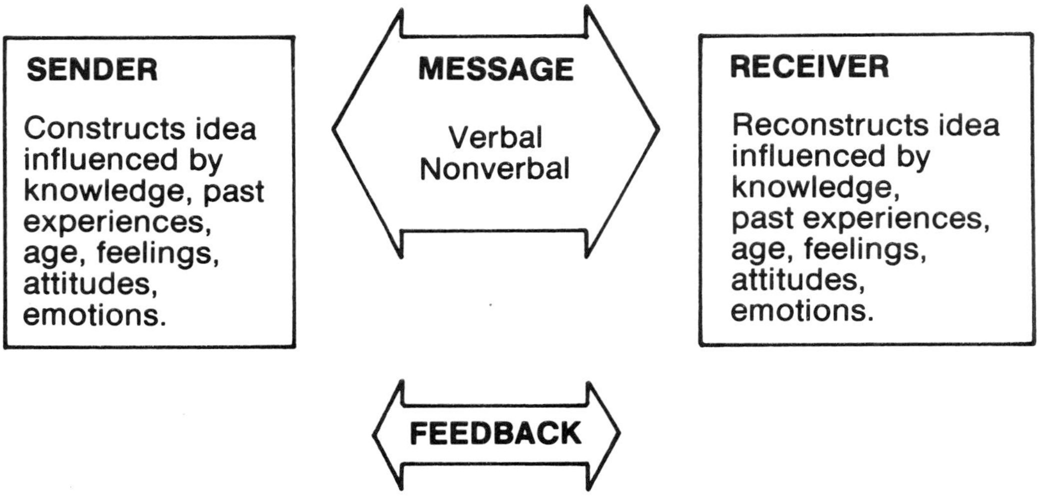

SENDER	MESSAGE	RECEIVER
Constructs idea influenced by knowledge, past experiences, age, feelings, attitudes, emotions.	Verbal Nonverbal	Reconstructs idea influenced by knowledge, past experiences, age, feelings, attitudes, emotions.

FEEDBACK

FIGURE 13-1   Communication process

if you are to be therapeutic. Idle, nonpurposeful conversation can actually be nontherapeutic and even destructive. The nurse utilizes the communication process for multiple purposes, including social reasons. For extended periods you may be the only family that an elderly person in the nursing home has. In that instance you are being therapeutic by spending some time talking to the individual.

COMMUNICATION AND THE NURSING PROCESS

The nurse uses communication skills during each step of the nursing process. Communication between the client, the client's family, and the health care team is essential to the effectiveness of the nursing process (Potter, 1989). Assessment involves the collection of data, which requires completeness and accuracy. Communication skills greatly affect the ability of the nurse to collect reliable, accurate, and adequate data.

The licensed practical nurse's role is to collect data that the registered nurse combines with other collected data to assess a client's status and to develop nursing diagnoses. If the data collected are not accurate and/or are not complete, the nursing care plan could be inappropriate for the client and consequently will lead to inappropriate, ineffective, or unsafe care. The implementation of care requires cooperation from the client. The nurse must use communication skills to explain what needs to be done and to solicit the client's consent and cooperation. The evaluation part of the nursing process requires that the nurse validate effectiveness of care through communication (verbal and nonverbal) with and observation of the client. The licensed practical nurse also collects data to assist in the evaluation of care provided.

NONVERBAL COMMUNICATION

What is nonverbal communication? What is its significance in the communication process? Without words people can show feelings: love,

pain, joy, contentment, peacefulness. Have you ever noticed that sometimes what a person says verbally does not match what is being communicated nonverbally? For example, you ask a person how things are going and the reply is "Great, things are great." However, you get the idea that things are not so great by the tears and the clenched teeth.

Nonverbal behavior does not always have the same meaning for all people. Cultural differences, age, sex, past experiences, and individual responses to situations can vary the meaning. For example, men in many societies have been conditioned to feel that they need to be strong both physically and emotionally. Some men and some women will have difficulty admitting that they are in pain or have other physical or emotional problems. Consequently, they may not seek assistance when needed and may mask nonverbal expressions of pain as much as possible. In this situation, you need to be attentive to subtle nonverbal communication. What, specifically, should you observe or collect data about to assess nonverbal communication? What precautions can you take to avoid miscommunication of nonverbal cues, and what can you do to avoid sending undesirable or nontherapeutic nonverbal messages? Body language is another term for nonverbal communication. The following represent body language.

Eye Contact

Eye contact suggests a willingness to communicate. Eye contact is an important step in the development of a relationship. It tells another person you are giving them your attention and are ready to listen. Lack of eye contact may suggest that a person is shy, embarrassed, nervous, about to tell you something that is emotionally difficult for them to say, anxious, or defenseless, or has low self-esteem or does not wish to communicate. The eyes carry other messages, such as sorrow when crying, anger by means of a fixed stare, and disgust when a narrowing of the eyes is noted. In some cultures, eye contact may be a sign of respect, and in other cultures it is a sign of disrespect or implies sexual consent. Therefore, the actual meaning should be checked out verbally.

Facial Expressions

The face tells others much of what we are feeling. The complex and unique musculature of the face enables us to smile, frown, and express joy, sorrow, surprise, anger, frustration, disbelief, preoccupation, anxiety, fear, suspicion, pain, and contempt. The facial expressions used to communicate these different feelings and emotions are unique so that many times you can recognize what the other person is feeling without asking them to verbalize. To be certain, you need to check out nonverbal communication in a verbal manner to ensure clarity. Nonverbal cues are indicators to the nurse but are not always clear as to exact meaning.

Posture, Gestures, and Gait

A person's posture reveals a great deal about his or her attitude, how he or she feels, and how he or she is getting along both physically and emotionally. A person with high self-esteem, in good physical and emotional health holds his or her body erect and in good alignment. A slouched body position may indicate physical pain, a disability, depression, or boredom. Holding the body tensely suggests that the person is in pain, extremely shy, or closed to communication.

Feelings of authority and domination are expressed through body position, such as standing above another person or leaning back in a chair with hands behind the head (Note Figure 13-2.). To avoid giving this impression, seek the other person's level when talking. In the patient situation, you could sit on a chair. To minimize the feeling of subservience that occurs when someone else is nonverbally communicating authority and dominance, and the desired relationship is that of colleague or peer, stand up if the other person is standing, so that you are at or close to eye level. Many times, short people have problems achieving eye level and need to use other means to achieve equality. Refer to Chapter 11 on assertiveness for suggestions.

Provide space so as not to intimidate the person with whom you are communicating. Give consideration to the idea that because of cultural and personal differences, some people prefer closeness and others need more space between you and them.

Body gestures carry messages. Some examples are tapping the fingers on a table or feet on the floor and twitching feet or legs. These gestures indicate boredom, impatience, discomfort (physical or emotional), anxiety, or anger. Wringing of the hands may communicate pain, fear, or anxiety. A clenched fist frequently communicates anger or pain. Since one gesture can

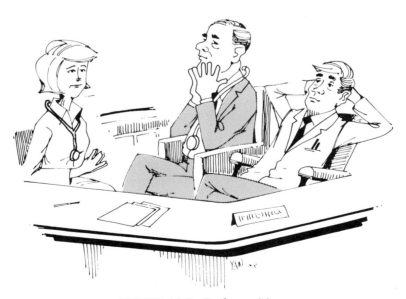

FIGURE 13-2   Body position

communicate two or more messages, you need to check out your observation verbally with the other person. The steepled hands of the man (high position) in Figure 13-2 communicate authority, domination, and superiority. The steepled hands of the nurse (low position) indicate feelings of low self-esteem. A slouched posture also indicates feelings of low self-esteem. What can you do regarding your posture and body gestures to give an impression of high self-esteem when you do not really feel that way?

The manner in which a person moves about (gait) carries a message of wellness or illness and high or low self-esteem. A deliberate, brisk gait communicates a different message from a slow, aimless one. The former indicates wellness and high self-esteem, while the latter indicates illness and/or low self-esteem.

Personal and General Appearance

A person's (the patient's or the nurse's) physical appearance, personal hygiene, and grooming convey significant nonverbal messages. Healthy persons with good self-esteem tend to be concerned about their general appearance and consequently attend to details of nutrition, hygiene, dress, and grooming. Persons with low self-esteem frequently convey their feelings about themselves through inattention to general appearance. Sometimes very ill persons will not have the energy to attend to these needs and depend on the nurse for assistance. Attention to or concern about personal appearance is one indicator of improving wellness. An emotionally ill person's progress can be measured by the degree to which the person attends to the aspects of general appearance.

Frequently, illnesses and therapies cause general changes such as skin changes (dryness, rashes), loss of muscle tone, and changes in awareness and alertness. These changes need to be detected and evaluated to determine the progress of the patient and the illness and the effectiveness of the therapies. The person's body response is communicating significant messages to you, the nurse.

Vocal Nonverbal Communication

Sounds such as crying, sobbing, sniffling, and sighing are considered nonverbal communication. Their meanings are not specific. Crying could be tears of sadness, joy, or fear. A sigh could indicate relief or reluctance. However, these sounds are significant and need to be attended to by the nurse. The patient is communicating. The loudness and the pitch of the voice (inflection) carry messages of joy, fear, discomfort, and excitement.

Touch

Touch communicates feelings of acceptance or nonacceptance. Failure to touch in appropriate situations, such as in care giving, can communicate rejection by the nurse.

Healing through touch is an ancient belief—"the laying of hands." Western culture socializes us not to touch others, particularly strangers. Therefore, touching when inappropriate in care giving can be viewed as an invasion of privacy or a sexual advance by the patient or the nurse. People who are anxious, dependent, or lonely generally need to have verbal support before nonverbal support is welcomed. Since all people need personal space, being touched can at times be threatening and not appreciated. Again, you need to establish a rapport or a relationship with a person prior to use of touch.

Touch is therapeutic. To touch and be touched is a human need. Holding and touching an infant is important because it can communicate love and caring. Infants who are not touched and held in a loving, caring manner fail to thrive, causing retardation in growth and development. The elderly have a great need for human touch and communication of acceptance. The skin is our outer boundary and receives messages from and is in constant communication with the environment. In some cases, touch may be the only sensation a patient is aware of and will arouse and stimulate the other senses. The skin also communicates outwardly in the form of rashes, goose bumps, warmth and coldness, and moistness and dryness. Therapists have found that touch is sometimes the most effective therapy for patients who are mentally ill or retarded.

Touch can communicate affection and closeness by hugging, kissing, handshakes, and touching the arm. Again, the form of touch used should be appropriate for the situation. Some people are comfortable with touch and others are uncomfortable. Some family members or entire families do not feel comfortable hugging and kissing, whereas others kiss and hug anytime they see one another. Touch can also convey dislike, anger, and physical aggression depending on how it is done. This form of touch is never appropriate and certainly never therapeutic.

Studies indicate that people who have been or are deprived of touch and physical affection have more physical and emotional illnesses. Hospitals and long-term care facilities are sensory-deprivation situations, since patients are being cared for by strangers, and their loved ones sometimes tend to touch them less. Patients who tend to be touched less by nurses are the seriously ill, those with communicable illnesses, those over 65 years of age, and adolescents. Lack of touching generally makes them feel less worthwhile. In seriously ill or semicomatose patients, touch is their only contact with the outside world. If you deprive them of touch, they may not progress as rapidly as they may with the stimulation of touching.

Smell

How does the sense of smell affect our personal relationships with others and our therapeutic relationships with patients? Americans, unlike many other cultures, are embarrassed and offended by various body odors. We use a great deal of hygiene products and colognes to ward off offensive odors. Advertisements tell us we can improve our relationships with others if we use their products.

Have you ever moved away or avoided someone with body odor or bad breath? The patient frequently cannot avoid the care giver. Therefore, it is obvious that you the nurse need to eliminate body odors and perfumes and strong colognes that are offensive to the patient. It will help you establish a therapeutic rapport and increase the patient's comfort. Body odors are interpreted as poor self-hygiene, and communicate to the patient that cleanliness and medical asepsis are not important to you. This makes patients reluctant to accept you as their nurse and to allow you to treat them. Patients have the right to refuse care from individuals they feel do not act in their best interest. The smell of smoke in the nurse's clothing is offensive to most patients. Some patients actually have an allergic response to "second-hand" smoke.

Patients frequently emit disagreeable odors due to their illnesses, treatments, or body responses. You need to be prepared psychologically so that you do not react negatively, either verbally or nonverbally. When odor is present, patients who are alert also smell the odor and are embarrassed. You can best help the patient by accepting the odor as part of the process of illness and by communicating that you recognize that the situation is distressing to him or her.

VERBAL COMMUNICATION

The ability to use language skills accurately in the form of speaking, reading, and writing is essential to the business of giving care and is as important as nonverbal communication skills. You need to assess your skills in these areas and make the necessary improvements. The following discussions include suggestions for improvement.

Speaking

Careful thought should be given to what you should say and how you should say it. Avoid set speeches, since they are impersonal and not individualized. Set speeches do not communicate concern or caring. Address people by title such as Doctor, Mr., or Mrs., unless the person prefers that you do otherwise.

The manner of delivery of the communication is important in its quality, acceptance, and understanding. Voices vary as to quality, tone, rhythm, and stress. Control a loud, raspy, or whiny voice. Avoid slurring: speak clearly and distinctly. The following are seven keys to effective speaking:

1. Speak with enthusiasm by varying tone, rhythm, and loudness.

2. Enunciate. Pronounce vowels and consonants clearly. Some medical terms sound very similar.

3. Use inflection to amplify the meaning of your message.

4. Avoid words that antagonize. For example, the word "contaminated" to a lay person may mean "dirty" or "filthy" and to the nurse means "unsterile" or "lacking medical asepsis."

5. Use short, simple sentences.

6. Adjust volume, rate, and speed of voice to the situation. If the receiver is knowledgeable of the situation, you can go faster.

7. Keep door open for feedback. Allow the receiver time to ask questions.

Evaluate your speaking skills through use of a recording device such as a tape recorder or video recorder. A videotape will reveal your nonverbal communication skills as well as your verbal skills.

Reading

Reading is one of the most important tools in your present and future education. In your practice as a nurse, you will need to be able to understand with accuracy and sometimes with quickness the information in patients' records and in textbooks and professional journals. Textbooks and professional journals are frequently used in the care-giving setting to help answer questions and to solve problems. The literature contains the information required to remain updated on issues in everyday practice.

Reading is a skill and requires practice to improve speed and comprehension. Your speed will slow down when you read technical materials and literature that contains unfamiliar or complex terms. Your rate of reading also depends on the number of pauses your eyes make. If you read word by word your rate will be slower than if you read in whole phrases. It is usually easy to increase reading speed but more difficult to improve comprehension (Ross, 1981, p. 73). Developing a vocabulary is essential. Tools you should use are medical and general dictionaries and glossaries. Look up only words that prevent you from understanding the sentence, since stopping frequently will decrease speed unnecessarily. Note the pronunciation as well as the meaning of the word and state the meaning in your own words. Note prefixes and suffixes of medical terms. You can arrive at the meanings of new words that use similar or familiar prefixes and suffixes. Use the career skills or language-development centers at your particular school or in your community if you have reading problems.

Writing

Writing skills are essential to the student and the graduate practical nurse. You will be taking notes in class and during meetings and reports. You will constantly be making notes in patients' records or entering information on the computer. Many acute-care facilities use computers as a communication tool. Writing and spelling skills are essential when processing requisition forms or other communication forms. Considering the importance of communicating accurately in health care settings; the message or information must be correct, concise, and legible.

Provided it is accurate and legible, a written communication usually relays the message better than verbal communication only. You do need to select the correct words to communicate the message accurately. This necessitates knowing medical terminology as well as having a knowledge of the situation.

Your observations and nursing interventions will be recorded on a legal document that becomes the patient's record. Be specific about your documentation. Use only accepted or standard abbreviations. Your ability to communicate the patient's condition and response plays a vital role in his or her well-being, since medications, treatments, and nursing care are ordered accordingly. Record and report only that which is relative to recovery or treatment. In addition, protect the right to privacy by sharing information only with those involved in the care.

DEVELOPING A THERAPEUTIC RELATIONSHIP
Determine the Purpose of Communication

Social conversation can be used to initiate a more purposeful conversation. However, it should not be overutilized, since the topics of social conversation will usually not lead to the information-sharing needed by the nurse and the patient. It will, however, help to establish rapport with a new patient.

Gathering information is an essential everyday activity of the nurse. When patients enter the health care setting or the nurse enters the patient's home to give care, the nurse conducts an interview to formulate a history of individual characteristics, past and present illnesses, the events leading to present needs, and the specifics regarding the presenting complaint(s) or need(s). At this time you gather a great deal of information directly from the patient and/or the patient's family. This information will be used during the entire treatment phase to help direct the medical and nursing orders. Thus, accuracy is of utmost importance. This is when the nurse–patient relationship begins. First impressions are essential to the development of the relationship.

Receiving information is part of the therapeutic nurse–patient relationship. Validating and clarifying that information means that the nurse first checks with the patient to make clear the meaning or intent of the statement and then verifies or evaluates the results. These techniques will be discussed later in this chapter.

The nurse shares information and ideas when teaching the patient about the illness or treatment and the plan of care. The patient many times participates in the sharing by giving information or ideas about how the plan might best work for him or her. You share feelings about the patient by displaying warmth, support, and caring. The patient shares feelings about the illness and the care being given or to be given. Techniques that you can use to share observations regarding the perceived feelings of the patient will be discussed later in this chapter.

A trusting relationship is developed by demonstrating that you care about and respect patients and that you feel they are important. Many techniques have already been offered and will continue to be offered in this chapter that will aid you.

Factors Influencing Communication

The nurse who understands what might help or hinder the communication process will be a better communicator. Several factors influence the communication process and apply to three categories: the environment, the nurse, and the patient. Age will influence the vocabulary you use. A child has limited language skills as compared with an adult. You will need to have appropriate teaching information based on age and understanding. "Talking down" to a person of any age demonstrates disrespect.

Sex can influence the type of information that your patient or you will feel comfortable discussing. A female patient may feel more comfortable discussing intimate and sexual topics with a female nurse, and males tend to discuss such matters more openly with a male nurse. Some patients may feel uncomfortable discussing the topic of sex with anyone. You need to consider this and create an accepting, nonthreatening situation.

Privacy, quiet, and comfort are essential to providing an environment and situation that are conducive to effective and therapeutic communication. Avoid teaching and other lengthy conversations when the environment is full of interruptions and when the patient is too fatigued or is experiencing pain or anxiety.

The intelligence and educational levels of the patient need to be considered when communicating. You do not want to use vocabulary and terminology that is not understandable to the patient, nor do you want to risk insulting them by "talking down" to a knowledgeable, highly educated individual. Talking above his or her level endangers understanding and "talking down" communicates disrespect and may anger the person. A person's age, occupation, and interests often give clues to the amount of information he or she has on a particular topic. A person in a health occupation probably is knowledgeable about illness and treatment.

Other factors to be considered are mental or sensory impairments, attitudes and values of the nurse and the patient, past experiences with illness, and being a health care recipient or patient. Many times a patient is not capable of engaging effectively in the communication process or developing a rapport because of mental, hearing, speech, or touch disorders. Attitudes the nurse has regarding sex, race, role identification, and illnesses can affect the communication process. Acceptance of others is essential to effective communication.

Language barriers are obvious problems in effective communication. Nonverbal communication skills are especially important in these cases. Members of the family or a bilingual health care worker can provide assistance. Lack of communication can lead to frustration on the part of the patient and the nurse, as well as to ineffective, unsafe care.

Genuineness and Empathy

Genuineness (sincerity and honesty) and empathy are essential to the development of effective relationships. These qualities demonstrate caring and support. Empathy is the ability to momentarily enter the psychological state of another individual (Murray, 1980, p. 250). It is striving to understand exactly what the other person is feeling and experiencing. It is difficult

to put yourself in the same situation when in fact you are not experiencing the same pain and anxiety that the patient is. You will not be able to empathize equally with all patients because of limited personal experiences with illness and treatment. Most nurses have experienced some degree of pain and anxiety and can relate to those experiences.

It is possible to expand empathetic skills by the use of imagination. Imagine yourself having the same experience of feeling the pain, frustration, and the concern about the effects of the illness on your life. Be careful not to drain your physical and emotional energies by identifying too closely with the situation, as this will prevent you from being helpful to the patient when he or she needs your strength and support.

Caring

Caring is having a positive regard for another person. It is basic to a helping relationship. Nurses show caring by accepting clients as they are and respecting them as individuals. When clients feel cared for they feel secure, even though they may be in threatening or anxiety-producing situations. Caring also promotes trust (Potter, 1989). Accepting clients as they are may be difficult at times depending on the particular illness or illnesses or the problems they present. For example, it may be difficult to accept clients with criminal records, those with Alzheimer's disease, or those who are socially dysfunctional in some area.

The development of a trusting relationship with a client is sometimes a challenge to the nurse.

Trust

Trust is an essential component of caring. Trust is relying on someone without doubt or question. Confidence, dependability, and confidentiality result in a trusting relationship (Potter, 1989). Trust makes communication more effective as individuals become more open and can express their thoughts and feelings. The therapeutic nurse–patient relationship is greatly enhanced by the trust in the nurses providing care that may develop in the patient.

Commitment

Commitment means to pledge or promise to do something to the best of one's ability. It is the understanding that the nurse has pledged to the patient the provision of the best nursing care possible. This attitude is demonstrated by the skill with which the nurse cares for the patient (Atkinson and Murray, 1985, p. 107).

Listening

To hear is only a part of listening. Hearing is the sensory process of sound waves reaching the ears and being transmitted to the brain (Atkinson and Murray, 1985, p. 110). Listening is the interpretation of the sound.

The patient and his or her problems and feelings are the center of the nurse–patient communications. You must develop listening skills in order to help the patient—it is essential to establishing a therapeutic relationship. Most people will communicate openly if they believe they have an attentive, caring listener who does not impose his or her beliefs and values and does not give unwanted and unneeded advice. You must learn to listen not only to words but also to the tone in which the words are conveyed and to the attitudes and emotions behind them (Murray, 1980, p. 238). Listening skills can be developed.

Listening attentively or actively demands focusing in on what the other person is saying and feeling. The patient must know that you are interested and that you care before he or she will share personal, perhaps embarrassing, information. To communicate interest and caring you can start with eye contact, sitting down, and an alert body posture. The nurse is usually standing when providing care; you do not want to communicate that you are in a hurry. Sitting down implies that you are willing to take the time to listen. It also communicates equal status. Sit facing the patient rather than on the side, again indicating interest in the person. Sit

within a comfortable distance. Being close may intimidate the patient. For personal interaction and when discussing personal information, the range is approximately $1\frac{1}{2}$ to 4 feet, or near enough to shake hands. It also prevents people who should not hear from hearing. An intimate-interaction distance is 3 to 18 inches, and a social interaction is 4 to 12 feet.

Do not begin or continue significant conversations while hanging onto the door or door frame. Provide for privacy by shutting the door or moving to a private area whenever possible. Be certain the patient is comfortable. It is difficult to communicate clearly when in pain or in need of bowel or bladder elimination.

Try not to write a great deal during the interview. Writing communicates inattention and interferes with the patient's spontaneity and your ability to listen. If you need to take notes, take brief ones. Be attentive, concentrate, and show interest in what the patient is saying, so that you understand fully what is being communicated. Ask the patient for his or her perception of the problem. For example, what brought the patient to the hospital?

Active listening requires a willingness to devote time and energy to the process. The nurse must utilize an extensive knowledge base. You must first listen before you can respond appropriately. Nursing students frequently feel ill at ease and useless when they are talking to patients because they do not feel as though they are "doing" for the patient. Through communication, the nurse establishes the therapeutic relationship, relieves stress, does patient teaching, and identifies health care needs (Atkinson and Murray, 1985, p. 110). Listening is one aspect of observation and a means of developing a confidential relationship.

While you are listening you may express agreement with a smile or nod of the head and respond to cues, but do not interrupt. Ask questions when the patient is finished, to clarify or solicit more information. Try not to probe into areas that the patient does not wish to share. Being an attentive listener and allowing patients to talk helps to relieve anxiety.

One suggested activity to increase listening ability is to practice with fellow students or friends. The task is to be able to repeat verbatim what the first person has said before you are permitted to say something and to continue until all persons have had a chance to say something. This activity forces you to listen attentively. Your friend or fellow student is able to tell you if you are accurate.

Territoriality

Territoriality is the space or things that individuals believe belong to them (Kozier, 1989). Nurses need to recognize that the client's territory exists and must be sensitive to the need for privacy. Knocking before entering a patient's room and getting permission to enter communicates sensitivity to the need for privacy.

Personal space is related to territoriality. It is the distance a person feels comfortable with when relating to another person. Nurses frequently invade this space when providing nursing care. A trusting relationship needs to be developed before the nurse is permitted into this space. A child instinctively rejects someone with whom they have not developed a trusting relationship. Clients sometimes refuse care that involves invasion of their personal space. Permission needs to be sought and obtained prior to providing care. Patients give permission for treatment and care on admission. However, verbal permission needs to be sought for specific treatment and care.

Intonation

The tone of the nurse's voice can have a dramatic effect on the meaning of a message. Depending on intonation, the phrase "How are you?" can express enthusiasm, concern, indifference, and even annoyance. A nurse's emotions can directly affect tone of voice. Often this is unconscious, and the words send one message while voice tone conveys something different.

Clients may question a nurse's credibility and caring if there is a discrepancy between the message and the tone of voice used in sending the message. The nurse must be aware of any emotions that send messages that negatively affect the development of a helping relationship.

The nurse should be aware that voice tone and pitch communicate the client's emotional and physical states such as fear, anger, grief, and energy level. A rested, healthy person's voice has clarity, inflection, and variations, whereas a fatigued, ill person sometimes has a weak, monotonic, unclear voice. Sensitivity to voice tone, facial expression, and other nonverbal cues enhance the nurse's assessment skills.

TECHNIQUES OF THERAPEUTIC COMMUNICATION
Encouraging Communication

Some communication techniques are designed to encourage communication. These techniques are broad opening statements, open-ended questions or statements, reflecting, selective reflecting, general leads, and silence.

Broad opening statements or questions allow the patient to select the direction of the conversation and the opportunity to express what his or her concerns are. Examples:

NURSE: "How are things going?"
NURSE: "How are things today?"
NURSE: "Tell me about yourself."

Open-ended questions and statements are identical to broad opening statements. You may hear or read both terms. Both terms allow the patient to expand or elaborate on a topic he or she selects.

Reflecting leads the patient to consider fully and to expand on his or her remark. It is a form of feedback or response that encourages the speaker to continue talking about a subject. It may include all or part of the speaker's statement. The following are examples:

PATIENT: "I was awake all night because I was so nervous."
NURSE: "You were nervous?" or "You were awake all night?"

Be careful not to overuse this technique as it may sound like you are parroting or echoing, and that could be annoying.

Selective reflecting encourages further exploration of a part of the patient's statement. Though similar to reflecting, the nurse selects the part of the statement that seems most significant and repeats or restates. For example:

PATIENT:	"This brace is giving me a bad time, I was awake all night."
NURSE:	"The brace is giving you a problem?"
PATIENT:	"I can't go home, not like this."
NURSE:	"You think you can't go home?"

General leads are one- or two-word responses by the nurse that encourage the patient to continue. Such words include "go on," "and then," "yes," and "oh."

Silence slows the pace of the conversation and gives the patient time to reflect on what has been said. This usually encourages further conversation. It allows the nurse time to observe for nonverbal cues. You will need to practice feeling at ease during silence.

Other communication techniques are designed to ensure mutual understanding and include clarifying and validating.

Clarifying helps to make meanings clear and to avoid misunderstanding. Sometimes it is difficult to identify feelings or to understand what is intended. When you speak to another person, there are at least six messages involved in the conversation: what I mean to say, what I actually say, what he hears, what he thinks he hears, what he says, and what I think he says. You must recognize these different messages and attempt to clarify. Examples of clarifying are

NURSE:	"I am not sure I understand."
NURSE:	"I am not sure I follow."
NURSE:	"Is this what you are saying?"

Validating means checking to see if a patient need has or has not been met. Evaluation statements are attempts at validating. Examples are

NURSE:	"How are you feeling after your pain medication?"

NURSE:	"Has your nausea subsided since I gave you the injection?"
NURSE:	"How did you sleep last night?"

Still other communication techniques are designed to encourage expressions of thoughts and feelings. These techniques are sharing observations, acknowledging thoughts and feelings, and verbalizing implied thoughts and feelings. The above are clarification techniques.

Sharing observations tells the patient that you have noted his or her response (physical or emotional) and are concerned and interested. Examples are

NURSE:	"You appear restless."
NURSE:	"I noticed you pacing the floor."
NURSE:	"I see that you are eating more today."

Acknowledging thoughts and feelings communicates to the patient that you understand and accept his or her feelings. Examples are

NURSE:	"This must be difficult for you."
NURSE:	"It must be difficult to be on bedrest."

Verbalizing implied thoughts and feelings helps the nurse to verify impressions and helps the patient to recognize or explore his or her feelings. Examples are

PATIENT:	"What is the point in talking about it?"
NURSE:	"Do you feel I won't understand?"
PATIENT:	"One thing after another, always something going wrong."
NURSE:	"Are you concerned about your progress?"

Giving information means sharing with patients regarding their illness, hospitalization, nursing care, and treatment. *Direct questioning and exploring* are used to obtain information from the patient. Exploring is seeking information to get details of a situation.

The following are practice questions. The correct answers are included at the end of the exercise. Determine if you can identify the technique being used.

NURSE: "You seem restless since your doctor was here."

PATIENT: "Why is this happening?"

NURSE: "I am not certain I understand. Are you referring to your wound?"

NURSE: "How are things right now?"

PATIENT: "This I.V. sure is bothering me."

NURSE: "Bothering you?"

PATIENT: "Things are a real mess today."

NURSE: "Oh."

PATIENT: "My mother should be here."

NURSE: "Your mother?"

NURSE: "When was your last bowel movement?"

NURSE: "Are you more comfortable since your brace was adjusted?"

PATIENT: "My husband has been too attentive lately."

NURSE: "Do you think he is overly concerned or anxious about you?"

Answers: Sharing observations; clarifying; broad opening statement or open-ended question; selective reflecting; general lead; reflecting; obtaining information or direct questioning; validating; verbalizing implied thoughts and feelings.

BLOCKS TO THERAPEUTIC COMMUNICATION

Responses, questions, or statements that hinder the flow of conversation and the development of a therapeutic relationship with the patient should be avoided. The nurse must be aware of the blocks and avoid them by using therapeutic communication techniques. Blocks include reassuring clichés, stereotyped comments, questions that require a "yes or no" answer, probing, leading questions, giving advice, belittling, changing the subject, and hostility.

Reassuring clichés are trite or pat answers and tend to minimize the significance of the patient's feelings and convey a lack of understanding or interest. Examples are

NURSE: "Everything will be okay."

NURSE: "You will be just fine."

NURSE: "Things always work out for the best."

NURSE: "Don't worry, it will be all right."

Comments such as these convey that the nurse is denying that the patient has a problem. The patient is interested in his or her own feelings and problems and not in how everyone else feels. Procedures that are routine and simple to the nurse may be problematic to the patient (DuGas, 1983, p. 183). Clichés give false reassurances. Maybe everything is not going to be all right.

Stereotyped comments lead the patient to respond in a like manner, thus keeping the conversation at a superficial level. Important information is not sought or given regarding the patient's condition or concerns. This tends to convey to the patient that you were not listening or not interested and were answering automatically. Examples are

PATIENT: "I am concerned about tomorrow."

NURSE: "Everyone is afraid of surgery." or "Everyone feels that way."

These comments also communicate to the patient that his or her concerns are not unique and are not important.

Closed questions or questions that can be answered by one word, such as yes or no, should not be used when you are seeking information that is more involved. For example, do not ask "Did you take your medication?" when you want to know if the patient is having any difficulty taking the medication or having any side effects. Do not ask "Did you have a good day?" when you want specific information about the nature of the patient's comfort or discomfort.

Probing may cause patients to become resentful and they will usually respond by avoiding conversation with you. Probing may be interpreted by the patient as an invasion of privacy. As the nurse, you are given private, privileged information. Use the therapeutic techniques to encourage conversation. Explain why you need certain information and do not seek information that you do not need. For example:

NURSE: "Now, let's find out what the real problem is."

NURSE: "Is that all you are going to tell me?"

NURSE: "Tell me why you feel that way."

Requesting an explanation could be viewed as probing. Often the person does not know the answer and, if he or she does, may resent your asking. It makes the patient uncomfortable when he or she has to explain feelings or actions.

Leading questions suggest a response that the nurse wants to hear. Leading questions tend to produce answers that may please the nurse but are unlikely to encourage the patient to respond without feeling intimidated. Consider the following two examples:

NURSE: "You are not going to smoke that cigar, are you?"

NURSE: "You have been well cared for by your nurses, haven't you?"

These questions prompt the patient to give an answer that pleases rather than to express his or her thoughts and feelings (Wolff et al., 1983, p. 232).

Giving advice indicates that the nurse knows what is best for the patient and is imposing her own values and judgments rather than seeking and acknowledging the patient's rights to his or her feelings. It tends to encourage dependency. Advice should be given by the nurse when requested. Examples of giving inappropriate advice are

NURSE: "You should take up golf. It is good exercise and will take your mind off your worries."

NURSE: "You should not worry about that. It only increases your blood pressure."

Belittling the patient's feelings or actions encourages resentment. It implies that the patient's feelings are not unusual or important and are not being accepted. It conveys that something must be wrong with the patient for having these feelings or concerns. Examples are

PATIENT: "I can not believe I still have this pain."

NURSE: "Most people have more pain than you have."

NURSE: "You are acting like a baby. Keep your chin up."

NURSE: "Most patients do better than you are doing at this point."

Disagreeing with the patient and expressing disapproval produce the same responses as belittling.

Changing the subject quickly stops a conversation. It takes the lead away from the patient, thereby blocking attempts to discuss his or her feelings or concerns. Furthermore, it prevents the patient from asking questions and causes frustration. The nurse frequently uses this block unconsciously when she is not knowledgeable of the topic and when the topic is embarrassing or uncomfortable, such as sex or chronic or terminal illness. Examples are

PATIENT: "I understand that the operation I need is pretty serious."

NURSE: "Yes. Would you like to eat now?"

PATIENT: "When will I be able to get off bedrest? I am really tired of lying in bed."

NURSE: "Soon. Let's talk about your medication now."

Hostility is obviously destructive to the patient–nurse relationship. Anxious patients frequently react with anger or hostility. Nurses and other health care workers frequently bear the brunt of this anger from patients and families, and it is difficult not to feel defensive and hostile in return. A hostile comment from the nurse can humiliate the patient and will hinder the nurse–patient relationship (DuGas, 1983, p. 183). Hostile comments may infringe on a patient's rights and lead to legal problems. Threatening or abusive comments violate patients' legal rights. Examples of hostile comments are

NURSE: "You have no right to say that."

NURSE: "Don't ever do that again."

NURSE: "I will not bring your pain medication if you behave that way."

The following are practice questions. Determine if you can identify the block being utilized. The correct answers are included at the end of the exercise.

> NURSE: "Of course you are going to be okay."
> NURSE: "Did you have a good breakfast?"
> NURSE: "Let's talk about your sexual problem."
> NURSE: "You should take up swimming; it will take your mind off your problem."
> NURSE: "Everybody is afraid before surgery."
> NURSE: "You have to expect some pain."
> PATIENT: "This lump is serious, isn't it?"
> NURSE: "Maybe. Do you want your bath now?"
> NURSE: "You are not going to get out of bed alone, are you?"
> NURSE: "Don't talk to me in that tone of voice."

Answers: Reassuring cliché; closed question or question with one-word answer; probing; giving advice; stereotyped comment; belittling; changing the subject; leading question; and hostility.

COMMUNICATIONS WITH COLLEAGUES

Communication with other members of the health team is an important aspect of the nurse's role. Few nurses work independently, and most nurses work in a complex information-gathering and information-sharing system. Communication is essential to the accurate planning, coordination, delivery, and evaluation of care and documentation of that care. The planning and delivery of care is a coordinated effort by a team. The nurse works and communicates closely with a variety of health care workers other than nurses. These other health care workers include the physician, respiratory therapist, physical therapist, laboratory technologist, dietitian, social worker, various types of technicians and business office personnel.

Transactional Analysis

Communication takes place in many ways. The most frequent channels are face to face, on the telephone, and written, such as the patient's record. It is essential to communicate effectively. Communication becomes more effective when people are aware of their effect on others and how to avoid poor communication. Transactional analysis is a method developed by Eric Berne (Grasha, 1983) that can help you interpret the verbal and nonverbal messages between two or more people. The theory is that each personality has three parts, the parent, the adult, and the child (P–A–C). Each of these parts influences our interactions and it is possible to analyze our communications in terms of P–A–C.

The parent part of our personality develops from characteristics of our real parents that we internalize and use in our daily interactions. This part includes the nurturing and critical parts, the dos and don'ts. The nurturing parent part supports, listens, and comforts, while the critical parent punishes, evaluates, demands, ridicules, and is intolerant. One of the best ways to improve communication is to eliminate the critical parent.

The function of the adult part is to help us solve problems and make decisions. It operates like a computer and takes in, considers, and analyzes information from the environment. The adult helps you deal with reality in productive and useful ways. The adult can be found in statements such as "What?" "Why?" "When?" "Who?" "How?" "I think," and "In my opinion."

The child part contains emotions, beliefs, and behaviors based on what we experienced early in life. We might behave as we did as a child in certain situations. We may become angry and have a temper tantrum or get into "fights" or become happy and excited depending on childhood reactions to similar situations. The child is also carefree, spontaneous, uninhibited, affectionate, and creative (Grasha, 1983, pp. 234–239). The positive aspects of each part should be used to develop effective communication skills.

Think about how you would feel and respond if your supervisor or instructor said to you, "Make certain this medication is given on time; you've made enough mistakes already." You would probably not feel very good about yourself or the person who made the statement. Another statement that is not effective is "You are not allowed to do that without checking with me first" or "You can't do anything right today." Think about how these messages could be delivered without destroying relationships.

An example of an effective interaction is as follows: "I see you are having difficulties with that procedure. Would you like help?" It is important to address others as your equal and with respect. When you feel bad after an interaction at home, at school, or as the nurse, evaluate the transaction to determine why it went poorly. You need to be able to "read between the lines." You or the person communicating with you may have used the negative parts of the child or parent. Analyze the following interactions and reconstruct them, if necessary, to get positive results.

YOU:	"I am feeling anxious, I don't think I can give this injection."
YOUR SUPERVISOR:	"In my opinion, you usually do things well."
YOU:	"I am sick and tired of all the work I have to do."
YOUR SUPERVISOR:	"If you don't do it, you will be fired."
YOU:	"I've had it, everybody is yelling at me today."
YOUR SUPERVISOR:	"How about taking a few minutes in the lounge to collect yourself and then let's talk about it."

"I" Messages

"I" messages are utilized in assertive responses and therapeutically with patients in mental health settings. Assertiveness is covered in Chapter 11. "I" messages can and should be utilized when the patient or a colleague is infringing upon your personal rights, you are explaining how you see the situation, or you are asked for your opinion. Overuse of "I" messages fo-

cuses on the nurse, not the patient, and gives the impression that the nurse is self-centered and not interested in the patient. Avoid overuse of "I" messages in social conversations for the same reasons.

COMMUNICATING WITH PATIENTS WITH SPECIAL NEEDS
The Elderly

The elderly frequently have communication problems due to sensory or motor impairments. Sensory refers to the senses: sight, hearing, touch, taste, and smell. Motor refers to muscular function. Muscles used in speech are sometimes affected by some diseases. Many elderly persons adapt to these losses and can learn to communicate effectively. The nurse needs to use nonverbal and written communication when necessary and appropriate.

If a patient has a hearing deficit, speak slowly and clearly, stand in front of the patient to provide an opportunity for lip reading, talk toward the patient's best ear, and reduce background noise (Potter, 1989). Be certain only one person is talking at one time. If the patient has a hearing aid, be certain the aid is clean, inserted properly, and has a functioning battery. Adjust the volume of the aid to a comfortable level or help the patient to do so. Keep eyeglasses clean. This helps the patient to see nonverbal cues (Potter, 1989).

Sometimes the patient's only means of communication are nonverbal messages. The nurse needs to be alert to the cues patients are communicating. For example, a patient with Alzheimer's disease may use an inanimate object such as a doll to communicate a need such as hunger, pain, or fatigue.

The Child

Communication with a child requires the nurse to develop a relationship with both the child and parents. The nurse receives much information from the parents. To communicate effectively with children, the nurse must understand the development of language and thought processes (Potter, 1989).

Young children communicate mainly through nonverbal messages. It is important to be honest with children. Explanations are always necessary when doing procedures and should be simple, short, and direct. Sometimes play is necessary to communicate at some age levels. Pictures, drawings, stuffed toys, and dolls are helpful to relate a message.

Crying is an important nonverbal communication used frequently by children. Children use crying to communicate a need or problem such as pain, hunger, or the need to be comforted.

COMPUTER COMMUNICATION

Computers have long been a part of our everyday lives. Computers entered the health care system during the 1950s. At first they were used primarily for financial purposes. As technology advanced, many departments in health care facilities became aware of the possibilities of the computer and began to use it as a tool to increase the effectiveness and efficiency of health care delivery. Today, many acute-care facilities have automated nursing documentation or use computers in some form. Nurses now recognize the potential for computers in improving nursing care practice and delivery of quality patient care. Computer systems are available to help facilitate documentation of patient data, prepare care plans, do patient monitoring, and facilitate scheduling of staff. Computers are used to manage diagnostic procedures such as scanning, radiologic studies, and clinical laboratory tests. The result is that the mundane, routine tasks are performed by the computer and the professional is reserved for creative skills and those unable to be performed by computers or robots. Computers are helpful tools for nurses.

At first, computers were used for calculation of numbers. Today, they can measure pressures and temperatures as well as control sophisticated equipment such as chemical analyzers and computerized axial tomography (CAT) scanners. Computers are also used as word processors or office automation equipment.

There are basically four types of computers:

1. Mainframe—the largest; controls and performs many functions.

2. Minicomputer—a smaller computer used to manage a limited number of functions.

3. Microcomputer—a small unit that links with the mainframe, permitting a large number of functions.

4. Personal computer—the smallest, having the least amount of functions, presently used in the home and in office settings.

Nurses use the microcomputer in the nursing department. The same confidentiality is required regarding the information entered and received via the computer as is required using the manual method of documentation. Nurses receive a computer code after successfully completing a computer course, usually provided by the employing facility. The computer code allows nurses access to the computer system. This code is known only to the individual nurse and the person in charge of assigning codes. This code is secured and cannot be shared with anyone else. Any break in security is basis for dismissal from the job. The reason for the tight security is patient safety and privacy, the legal protection of the nurse and the facility, and accountability. The facility must be confident that the person who entered the data regarding care is truly the person identified by the code.

The nurse does not need to know the mechanics of the computer, but should be computer literate. This means that you should understand some terms used and have a basic understanding of the way a computer functions. Two terms frequently used are *computer hardware* and *computer software.* The hardware is the machine itself. Computer hardware is comprised of four essential components: devices for receiving input, processing data, storing data, and processing output. The most common input device is the keyboard, which functions very much like a typewriter, with some modifications. A device resembling a pen light is sometimes used to enter information on the computer screen. The central processing unit directs information to the appropriate area in the system and processes the data, such as calculations. Devices for storing data or information are called memory. The two types of memory that exist are permanent internal factory-installed memory or read-only memory (ROM) and temporary or random-access memory (RAM), which is generated by the user and deleted when the machine is turned off. Permanent storage of data and information can be done by using floppy or hard disks (Ball and Hannah, 1984, pp. 55–56).

Computer software is the programmed instructions that direct and permit the computer to carry out functions. A programmer develops the program or a set of instructions. The complexity of the particular set of instructions determines the capacity and function of the computer. A patient-care documentation system would be programmed considerably differently from a CAT scanner. However, the same computer can be programmed for multiple functions.

What does this mean to the person entering nursing? Familiarity with computers helps you adapt to and understand how high-technology information systems can assist you. Computer-aided instruction is used in many schools of nursing to enhance your learning and to familiarize you with computer use.

Summary

Effective communication between patients and nurses and between nurses and other health care workers is essential, because it contributes to the quality of care and the patient's well-being. The nurse must develop effective verbal and nonverbal skills for the purpose of helping the patient meet his or her health care needs. It is essential that the nurse understand the communication process and barriers or factors influencing the process.

Communication skills such as listening, nonverbal and verbal therapeutic techniques, and the recognition of the effects of blocks all help the nurse to establish a rapport with the patient. This rapport and these skills enable the nurse to conduct the interview effectively, for the purpose of receiving information, giving, clarifying, or validating information, and establishing patient-care goals. Understanding transactional analysis will further enhance the nurse's ability to communicate effectively with patients and colleagues.

Process recordings of actual communication with patients and colleagues in clinical settings help the nurse to analyze interactions and the effectiveness of communication techniques. These recordings help the nurse recognize and identify when blocks to communication are being used. The nurse can then improve communication skills by reconstructing ineffective responses, statements, and questions to be more effective in a similar future situation. Computer literacy and a beginning understanding of the value and use of a computer will further develop the nurse's communication skills.

*R*EFERENCES

Atkinson LD, Murray ME. *Fundamentals of Nursing: A Nursing Process Approach.* New York: Macmillan, 1985.

Ball MJ, Hannah KJ. *Using Computers in Nursing.* Reston, VA: Reston Publishing, 1984.

DuGas BW. *Introduction to Patient Care: A Comprehensive Approach to Nursing.* 4th. ed. Philadelphia: WB Saunders, 1983.

Grasha AF. *Practical Applications of Psychology.* 2nd. ed. Boston: Little, Brown, 1983.

Kozier B, Erb G, Bufalino PM. *Introduction to Nursing.* Redwood City, CA: Addison-Wesley, 1989.

Murray M. *Fundamentals of Nursing.* 2nd ed. Englewood Cliffs, NJ: Prentice-Hall, 1980.

Potter PA, Perry AG. *Fundamentals of Nursing Concepts: Process and Practice.* 2nd ed. St. Louis, CV Mosby, 1989.

Ross CF. *Personal and Vocational Relationships.* 5th ed. Philadelphia: JB Lippincott, 1981.

Wolff L, Weitzel MH, Zornow RA, Zsohar H. *Fundamentals of Nursing.* 7th. ed. Philadelphia: JB Lippincott, 1983.

CHAPTER
14
Cultural Differences

Learning Objectives

Upon completing this chapter, you will
1. Explain, in your own words, nine basic daily needs of all persons.
2. Explain, in your own words, the philosophy of individual worth as it applies to health care.
3. Describe your culture in the areas of
   a. family
   b. religion
   c. communication
   d. educational background
   e. economic level
   f. wellness and illness beliefs and practices
4. Identify various groups in your geographic area that are culturally different as compared with your culture.
5. Describe specific differences of cultural groups in your geographic area that may have importance in patient-care situations.

INTRODUCTION

You have chosen a career that will give you the opportunity to meet people from many different backgrounds. Some of these people will belong to a different social class and/or cultural group. Some will have different values than you have. Some will have a different lifestyle. Sometimes it comes as a surprise when you discover that people think, feel, believe, and act differently from you and your family and friends and actually see the world differently than you do.

The purposes of this chapter are to encourage you to identify how all persons are alike and to discover how all persons are different.

BASIC DAILY NEEDS

Before you start to think about people and their differences, a good place to start is to think about how people are the same. Because of genes, each individual in the world, perhaps with the exception of identical twins, is different from the next person. But all people share the same basic daily needs regardless of age, sex, economic status, lifestyle, religion, country of origin, or culture. Chapter 18 will discuss human needs as understood by the psychologist Abraham Maslow. However, many years ago, Vivian Culver, a registered nurse (1974, p. 375–376) listed nine essential daily needs of all persons. Although more needs can be added to this list, these needs are a good place to start.

1. Personal care and hygiene
2. Sleep and rest
3. Nutrition and fluids
4. Elimination
5. Body alignment and activity
6. Environment
7. Emotional and spiritual support
8. Diversion and recreation
9. Mental hygiene

These nine needs can form the basis for planning patient care. However, you must under-

stand their meaning for well persons, including yourself, before you can apply them to individuals in the clinical area. Once you gain understanding, the application to patients will be easy.

Personal Care and Hygiene

Clean hair, skin, nails, teeth, and clothing serve two general purposes: protection from illness and promotion of well-being. Skin constantly secretes sebum, the cold cream–like substance of the body, to keep skin supple. Skin eliminates fluid in the form of perspiration to help keep body temperature stable. Sebum and perspiration are odorless substances. Ever-present bacteria on the skin are responsible for the body odor we associate with the body's oils and perspiration. We meet personal care and hygiene needs by bathing, shampooing, hand washing, oral hygiene, and grooming.

Sleep and Rest

Sleep is needed in order to refresh ourselves, yet the actual number of hours of sleep required is individual. Rest or periodic relaxation is just as important, as it too helps the body restore itself.

Nutrition and Fluids

To stay healthy, we all need to eat a diet made up of a variety of foods as you learned in Chapter 10. A minimum of six to eight glasses of water each day, in addition to the food and other beverages we eat and drink, is recommended to help our body complete its many chemical reactions, transport nutrients, regulate temperature, and lubricate various body parts.

Elimination

Elimination of wastes from the body is primarily accomplished by the kidneys for urine and the large intestine for feces. The skin, although not as good at elimination as the above two organs, does eliminate some body wastes through perspiration.

Body Alignment and Activity

Body alignment, or the relationship of body parts to one another, is better known as posture. When posture is "good," the body can be used in a comfortable manner without danger of injury; good posture also enhances the functioning of the respiratory, gastrointestinal, and circulatory systems. Also, you will not get tired as quickly if good posture is maintained. The function of the above body systems can also be enhanced by exercising the body daily. Exercise also helps maintain muscle tone.

Environment

Environment refers to the space that surrounds us and changes many times during a day. Regardless of our specific environment, the most essential component of our surroundings is oxygen. After that environmental need is met, the focus is on safety. When oxygen and safety needs are met, the individual can focus on changing his or her environment for comfort and taste.

Emotional and Spiritual Support

Our emotions greatly influence our health, because the body and the mind are linked. This linking enables the body to influence the mind and the mind to influence the body. All emotions, including excitement, fear, anger, worry, grief, joy, surprise, and love, can influence our bodies positively or negatively. Become aware of your emotions and learn to handle them for your own benefit. Spiritual and emotional needs are closely related, yet different. Persons meet their spiritual needs in a variety of ways that are unique to personal beliefs.

Diversion and Recreation

We all need to turn aside from our usual activities (diversion) and refresh our body and mind with activities other than work (recreation).

Mental Hygiene

This need involves the care and hygiene of the brain. Just as there are health habits of the body, so should you strive for daily health habits of the mind. You should strive to understand and accept yourself, be happy, work well with others, accept criticism, know your abilities and inabilities, trust and respect others, and accept responsibility for yourself.

CULTURE
Definition of Culture

Culture is the total of all the ideas, beliefs, values, attitudes, and objects that a group of people possess and the ways they have of doing things. Culture also includes standards of behavior and sets of rules to live by. The generally accepted ways of doing things common to all people who share the same culture are called customs.

Characteristics of Culture

An important point about culture is that it is learned behavior. From the moment you were born you began to learn about the culture of the group into which you were born. The process of learning your culture (the way your group does things) is called *socialization*. Right now you are being socialized into the career of practical nursing. You are learning how to think and act as a nurse. The same thing happens when the culture of your group is passed on from generation to generation.

Cultural Diversity

The existence of many cultures in a society is called *cultural diversity.* The United States has many groups that possess social and cultural differences when compared with each other. Some of these groups include single parents, people who live in poverty, homosexuals, bisexuals, the wealthy, and members of different ethnic groups. An ethnic group is made up of people who are members of the same race, religion, or nation, or speak the same language. They derive part of their identity through membership in the ethnic group. Examples of ethnic groups in the United States include Native Americans, African Americans, Asian Americans, Hispanic Americans, German Americans, and Jews. People who belong to the same cultural group may develop the attitude that their way of doing things is superior to groups with different cultures (ethnocentrism). This attitude develops when persons hold their customs and ways as the norm against which to measure and evaluate the customs and ways of others. When intolerance of another cultural group occurs, prejudice is experienced. When rights and privileges are withheld from those of another cultural group, discrimination is the result.

Importance of Cultural Differences

As a practical nurse, you need to be aware that cultural differences often exist between you and your patients. To fail to develop cultural awareness could lead to misunderstandings, stress for the patient and you, and confusion. You could make false assumptions, labeling the patient as difficult or uncooperative. It is probable that less-than-adequate care could be experienced by patients when their cultural differences are overlooked or misinterpreted.

PHILOSOPHY OF INDIVIDUAL WORTH

The philosophy of individual worth is the belief shared by all members of the health team of the uniqueness and value of each human being who comes for care, regardless of differences that may be observed in that individual. As a practical nurse, you need to realize that each individual has the right to live according to personal beliefs and values, and deserves respect as a human being. Many factors are responsible for patients being different from you. They may think and behave differently because of social class, religion, ethnic background, or personal choice. Regardless of differences, all patients have the right to quality nursing care, and as a practical nurse you cannot decrease the quality of care because of differences you have observed. Practical nurses need to guard against making judgments about people who are culturally different. This does not mean you must accept for yourself or approve the differences you observe. It means taking the difference at face value, accepting people as they are, and giving quality care regardless. Be aware of your own attitudes, beliefs, and values as they affect your ability to give care. If you do identify biases, see them for what they are. Become aware of cultural differences, acknowledge that they exist, and then gather knowledge about them so that you may work on trying to modify your biases. If it is impossible for you to eliminate biases, work around them without compromising patient care.

LEARNING ABOUT DIFFERENT CULTURES
How to Begin

The area of cultural differences is a vast area to investigate. One way to learn about different cultures is to read as much material as you can about the different cultures to which you are personally exposed. The list of suggested readings on pages 184–186 can help you get started. A helpful class activity could be a report from peers who represent various cultural groups. Regardless of the method used to gather information about different cultures that would be helpful to you as a practical nurse, it is important to remember not to apply that information automatically to all individuals in that group. To do so would make you guilty of stereotyping individuals—that is, having a fixed notion that everyone in that cultural group is the same. It can lead to classifying people as being the same just because they share the same religion, lifestyle, or ethnic background.

Avoiding False Assumptions

Personal experiences, geographic locality, economic level, and educational background are a few of the conditions to be taken into account when trying to understand differences displayed by various cultural groups as compared with your culture. To fail to do so could result in false assumptions that may lead to embarrassment and misunderstandings. The best you can do with your information is to apply it to groups in a general way. This indicates that the values, attitudes, beliefs, and customs you read about generally describe the group, but not each individual in that group. For example, immigrants may quickly begin to acculturate, or adopt the ways of the new culture. But no matter how much people acculturate, old ways may never be given up completely, and an interesting blend of cultures may emerge.

AREAS THAT MAY DIFFER CULTURALLY

Brownlee (1978) offers a method to help health care workers tackle the problem of acquiring knowledge of cultural differences by developing an awareness in themselves that differences exist in areas that might ordinarily be taken for granted. General information follows about family, religion, communication, educational background, economic level, and wellness and illness beliefs and practices. After reading about each area, you will be given an opportunity to develop awareness of your own cultural patterns in these areas. Sharing this information with peers, if desired, can be a good learning experience.

Family

The family is the basic unit of society, no matter what culture is being discussed. The role of the family is to have children, if desired, and raise them to be contributing members of the group. Actual child-rearing practices will vary from culture to culture, but families will generally socialize the young to the culture of the group and meet their physical and psychological needs. Some cultures expect the nuclear family (mother, father, and children) to live in the same house, while others may expect the extended family (the nuclear family plus grandparents and other kinsmen) to do so. Some Vietnamese families are examples of extended families, with three or more generations living in the same house. In many of these families, ties are strong, and behaviors that enhance the family name are encouraged, for example, obedience to parents and those in authority.

The traditional nuclear family is being challenged by the single-parent family. According to 1990 statistics of the U.S. Bureau of the Census, approximately 25% of all households in the United States were single-parent families. Although a parent can become a single parent by the death of a spouse or by electing not to marry at time of pregnancy, divorce accounts for a large number of single-parent families. Health care workers who have not been in the same situation may be unaware of and insensitive to the special way of life of this type of family. Respond to the following statements; your responses will help you discover your own cultural patterns regarding the family.

1. Describe your family structure (nuclear, extended, or alternative lifestyle).

2. Describe the role of children, if any, in your family.

3. Discuss who gives permission for hospitalization in your family.

4. List factors that influence the decision of your family members to visit or not to visit when a member is ill.

5. Describe the effect of your hospitalization today at 4 P.M. for surgery tomorrow would have on you and your family.

Religion

Religious beliefs are very personal to the individual. Religion is an important aspect of culture, but can have different meanings in people's lives. For some, religion is a brief, momentary, and sporadic part of daily life. For others, it may influence every aspect of life and have a profound effect on personal outlook and how they live. Although Chapter 15 deals with religious differences, this aspect of life cannot be excluded from the present chapter because of the close relation between religious beliefs and the concept of wellness and illness for some groups. Also, practical nurses should be aware of their own religious beliefs, obligations, and attitudes and be aware if they influence care that is given to patients. The questions that follow give you the opportunity to discover your own cultural patterns regarding religion.

1. Do you have a religious affiliation?

2. What role does religion play in your life?

3. Is prayer helpful to you?

4. What is your source of strength and hope?

5. What religious practices or rituals are important to you?

6. What religious books or symbols are helpful to you?

7. What dietary inclusions/restrictions are part of your religious beliefs?

8. How does your religion view the source of and meaning of pain/suffering?

Communication

Chapter 13 introduced you to types of communication and some barriers to the communication process. A major barrier to communication in health care is when the patient or nurse speaks a different language. A person's language gives a view of reality that may differ from yours. For example, in English the clock runs but in Spanish it walks. This illustrates the different concept of time between two cultures. For a person with English as a first language, time could move quickly, and there may be a rush to get things done. For those with Spanish as a first language, time may move more slowly. The following is a list of areas of communication that may vary for people who are culturally different.

Forms of Greetings and Goodbyes

You may greet your patient and want to get right down to business, but the patient might expect some light conversation before getting down to the matter at hand. Some cultural groups take an hour to say good-bye while others get up and leave without saying anything.

Appropriateness of the Situation

Some groups prefer people to sit, not stand, while conversing. For some, the sharing of food is a good way to relate to others and get them to verbalize.

Confidentiality

All information the patient gives the nurse is considered confidential and cannot be divulged. Some patients do not want their spouse questioned or kept informed about their problems of the reproductive organs for fear the spouse will think they are less desirable sexually.

Emotions and Feelings

Emotions are universal, but the cues to those emotions vary considerably. A lack of awareness of this fact can cause unnecessary emotional trauma on the part of the patient and the nurse. Some cultural groups cannot display affection in public, show disapproval or frustration, or vent anger in public. Some cannot take criticism. You may show dissatisfaction with team members by directly approaching them. Some team members may show dissatisfaction with you by being polite to your face and then complaining about you to the rest of the staff.

Pain Expression

Pain has two parts, sensation and response. All individuals experience the same sensation of pain. However, one's culture might provide guidelines for approved ways of expressing one's response to the pain. Some cultures teach individuals that it is acceptable to cry, moan, and exhibit other behavior that calls attention to the pain. Other cultures encourage uncomplaining acceptance of pain and passive, behavior when pain is experienced (stoic behavior). Discuss some nursing situations in which the above two different reactions to pain could have negative consequences if a practical nurse lacked knowledge of cultural differences in pain expression.

Tempo of Conversation

You may tend to speak with speed and expect a quick response. The patient may be accustomed to pausing and reflecting on a response.

The Meaning of Silence

Silence can mean anything from disapproval to warmth, but generally does not indicate tension or lack of rapport. Silence can be difficult for some persons to tolerate. Resist the temptation to jump in at a pause by forcing yourself to meditate or even bite your tongue (hopefully, not literally).

Now develop an awareness of your own cultural patterns regarding communication by answering the following questions.

1. What facial or body habits are you aware of in yourself while talking?

2. How do you greet people and how do you say good-bye?

3. How do you express
   a. love?
   b. hate?
   c. fear?
   d. excitement?
   e. disappointment?
   f. dissatisfaction?
   g. humor?
   h. anger?
   i. sadness?
   j. happiness?

4. Do you make eye contact when you talk to people?

5. Do you touch people while talking?
   a. If so, how do they react?
   b. How do you react when people touch you while they are talking to you?

6. How do all of your personal habits fit with those of the cultural group to which you belong?

Educational Background

Federal studies estimate that about 25 million adults have literacy skills below the fourth-grade level; these persons are called functionally illiterate (Kozol, 1985, p. 8). These Americans have trouble reading and understanding simple directions. Another 35 million have skills below the eighth-grade level (Kozol, 1985, p. 6). Differences in educational background need to be taken into consideration when conducting patient teaching. The above statistics indicate that one out of every three Americans have some difficulty with reading or writing, so adapt your explanations to the patient's level of understanding. Responding to the following statements will help you to identify your own beliefs and practices regarding education.

1. Calculate the number of years of education you have had.

2. State your ultimate educational goal.

3. Discuss the role education plays in your life.

4. Describe your feelings regarding a person who has less education than you have.

5. Describe your feelings regarding a person who has more education than you have.

6. Describe what your feelings would be if you were referred to your school's skills center.

7. Discuss what impact you think your cultural background has on your values and practices regarding education.

Economic Level

Economic level is frequently related to educational background, and sociologists use these two factors to determine the social class of individuals. As a practical nurse, you will take care of patients who are very wealthy and some who are at or near the poverty level, as well as those who have midlevel incomes. A patient's annual income will determine the type of house he or she lives in, the neighborhood where he or she lives, the availability of food, and the ability to participate in certain types of preventive health care. Practical nurses need to take economic level into consideration when they make suggestions during patient teaching and adapt the suggestions accordingly. Identify your personal patterns regarding economic level by responding to the following statements.

1. Describe how your economic background affects your daily life in the following areas:
   a. availability of food
   b. availability of shelter
   c. availability of clothing
   d. amount and type of recreation

2. Discuss your feelings toward a person who has less money than you have.

3. Discuss your feelings toward a person who has more money than you have.

4. Describe how your feelings fit with those of your cultural group?

Wellness and Illness Beliefs and Practices

Wellness and illness can have different meanings for persons who are culturally different. Wellness and illness are relative terms, and what is good health to one person can be sickness to another. Wellness may not be a priority item to some patients. As far as prevention of disease is concerned, some patients will believe illness can be prevented and have elaborate rituals and special persons to carry out those rituals, not only to cure disease, but to prevent its occurrence in the first place. Others will look at prevention as an attempt to control the future, an impossible feat in the way they view their lives. When disease does strike, some will blame pathogens (germs), some spirits, and others an angry god. Generally, death and dying will bring out strong emotions in people. Be aware that some cultures can have special taboos and prohibitions when death occurs. Roles that family and friends carry out at the time of death may vary.

Many cultural groups attach stigma to mental illness and psychiatrists, but do not attach the same stigma when physical health is impaired. Some groups may feel that the symptoms manifested are a healthy reaction to an emotional crisis. Some cultural groups have the understanding that the mind and body are united and are not separate entities. These cultures may have traditional healers that are expert at healing both the mind and the body.

In the area of nutrition, some groups will have special foods or food combinations that can prevent or cure illnesses, while others pay little attention to what is eaten in a day's time.

Individuals in some cultures will be embarrassed when they have to discuss bodily functions or have certain body parts examined; others will not be bothered by this. Hygiene practices will vary according to beliefs, living conditions, personal resources, and physical characteristics. To assist you in identifying your own cultural patterns regarding wellness beliefs and practices, respond to the following.

1. Describe what it means to you to have good health.

2. What are some practices or beliefs that you have regarding staying well?

3. Describe what it means to you to be sick.

4. List some foods in your diet that help you prevent illness.
   a. How does eating these foods prevent illness?
   b. What are some foods you must avoid in order to prevent illness?

5. How do you care for your skin and hair?

6. Describe the customs you have when there is a death in your family.
   a. Who makes burial arrangements?
   b. Who should be present when the death occurs?
   c. Describe what you believe happens to a person after death.
   d. Do you have a get-together after the ceremony? If so, for whom?

7. Describe your attitude toward mental illness.

8. Describe what you think causes mental illness.

9. Who do you think should treat mental illness?

It is hoped that this overview has started you thinking in terms of cultural differences. And along with that awareness, hopefully a respect has developed for ways of doing things that may be different from your way. The varied cultural backgrounds of your classmates and patients can result in interesting learning experiences for you. Your developing cultural sensitivity will be invaluable in patient care. When you find a patient who is "difficult" or "uncooperative," be ready to ask yourself, "Is there something about the patient being culturally different that is responsible for the behavior?" When cultural differences are identified, you are more likely to see the value of the other person's way and will be on your way to clearing your mind of cultural prejudice.

Summary

A good place to start learning about how people are different is to remind yourself that all persons have similarities. The nine basic daily needs are shared by all persons. How individuals meet these needs varies with their cultures, the learned ways they have of doing things.

Awareness of cultural differences is important for practical nurses so that they can avoid false assumptions and misunderstandings about the patients for whom they care. It is important to be aware of your personal beliefs and practices in the areas of family, religion, communication, educational background, economic level, and wellness and illness beliefs and practices. Some ways to learn about cultural differences include reading about different cultures, especially those found in your geographic area, and having reports from peers who are culturally different.

A guideline in health care is the philosophy of individual worth, the belief that all persons are unique and have value, regardless of the way they do things, and deserve the best nursing care you can give.

*R*EFERENCES

Baker C, Mayer G. One approach to teaching cultural similarities and differences. Nurs Educ 1982; 21(4):17–22.

Brink P. Value orientations as an assessment tool in cultural diversity. Nurs Res 1984; 33:198–203.

Brink P. *Transcultural Nursing: A Book of Readings.* Prospect Heights, IL: Waveland Press, 1989.

Brownlee A. *Community, Culture and Care: A Cross Cultural Guide for Health Workers.* St Louis: CV Mosby, 1978.

Clinton J. Ethnicity: the development of an empirical construct for cross-cultural health research. J Nurs Res 1982; 4:281–300.

Culver V. *Modern Bedside Care.* 8th ed. Philadelphia: WB Saunders, 1974:374–384.

deWitt S. *Keane's Essentials of Medical-Surgical Nursing.* 3rd ed. Philadelphia: WB Saunders, 1992.

Fitzgerald F. Patterns from other cultures: how they view you, themselves, and disease. Consultant 1988; 28(3):65–67.

Fulton C. Integrating cultural content into the nursing curriculum. Nurs Educ 1985; 10(1):26.

Hall E. *The Hidden Dimension.* New York: Peter Smith, 1992.

Idem. The Silent Language. New York: Doubleday, 1990.

Hamilton E, Whitney E, Sizer F. Cultural and religious cuisines: which ethnic group has the best way to eat? In: Hamilton E, Whitney E, Sizer F. *Nutrition Concepts.* St Paul, MN: West Publishing, 1991.

Hartog J, Hartog E. Cultural aspects of health and illness behavior in hospitals. West J Med 1983; 139:106–112.

Kozol J. Dehumanizing the humanities: scholars and adult illiteracy. Educ Digest 1985; 51(4):6–9.

Kuhni C. When cultures clash at the bedside. RN 1990; 53(1):23–26.

Leininger M. Transcultural care diversity and universality: a theory of nursing. Nurs Health Care 1985; 6:209–212.

Idem. Transcultural Nursing: Concepts, Theories and Practices. 2nd ed. New York: Wiley, 1988.

Low S. The cultural basis of health, illness and disease. Social Work Health Care 1984; 9(3):13–23.

Marchione J, Stearns S. Ethnic power perspectives for nursing. Nurs Health Care 1990, 11:296–301.

Milliken M. *Understanding Human Behavior: A Guide for Health Workers.* 4th ed. Albany, NY: Delmar Publishers, 1987.

Neiderhauser V. Health care of immigrant children. Pediatr Nurs 1989; 15:569–574.

Randall DE. Strategies for working with culturally diverse communities and clients. 1st ed. Bethesda, MD: Association for the Care of Children's Health, 1989.

Tripp-Reimer T. Research in cultural diversity. West J Nurs Res 1984; 6:130–132.

Tripp-Reimer T, Brink P, Saunders J. Cultural assessment: content and process. Nurs Outlook 1984; 32:78–82.

U.S. Bureau of the Census. *Statistical Abstract of the United States 1990.* Washington, DC: US Department of Commerce.

SUGGESTED READINGS

Asian Americans

Chow E. Cultural health traditions: Asian perspectives. In: Branch M, Paxton P, eds. *Providing Safe Nursing Care for Ethnic People of Color.* New York: Appleton-Century-Crofts, 1976:99–114.

Dobbins E, Lynch B, Fischer D, Santopietro-Smith M, Laine C. A beginner's guide to Vietnamese culture. RN 1981; 44(1):44–45.

Gallo A, Edwards J, Vessey J. Little refugees with big needs. RN 1980; 43(12):45–48.

Koval D, Brennan AM. Exotic diseases you're sure to see more of. RN 1980; 43(9):73–80.

Moccke M. In search of healers—Southeast Asian refugees in the American health care system. West J Med, 1983; 139:835–840.

Orque M. Nursing care of South Vietnamese patients. In: Orque M, Block B, Monrroy L, eds. *Ethnic Nursing Care.* St Louis: CV Mosby, 1983:245–269.

Santopietro M, Lynch B. What's behind the inscrutable mask? RN 1980; 43(10):57–61.

Tien-Hyatt J. Keying in on the unique care needs of Asian clients. Nurs Health Care 1987; 8(5):269–271.

When the patient is from Southeast Asia. Emerg Med 1983; 15(5):111–112, 115, 116, 120.

African Americans

Block B. Nursing care of black patients. In: Orque M, Block B, Monrroy L, eds. *Ethnic Nursing Care.* St Louis: CV Mosby, 1983:81–113.

Block B, Hunter M. Teaching physiological assessment of black persons. Nurse Educ 1981; 6(1):24–27.

Friedman M. Transcultural family nursing: application to Latino and black families. Pediatr Nurs 1990; 5:214–222.

Grier M. Hair care for the black patient. Am J Nurs 1976; 76(11):1781.

Jacques G. Cultural health traditions: a black perspective. In: Branch M, Paxton P. *Providing Safe Nursing Care for Ethnic People of Color.* New York: Appleton-Century-Crofts, 1976:115–124.

Roach L. Color changes in dark skins. Nursing 77 1977; 7(7):48–51.

Hispanic Americans

Anthony-Tkach C. Care of the Mexican-American patient. Nurs Health Care 1981; 2:424–427, 432.

de la Vega. Considerations for reaching the Latino population. SIECUS Rep 1990; 18(3):1–8.

Friedman M. Transcultural family nursing: application to Latino and black families. Pediatr Nurs 1990; 5:214–222.

Gonzalez-Swafford M, Gutierrez M. Ethno-medical beliefs and practices of Mexican-Americans. Nurs Practitioner 1983; 8(10):29–30, 32, 34.

Lasater T, Montalvo F. Understanding Mexican-American culture: a training program. Children Today 1982; 8(10):23–25, 35.

Pasquale E. The evil eye phenomenon: its implications for community health nurse. Home Health Care Nurse 1984; 2(3):32–35.

Homosexuals

Baptiste DA. The gay and lesbian stepparent family. In: Bozett F, ed. *Gay and Lesbian Parents.* New York: Praeger Publishers, 1987.

Brossart J. The gay patient—what you should be doing. RN 1979; 42(4):50–52.

Hall M. Lesbian families: cultural and clinical issues. Social Work 1987; 23:380–385.

Pogoncheff E. The gay patient—what not to do. RN 1979; 42(4):46–50.

Varcarolis E. *Foundations of Psychiatric–Mental Health Nursing.* Philadelphia: WB Saunders, 1990.

Native Americans

Backup R. Health care of the American Indian patient. Crit Care Update 1980; 7(2):16–22.

Handy M, Burkhardt M. Nursing the Navajo. Am J Nurs 1977; 77(1):95–96.

Primeaux M. Caring for the American Indian patient. Am J Nurs 1977; 77:91–94.

Rowell R. Native American stereotypes, and HIV/AIDS. SIECUS Rep 1990; 18(3):9–15.

Wilson U. Nursing care of American Indian patients. In: Orque M, Block B, Monrroy L, eds. *Ethnic Nursing Care.* St Louis: Mosby-Year Book, 1983:271–295.

The Family

Bobak I, Jensen M, Zalar M. The family, a unit of care. In: Bobak I, Jensen M, Zolar M. *Maternity and Gynecological Care, the Nurse, and the Family,* 4th ed. St Louis: CV Mosby, 1989.

Van Brede A. Health issues facing American children. Pediatr Nurs 1989; 15:575–577.

Single Parents

Burns C. The hospitalization experience and single parent families: a time of social vulnerability. Nurs Clin North Am 1984; 19:285–293.

Dresen S. The young adult: adjusting to single parenting. Am J Nurs 1976; 76:1286–1289.

Norton A, Glick P. One parent families: a social and economic profile. Fam Relat 1986; 35(1):9.

Profile: the single parent family. The Communique: Quarterly Publication of the Wisconsin League for Nursing 1982; 1(4):171–173.

Varcarolis E. Blended families. In: Varcarolis E. *Foundations of Psychiatric–Mental Health Nursing*. Philadelphia: WB Saunders, 1990.

Whaley L, Wong D. Social, cultural and religious influences on child health. In: Whaley L, Wong D. *Nursing Care of Infants and Children*. 4th ed. St Louis: Mosby-Year Book, 1991:29–63.

Idem. Family influences on child health promotion. In: Whaley L, Wong D. *Nursing Care of Infants and Children*. 4th ed. St Louis: Mosby-Year Book, 1991:64–104.

CHAPTER
15
Spiritual Needs and Religious Differences

Learning Objectives

After completing this chapter, you will
1. Discuss the practical nurse's role in meeting spiritual needs of the patient and the family.
2. List members of the health team who can help meet patient's spiritual needs.
3. Discuss personal religious beliefs, or absence of them, and discuss how this will influence nursing practice.
4. Discuss the general beliefs that account for the differences between non-Christian religions and Christianity.
5. Describe specific nursing actions that can be used to meet the needs of patients with different religious backgrounds.

INTRODUCTION

Spiritual needs are not given the emphasis that other daily needs of the patient are given. However, only when spiritual needs are met, can nurses say they have directed care to the total person. Spiritual needs arise out of humans' desire to find meaning and purpose in life, suffering, and death. An individual's spiritual dimension is a very private and personal area and includes the beliefs and value system that are his or her source of strength and hope. Whereas emotional needs refer to the relationship of individuals within themselves, spiritual needs refer to the relationship of individuals to a higher being. Therefore, spiritual help differs from emotional support. The practical nurse learns to recognize the need for spiritual help in patients and develops ways to offer this help. Although many persons have a spiritual dimension, needs arising in this area depend on a variety of situations and the individual's ability to cope with them. A crisis situation such as illness or injury can intensify spiritual needs and, depending on an individual's beliefs, can profoundly affect his or her response to illness, rate of recovery, and attitude toward treatment. Be especially alert to the need for spiritual help in patients who are in pain, have an incurable disease, are dying, or have experienced the death of a loved one. Patients who are facing an undesirable outcome of illness (such as an amputation) or are not in control of themselves, also may need spiritual help.

HOW DO I MEET SPIRITUAL NEEDS OF MY PATIENT?

The pastoral care team is comprised of ministers, priests, rabbis, nuns, and lay persons who are educated to meet spiritual needs in a health care setting. If an institution does not have a pastoral care team or chaplain on staff, a listing of religious representatives of area churches will be available. The practical nurse also has the responsibility to help meet spiritual needs of patients.

Perhaps the best place to start in meeting spiritual needs is to be aware of your personal spiritual beliefs and relationship to a higher being. When you acknowledge that your own beliefs are effective for you but not necessarily for others, you can set them aside when helping patients meet their spiritual needs. Ask questions to help the patient verbalize beliefs, fears, and concerns. Show interest through supportive statements, listen with an understanding attitude, and respond as naturally to spiritual concerns as you do to physical needs. It is always a delicate matter to help patients face the reality of a terminal illness without abandoning hope. Encouraging active involvement in care can help to uphold hope. When a patient faces death, you can help make his or her remaining days meaningful by attending to needs and approaching the patient in a supportive and empathic manner. When the priest, rabbi, or minister does come to your unit, inform him or her of the patient's background and condition and what interventions you have incorporated into the plan of care.

HOW THE PATIENT MEETS SPIRITUAL NEEDS

Many patients will help meet their spiritual needs by belonging to specific religious denominations. A denomination is an organized group of persons who share a philosophy that supports their particular concept of God. The different rituals and practices that religions exercise are stabilizing forces for the patient. Rituals can bring the security of the past into a crisis situation. Concrete symbols, such as pictures, herb packets, rosaries, statues, various jewelry, and other objects can affirm connection with God. Prayer is a spiritual practice of some individuals whether or not they are members of an organized religion. Prayer can put a patient in touch with a personal God and sometimes decrease anxiety with the same success as a drug.

The value of these rituals and practices is determined by the faith of the patient and not by scientific proof as to their benefit. When a patient expresses interest in praying, ask what prayer he or she would like to say and try to accommodate the request. When patients are not allowed to practice their religious rituals, practices, and responsibilities, they can feel guilty and uneasy. As a practical nurse, you need to develop an awareness of the general religious philosophy of the patient's particular denomination. If membership is claimed in a specific denomination, be aware of the rituals and exercises that the patient believes in and practices. Spiritual distress can be observed in patients who are unable to practice their religious rituals and/or experience a conflict between their religious and spiritual beliefs and the prescribed health regimen.

Agnostics hold the belief that the existence of God can be neither proved nor disproved. Atheists do not believe that the supernatural exists, so they do not believe in God. Whereas Christians may find comfort and solace in their refuge in God, including passing over into another life after death, the atheist does not have this belief to sustain him or her. It may be difficult for the nurse who believes in the supernatural to relate to atheistic beliefs. The nurse may feel unsuccessful in meeting the total needs of the patient who is an atheist. However, since atheists do not believe in the supernatural, they do not have this need. The nurse should allow this patient to express personal feelings about life, death, separation, and loss and not impose personal beliefs and values on the patient.

The remainder of this chapter will present beliefs and practices of various religions that are found in the United States and Canada and their nursing implications. This information will serve as a reference to be used in meeting spiritual needs of specific patients during your time as a student practical nurse and in your nursing career after you graduate. Although each religion has beliefs and practices, sometimes an individual will adapt them to fit his or her own circumstances. Do not assume that all Protestants, Catholics, Jews, etc. actually believe in all the aspects of their formal religion. Do not judge a patient if variations in his or her beliefs exist. Clarify with the patient when health issues and decisions involve religious beliefs. The references at the end of the chapter can be used to learn more about a specific religion when that information is needed.

Table 15-1 lists features of the major non-Christian religions.

Table 15-1 Major Non-Christian Religions

RELIGION	SPECIAL FEATURES	NURSING IMPLICATIONS
Judaism	Observation of Sabbath	Provide time for rest, prayer, and/or study from sunset on Friday till after sunset on Sunday, if desired.
		Provide yarmulke (skullcap) or prayer shawl, if desired. Inform family of need for these items.
	Observation of dietary rules (Kosher). Clarify if patient follows these dietary rules.	Make arrangements for separate utensils for preparing and serving meat and milk dishes, if desired.

Table continued on the following page.

		If separate dishes not available, these foods can be served in the original containers or on paper plates.
		Meat may be consumed a few minutes after drinking milk, but six hours must pass after eating meat before drinking milk (Carpenito, 1983, p. 457).
		Do not serve pork, ham, Canadian bacon, eel, oysters, crab, lobster, shrimp, or eggs with blood spots.
	The dying Jewish patient	Family and friends may want to be with the patient at all times.
		Some Jews do not believe in autopsies, embalming, or cremation.
		Some Jews may not want the nurse to touch the body of a deceased Jew and may request that the nurse notify the Burial Society for preparation of the body for burial.
Islam	General beliefs	Some Muslims, members of the Islam religion, may desire to pray to their God (Allah), five times a day (after dawn, at noon, in midafternoon, after sunset, and at night). If patient requests to face Mecca, the holy city of Islam, a bed or chair may be positioned in a southeast direction.
		If a Muslim brings the Koran, the holy book of Islam, to the health care

institution, do not touch it or place anything on top of it.

If a Muslim wears writings from the Koran on a black string around the neck, arm, or waist, these writings should be kept dry and should not be removed (Henley and Clayton, 1982, p. 919).

Rules of cleanliness may include eating with the right hand and cleansing self with the left hand after urinating and defecating.

Observation of dietary rules	Some Muslims might not eat pork and pork products, eel, oysters, crab, lobster, shrimp, and meats from animals that have not been bled to death by a Muslim.
	Some Muslims might not drink alcoholic beverages.
Observation of female modesty	Some Muslim females prefer to be clothed from head to ankle. During a physical examination, they may prefer to undress one body part at a time.

MAJOR CHRISTIAN RELIGIONS
General Considerations

General features of the major Christian religions are given in Table 15-2.

The Bible

Many Christian patients will find comfort in reading or having someone read to them selected passages from the Bible. Treat the patient's Bible with respect. In addition to believing it contains the inspired word of God, some persons have received their Bibles as gifts commemorating special occasions such as a wed-

Table 15-2 Christian Denominations and Groups

DENOMINATION/ GROUP	SPECIAL FEATURES	NURSING IMPLICATIONS
Protestants	General practices to be clarified	Would patient like to be visited by personal minister?
		Does patient want Communion, anointing with oil, or time for bible reading?
		If patient is an infant and condition is serious, do parents desire Baptism if child is not baptized?
		If patient is dying, what are family's beliefs about death and dying?
Roman Catholics	General beliefs	If desired and condition allows, make arrangements for patient to attend Mass. Ill Catholics are excused from this obligation on Sundays and holy days.
		If desired, arrange for the sacrament of Reconciliation and provide privacy when the priest hears the patient's confession.
		If desired, arrange for the anointing of the sick, which offers hope and consolation and assists in physical, mental, and spiritual healing.
	The dying Catholic patient	Seriously ill Catholic patients may want to receive the Last Rites. Make arrangements for the priest to administer the sacrament of Reconciliation, the anointing of the sick, and Holy Communion.

	Observation of dietary rules	When sick, a Catholic is excused from fasting (giving up food for a specified period of time) and abstaining (giving up meat at certain times).
	Desire for religious objects	Catholic patients may request that religious pictures and objects be kept at the bedside or on their persons. These are reminders of God's presence in their lives and are sources of consolation.
Jehovah's Witnesses	General beliefs	Jehovah's Witnesses will refuse to receive blood products, including plasma. To receive such products is viewed as a violation of the law of God.
Seventh Day Adventists	Observation of dietary rules	Adventists generally do not smoke or drink. Some Adventist patients may avoid beverages with caffeine. Many Adventists are vegetarians and use soybean products as a protein source. These dietary practices are not mandatory.
	Observation of the Sabbath	Adventists observe the Sabbath from sunset on Friday to sunset on Saturday and do not pursue their jobs or worldly pleasures during this time.
Mormons	General beliefs	Mormon patients may avoid tobacco, alcohol, coffee, and tea.

Table continued on the following page.

Christian Scientists	General beliefs	Patient may believe that sickness can be eliminated through prayer and spiritual understanding. Healing is considered an awakening to this belief.
		Patient may want to have a Christian Scientist practitioner contacted to give treatment through prayer.
Amish	General beliefs and practices	The Amish do not believe in health insurance and social security and rely on mutual aid in time of need (Wiggins, 1983, p. 26).
		Patients may believe that sudden fright or blood loss may cause loss of the soul (Wiggins, 1983, p. 26).
		Female patients may not approve of cutting their hair.

ding, graduation, confirmation, anniversary, or jubilee. Sometimes Bibles list passages that can be used in specific patient situations, such as pain, sorrow, sleeplessness, etc.

Baptism

When a patient belongs to a religious group that believes Baptism is essential to salvation, requests the sacrament, and death is imminent, the practical nurse may baptize if the minister or priest has not yet arrived. When the dying patient is an infant, Baptism may be given if the religious beliefs of the parents include infant baptism. The procedure for Baptism is as follows:

1. If the patient is Protestant, have a witness for the Baptism, if possible. This is not necessary for a Catholic patient.

2. Allow water to flow over and contact skin while saying the words: "[name, if known], I baptize you in the name of the Father, and of the Son, and of the Holy Spirit."

3. If the patient is Catholic and it is uncertain if Baptism was received in the past, precede the above words with "If capable. . . ." These words indicate the desire for the sacrament if it has not been received before.

4. Report the Baptism to the chaplain or pastoral care team and the family.

5. Record the Baptism on the Nurses' Notes.

Table 15-3 summarizes the status of Baptism for various religious denominations and groups found in the United States and Canada.

Table 15-3 Baptism Beliefs and Practices

DENOMINATION/ GROUP	AGE OF ADMINISTRATION	METHOD	COMMENTS
Assembly of God	Age of accountability	Immersion	The person should understand the meaning of Baptism.
Bahá'í	—	—	No baptism.
Baptist	Adult	Immersion	Not a means of salvation. Opposed to infant baptism. The person should understand the meaning of baptism.
Christian Scientist	—	—	No baptism.
Eastern Orthodox Churches	Infant	Immersion	Age of infant differs by group.
Episcopalian	Infant	Sprinkle	Necessary for salvation.
Jehovah's Witnesses	Adult	—	No infant baptism. Necessary for salvation.
Lutheran	Infant or adult	Sprinkle or immersion	Infant baptism at 6 to 8 weeks.
Methodist	Infant and adult	Sprinkle or immersion	An outward and visible sign of an inward and spiritual grace.
Mormon	8 years or older	Immersion	Baptism causes remission of sins. Allows person to receive the gifts of the Holy Spirit. Required for salvation.

Table continued on the following page.

Presbyterian	Infant	Usually sprinkling	—
Quakers	—	—	No baptism. At birth, infant's name recorded in official book.
Roman Catholic	Infant or adult	Usually sprinkling, or immersion	Means of salvation and initiation into the community. Removes all sin. Person receives Holy Spirit.
Seventh Day Adventists	Adult	Immersion	Opposed to infant baptism. Makes one a church member.
United Church of Christ	Infant	Immersion	When baptized, become a church member.

Communion

Various groups differ in their interpretation of the meaning of Communion. Table 15-4 discusses the status of communion beliefs and practices for various denominations and groups in the United States and Canada.

Table 15-4 Communion Beliefs and Practices

DENOMINATION/ GROUP	DO THEY HAVE THIS PRACTICE?	COMMENTS
Assembly of God	Yes	—
Baptist	Yes	A remembrance of Christ's death.
Christian Scientists	No	—
Eastern Orthodox Churches	Yes	Belief same as Catholic.
Episcopalian	Yes	Considered a sacrament.

Lutherans	Yes	Considered a sacrament. Believe the presence of Christ is real.
Methodists	Yes	Open to everyone including children.
Presbyterian	Yes	Believe Christ is present in spirit.
Quakers	No	—
Roman Catholic	Yes	Believe the bread and wine are the Body and Blood of Christ.
Seventh Day Adventists	Yes	Practice washing of the feet in preparation.
United Church of Christ	Yes	Considered a sacrament.

Summary

The practical nurse has the responsibility to care for the total person: physical, emotional, and spiritual. Spiritual needs of patients arise out of their desire to find meaning in life, suffering, and death. In order to meet the spiritual needs of patients, you must be aware of personal spiritual beliefs, or the absence of them. Members of the health team who assist the practical nurse in meeting patient's spiritual needs are the minister, priest, rabbi, chaplain, and pastoral team. Many patients will help meet their personal spiritual needs by belonging to an organized religion. Spiritual distress can occur when patients cannot fulfill the rituals and practices of their religion and/or experience conflict between their spiritual beliefs and health regimen. For these reasons, you must develop an awareness of religious differences and an understanding of basic beliefs, rituals, and practices of the many religious denominations and sects that exist today. Although the majority of patients in the United States will be Protestant, Catholic, and Jewish, there are other denominations you will encounter, including individuals who have no religious beliefs. By learning about these groups, you will be able to accommodate their beliefs and practices and be able to say "I have met the needs of the total person."

REFERENCES

Abu-Saad H. Middle Eastern nursing students in the U.S. Nurs Educ 1982; 21(7):22–25.

Adams C. *A Reader's Guide to the Great Religions*. 2nd ed. New York: Free Press, 1977.

Anderson G. Medicine vs. religion: the case of the Jehovah's Witnesses. Health Social Work 1983; 8(1):31–38.

Assemblies of God. In: *World Book Encyclopedia.* Vol. 1. Chicago: World Book, 1983:781.

Bahá'ís. In: *World Book Encyclopedia.* Vol. 2. Chicago: World Book, 1983:25.

Bamberger B. Judaism. In: *Academic American Encyclopedia.* Vol. 15. Danbury, CT: Grolier, 1982:458–463.

Booty J. Anglicans. In: *World Book Encyclopedia.* Vol. 1. Chicago: World Book, 1983:439–440.

Burghardt W. Roman Catholic Church. In: *World Book Encyclopedia.* Vol. 16. Chicago: World Book, 1983:375–379.

Burkle H. Christianity. In: *World Book Encyclopedia.* Vol. 3. Chicago: World Book, 1983:406–407.

Carson V. *Spiritual Dimensions of Nursing Practice.* Philadelphia: WB Saunders, 1989.

Capps W. Religion. In: *World Book Encyclopedia.* Vol. 16. Chicago: World Book, 1983:206–216a.

Carpenito L. *Nursing Diagnosis: Application to Clinical Practice.* Philadelphia: JB Lippincott, 1983:451–466.

Conflict: religious belief vs. emergency care . . . patients who have refused to consent to life saving blood transfusions. Emerg Nurse Legal Bull 1982; 8(4):2–9.

DiMeo E. Rx for spiritual distress. RN 1991; 54(3):22–24.

Fielding WJ. *The Shackles of the Supernatural.* New York: Vantage, 1969.

Gershan J. Judaic ethical beliefs and customs regarding death and dying. Crit Care Nurse 1985; 5(1):32–34.

Henley A, Clayton J. Illness and the life cycle. Health Social Serv J 1982; 92:972–974.

Idem. Religion of the Muslims. Health Social Serv J 1982; 92:918–919.

Herbster B. United Church of Christ. In: *World Book Encyclopedia.* Vol. 20. Chicago: World Book, 1983:22.

Heywood-Jones I. Bearing witness. Nurs Times 1984; 80(6):47.

Idem. Nursing on the Sabbath. Nurs Times 1984; 80(9):47.

Hudson W. Baptists. In: *World Book Encyclopedia.* Vol. 2. Chicago: World Book, 1983:71–72.

Kamell M. *The Middle East: A Humanistic Approach.* Elizabeth, NJ: Andrews, 1973.

Marty M. Protestantism. In: *World Book Encyclopedia.* Vol. 15. Chicago: World Book, 1983:735–737.

McBride A. *Invitation: A Catholic Learning Guide for Adults.* Washington, DC: Paulist National Catholic Evangelization Association, 1984.

Melton J. *The Encyclopedia of American Religions.* Vol. 1 and 2. Wilmington, NC: McGrath, 1978.

Mormons. In: *World Book Encyclopedia.* Vol. 13. Chicago: World Book, 1983:662–665.

Murray R, Zentner J. *Nursing Assessment and Health Promotion Strategies Throughout the Lifespan.* 4th ed. East Norwalk, CT: Appleton & Lange, 1989.

Nichols JH. Presbyterians. In: *World Book Encyclopedia.* Vol. 15. Chicago: World Book, 1983:676–677.

Piepgrass R. The other dimension: spiritual help. Am J Nurs 1968; 68(12):2610–2613.

Quakers. In: *World Book Encyclopedia.* Vol. 16. Chicago: World Book, 1983:3.

Rabinowicz H. The Jewish view of death. Nurs Times 1979; 75(18):757.

Recognizing your patient's spiritual needs. Nursing 77 1977; 7(12):64, 66–70.

Saylor D. The spiritual self. J Pract Nurs 1977; 27(8):16–17, 30.

Stoll R. Guidelines for spiritual assessment. Am J Nurs 1979; 79(9):1574–1577.

Walker C. Attitudes to death and bereavement among cultural minority groups. Nurs Times 1982; 78(50):2106–2109.

When patients refuse blood. Emerg Med 1984; 16(18):65, 69.

Wiggins L. Health and illness beliefs and practices among the old order Amish. Health Values 1983; 7(6):24–29.

Wood E. Methodists. In: *World Book Encyclopedia.* Vol. 6. Chicago: World Book, 1983:358–359.

Zernov N. Eastern Orthodox Churches. In: *World Book Encyclopedia.* Vol. 6. Chicago: World Book, 1983:43–44.

part V
WHERE YOU ARE GOING

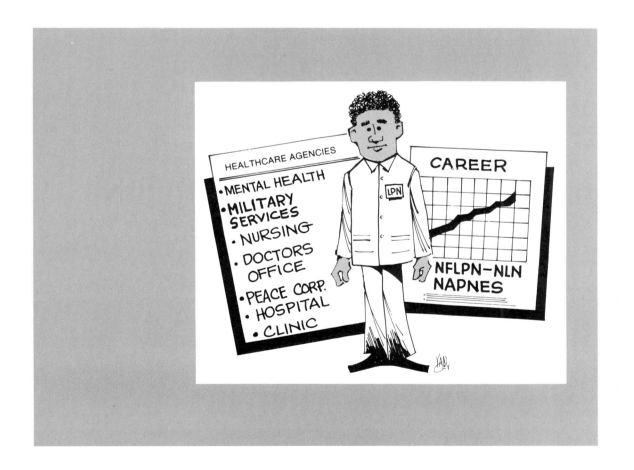

CHAPTER 16
Agencies That Deliver Health Care Services

Learning Objectives

Upon completing this chapter, you will
1. Compare public and private health care agencies according to the following criteria:
   a. source of funding,
   b. services provided,
   c. examples of agencies in your geographic area,
   d. possible place of employment for practical nurses.
2. Discuss the following methods of payment for health care services:
   a. personal payment (private pay),
   b. nongovernmental health insurance plans,
   c. government-sponsored health insurance plans.
3. Discuss the effects of the following trends on health care agencies and employment:
   a. changes in the nature of the population,
   b. shifting of nursing supply and demand,
   c. increase of health care costs,
   d. rise of alternative delivery systems of health care.

INTRODUCTION

It is difficult to discuss the American health care system because it is a very complex one, made up of many different agencies and individuals whose services sometimes stand alone and sometimes overlap. It is possible to understand the health care system in our country when the various services are put into two general categories—services delivered by the *public sector* and those delivered by the *private sector.* Knowledge of agencies that deliver health care services is necessary so that the practical nurse is aware of health resources available to the patient. The various health care agencies could also be a potential source of employment for persons in health care.

PUBLIC VERSUS PRIVATE HEALTH CARE AGENCIES

There are two types of public health care agencies—*official* and *voluntary.* Official health care agencies are government agencies that are supported by tax money, are accountable to the taxpayers and the government, and engage in services that are mandated by law. The primary emphasis of government (official) agencies is delivering programs of disease prevention and wellness promotion, but direct service of health care is sometimes provided.

Voluntary agencies are supported by voluntary contributions and sometimes by a fee for service. Although they are tuned in to public opinion, voluntary agencies are accountable to their supporters, and their activities are determined by supporter interest, not legal mandate. Their primary emphasis is research and education, but may also offer direct health services to the consumer. Some of the official and voluntary health care agencies operate at the local, state, federal, and international level.

Perhaps you are most familiar with private health care agencies because entrance to the health care delivery system in the United States is generally gained through these agencies. Although some voluntary or nonprofit agencies are found in the private sector, private health care agencies are generally proprietary, or for-profit, and a fee is charged for their services. Their primary emphasis has been curing disease and illness, although the past few years has brought about a change in emphasis to include disease prevention and wellness promotion. Table 16-1 outlines the major differences between public and private health care agencies. As you read about public and private health care agencies, think of them as potential sources of employment for the practical nurse.

Examples of Public Health Care Agencies

Local Level

The official health agency at the local level is the city or county health department, which is funded by local tax money as well as by subsidies from the state and federal levels of government. The local health department carries out state laws concerning community health, but can also establish its own laws.

State Level

Although the organization and name may differ, each state has a state health department, an official health agency that is funded from state tax money and sometimes receives money from the federal government.

Federal (National) Level

The official health agency at the federal level is the Department of Health and Human Services (HHS), which was created in 1980, when the former Department of Health, Education, and Welfare was reorganized. It is funded by federal taxes and is headed by a person appointed by the President of the United States, who advises the President in health matters. The division of the Department of Health and Human Services that is concerned primarily with health is the U.S. Public Health Service (USPHS). The six agencies that make up the USPHS are as follows:

Table 16-1 A General Comparison of Health Care Agencies in the Public and Private Sectors

	PUBLIC		PRIVATE
	OFFICIAL (GOVERNMENT)	NONOFFICIAL (VOLUNTARY)	
SUPPORT	Tax money	Voluntary contributions and fees for service	Fees for service
PRIMARY SERVICE	Programs of disease prevention and wellness promotion	Research and education	Curing disease and illness
ADDITIONAL SERVICES	Sometimes direct service of health care	Offer direct health services	Disease prevention and wellness promotion
ACCOUNTA-BILITY	Taxpayers and government	Supporters, boards, etc.	Owners
HOW PROGRAMS DETERMINED	Legal mandate	Supporter interest	Defined goals of the organization

- Food and Drug Administration (FDA)
- Centers for Disease Control (CDC)
- National Institutes of Health (NIH)
- Health Services Administration (HSA)
- Health Resources Administration (HRA)
- Alcohol, Drug Abuse, and Mental Health Administration

International Level

Health activities take place at the international level through the World Health Organization (WHO), an agency of the United Nations. The WHO is located in Geneva, Switzerland. The major objective of the WHO is the highest possible level of health for all people of the world. This organization defines health as a state of complete physical, mental, and social well-being and not merely the absence of disease or infirmity. The WHO is funded through fees paid by member nations of the United Nations.

Examples of Voluntary Health Care Agencies

Voluntary or nonofficial health care agencies are so named because they are not for profit. The health services they provide are complementary to official health agencies, and often meet the needs of persons with specific diseases (for example, heart disease) and certain segments of the population (for example, the handicapped). Although there are paid personnel working in voluntary health agencies, volunteers form a major support system. A few examples of voluntary health agencies follow. Refer to your local telephone directory for additional names and numbers of voluntary health care agencies.

Community Hospitals

These nonprofit hospitals are operated by community associations or religious organizations and provide short-term inpatient care for acute illnesses and injuries.

Visiting Nurse Association (VNA)

This public voluntary agency provides home nursing care for those with acute and chronic diseases; its members also make visits to mothers with newborns. Visiting nurses are engaged in health teaching and frequently involve the family in the care of their loved ones. Visiting nurses also assist with referrals for patients to other community services.

American Cancer Society

This voluntary agency, a national organization with state and local chapters, is involved in extensive cancer research, education of the public regarding cancer, and is a source of up-to-date information for health professionals in the prevention, diagnosis, and treatment of cancer. This association also assists patients with referrals and supplies as needed.

American Lung Association

This voluntary agency conducts research for respiratory and lung diseases, including asthma, and provides educational materials for the general public and health care workers. The Christmas seals you receive each fall help to support this organization.

Alcoholics Anonymous

This voluntary agency provides help for the alcoholic, if it is desired, and also provides help for families of alcoholics.

ALS Society of America

This voluntary organization gathers information about patients with amyotrophic lateral sclerosis (Lou Gehrig's disease) for research pur-

poses, provides information about this rare disease to lay persons and health care workers, and gives patient care tips to nursing personnel.

National Easter Seal Society

This voluntary organization conducts research and provides information about cerebral palsy to the public and to health care workers.

LaLeche League

This voluntary organization provides information and support for breastfeeding mothers and provides breast milk for infants who must have this form of nourishment, but do not have a source.

United Ostomy Association (UOA)

This voluntary organization provides education and support to patients who have had ostomy or urinary-diversion surgery.

Examples of Private Health Care Agencies

Private health care agencies also complement and supplement government agencies. Perhaps the most change in health services in the past few years has been noted in this area, as compared with public health services in general.

Family-Practice Physician

Primary care is a term used to describe the point at which an individual enters the health care system. Family-practice physicians are a source of primary care. These physicians provide diagnosis and treatment, and the patient is billed a fee for the services. If further diagnostic evaluation is needed, the patient is referred to a specialist. See Appendix C for a listing of specialists.

Health Maintenance Organization (HMO)

The HMO is an organized health care delivery system that is a form of prepaid group physician practice. The subscriber pays a fixed amount per year in advance to the HMO, and then receives all medical care with little or no additional payment each time the services of a doctor is provided. This prepaid plan establishes the incentive to contain costs and services. HMOs place emphasis on health promotion and illness prevention. Treatment services are also offered by HMOs.

Proprietary Hospitals

For-profit hospitals are operated for the financial benefit of the owner of the hospital, who can be an individual, a partnership, or a corporation. The profit is earned by running the hospital efficiently, using management techniques.

Outpatient Clinics

Outpatient clinics provide follow-up care to patients after hospitalization, and management of disease on an ambulatory basis for those who do not need to be hospitalized. Outpatient clinics are generally part of a hospital and function by appointment only. Patients are seen in specialty areas such as diabetes, neurology, allergy, and oncology. The number of specialized clinics depends on the size of the hospital, and a full-time staff is employed.

Ambulatory Care Facilities (Urgent Care Centers)

Facilities are available for walk-in patients who do not have an appointment. These clinics make available primary health care as an alternative to being seen by a family doctor and, therefore, are used by persons who do not have a family physician or who desire quick service outside of regular office hours. The names given to these services reflect the type of care they provide: Convenience Clinics, Express Care, Quick Care, etc.

Ambulatory Surgery Centers

One-day surgical care centers perform surgery at a scheduled date and time, and discharge the patient when he or she has recovered from the anesthesia, eliminating the need to be hospitalized overnight. These services are also known as outpatient surgery within an established hospital. Free-standing outpatient surgery hospitals provide outpatient surgery as their only service.

Free Clinics

Some communities have established free clinics as an alternative means of obtaining primary health care. These clinics are used by persons who cannot afford traditional health services or are reluctant to use more traditional services. The fee is minimal and the environment is as free of red tape as possible.

Long-Term (Extended) Care

Long-term–care units offer care for patients who need more time to recover than short terms of hospitalization would allow. These facilities offer nursing care with an emphasis on restoring individuals to their personal level of physical and emotional wellness and returning them to their homes and families. Extended care services can be found as part of existing hospitals or as separate facilities and as part of nursing homes.

Nursing Homes

Nursing homes are institutions that have taken the responsibility for the care of persons who are disabled, terminally ill, homeless, and/or helpless when their families cannot or will not care for them at home. Although the aged and elderly are frequently seen as nursing home residents, these health care agencies will also serve chronically ill persons of all age groups. The level of care required by residents is defined by the level of nursing care required—either skilled, intermediate, or custodial.

Home Health Care Agencies

Home care programs provide a variety of health services in the home, such as nursing, occupational therapy, and physical therapy. Some agencies also provide homemaker and companion services. Hospitals are developing home care agencies as adjuncts of care, and private agencies are offering services in an effort to keep people in their homes for treatment.

Adult Day Care Centers

Hospital-based and proprietary adult day care centers provide services for individuals who need supervision because of physical or safety needs, yet are not candidates for nursing home placement.

Wellness Centers

An emphasis on promoting wellness has resulted in a multitude of services in this area of health care. Not only have hospitals developed programs to detect disease in early stages, but they have also developed programs to promote wellness through nutritional counseling, exercise programs, stress reduction, and weight control. The private sector is also active in the wellness area. People have an interest in exercise and fitness clubs, weight-reduction programs such as Weight Watchers, and smoking cessation classes.

METHOD OF PAYMENT

It is helpful for the practical nurse to have a knowledge of the different methods by which hospitalized or ambulatory patients pay their health care bills. Health care is expensive, and cost containment, the holding of costs to within fixed limits, is a goal of most public and private health care agencies today. The practical nurse should remember that regardless of who pays the health care bill, equipment and supplies should never be wasted. All of us benefit when such an attitude is adopted. Knowledge of methods of payment for health care services will also help the practical nurse develop an awareness and understanding of the value of health insurance as a fringe benefit of employment.

Personal Payment (Private Pay)

Paying the cost of health care directly out of pocket was the primary method of payment of health care costs prior to the 1940s. This method of payment is used by some patients today, but the cost of health care services discourages the use of this method for the average person.

Private Group Health Insurance (Nongovernment)

Group health insurance is the pooling of individual contributions for a common group goal—protection from financial disaster due to health care bills. When insured, the individual is said to have third-party coverage, that is, a fiscal middleman, who will pay health care bills. Two examples of private group health insurance are

- Blue Cross and Blue Shield—Blue Cross covers hospital inpatient costs and Blue Shield covers inpatient physician costs. A major medical plan is available to include the cost of some outpatient services. Individuals can purchase coverage from Blue Cross and Blue Shield but the cost is higher than group plans.

- Health policies through commercial insurance companies—Many of the major insurance companies offer health insurance to individuals and groups.

Government-Sponsored Health Insurance Plans

Medicare

The aged generally find themselves ineligible for group insurance plans because they are unemployed, and they cannot afford private plans for the same reason; this occurs at a time when some individuals require more hospitalization and medical care because of their age. In 1965, a provision was added to the Social Security Act in the form of a federally sponsored and supervised health insurance plan that financed health care for all persons over age 65. Part A of the Medicare bill involves hospital benefits and applies to persons under age 65 who are permanently and totally disabled and to victims of end-stage renal disease. Coverage is also offered for posthospitalization convalescence in extended-care facilities and home health services. Part A is available without cost to those who meet eligibility requirements, but includes a deductible.

Part B of Medicare is similar to a major medical plan, as it includes inpatient and outpatient physician services and a wide range of other related services for people over 65. Part B is available for a monthly premium to those who are eligible for enrollment. Many persons over age 65 also carry some form of private supplemental coverage in addition to Medicare to cover deductibles, coinsurance, and limited-coverage situations that exist in the federal program.

Medicaid

The poor generally find themselves ineligible for private insurance coverage for the same reasons as the aged. Another provision that was added to the Social Security Act in 1965 was the Medicaid program, which expanded the financial assistance provided to states and counties to pay for medical services for the poor. The Medicaid system developed out of the welfare system to service low-income families. Medicaid is a system of federal grants to states to match their expenditures in the area of payment of health care costs for people eligible for the program.

WHAT TRENDS CAN TELL YOU

"What is in store for me in the area of job possibilities in practical nursing?" Although it is impossible to predict the future, it is possible to identify trends that generally affect your career in the present and to predict their possible influence on the direction of your career in the future. Health care in the United States is changing rapidly and dramatically. Each change may place new demands and restrictions on or present opportunities to those involved in health care careers. We have identified four trends involving health care today, the impact of these trends on health care in the present, and possible effects on nursing in the future, especially in the area of employment. The trends are

1. Changes in the nature of the population,

2. Shifting of nursing supply and demand,

3. Increase of health care costs,

4. Rise of alternative systems of delivery of health care.

Changes in the Nature of the Population

The population of the United States and Canada is getting older and living longer. Starting in the 1970s, the birth rate has decreased at the same time that the number of persons over age 65 has increased. By 2000, it is estimated that the number of persons over age 65 will continue to increase to 34.9 million persons. By 2030, projections state there will be 65.6 million persons over age 65. Clearly, these projections indicate that the population of the United States continues to get older (National Population Projections, 1989, p. 6). In addition, the National Commission to Prevent Infant Mortality reports that the infant mortality rate (the number of infants who die in the first year of life) has decreased to 9.8 infant deaths per 1000 live births in 1989 (*Green Bay Press-Gazette,* March 26, 1992). We have also experienced a decrease in the general death rate. Some of the causes for these changes are improved health care (especially in the area of public health), advances in medical science, increased standard of living, and prevention of illness and promotion of wellness.

At the turn of the century, a major cause of death was infection, especially pneumonia and communicable diseases. The development of immunizations and environmental health measures to prevent communicable diseases and antibiotics to cure infectious diseases have been responsible for decreasing the death rate from these conditions. People still die from pneumonia, but today, heart attack, stroke, and cancer are the major causes of death. Thanks to advances in technology and medical science, some people are having today's killer diseases diagnosed in the early stages. These diseases are becoming chronic diseases for some, the diseases they have to live with in the extra years they have gained in life expectancy. Also, in living longer, people are more prone to the development of degenerative diseases, such as arthritis, that become evident as the body declines or deteriorates with age. Emphasis on personal wellness in the areas of physical fitness, nutrition, and control of stress is helping some people live not only longer, but better.

Our population is getting older, but this does not mean that all people in the older age group are becoming invalids or dependent on others. However, this increase in the elderly population as a whole carries with it an increasing percentage of people who depend on others for assistance in meeting their daily needs.

Impact on Jobs for Practical Nurses

We have seen the increased emphasis on a lifestyle for wellness create jobs for practical nurses with weight loss programs, holistic health, nutrition, and aerobics. Nursing homes and adult day care centers help meet the needs of those in our aging population who are dependent because of chronic disease; this subpopulation is increasingly becoming a source of employment for practical nurses.

Shifting of Nursing Supply and Demand

Traditionally, all levels of nursing have been attractive choices for women. Since the late 1970s there continues to be an increase in the number of men who enter nursing school. The age of applicants to nursing programs has increased. However, during the 1980s, nursing school enrollments began to decline. The National League for Nursing documented more than a 26% decrease in applications to registered nursing programs over a several-year period (Morrissey, 1987, p. 198).

Reasons for Past Decline in Nursing School Enrollments

Reasons for the past decline in nursing school enrollments have included

1. A general decline in enrollments in all programs and courses of study in technical schools, junior colleges, and colleges and universities. New high school graduates have traditionally filled programs in higher education. The number of high school graduates has declined. There are more people in the United States over age 65 than there are teenagers (Choate and Linger, 1986, p. 27).

2. The women's movement has encouraged women to choose from a wider variety of career possibilities. Traditionally, when asked what they wanted to be when they grew up, little girls responded: a secretary, housewife, nurse, teacher, or librarian. Today, women are becoming cab drivers, business and management trainees, coal miners, nuclear engineers, lawyers, and anything else they want to be.

3. Potential students of programs of higher education were aware of the issues nursing faces, including the issue of entry into practice and the attempt to establish two levels of nursing in the 1980s. Nursing was not looked at as an attractive option because the scope of practice, educational programs, and licensing requirements for the potential two levels of nursing were undecided and unestablished.

4. Financial aid decreased at the same time that tuitions increased. Many potential nursing students were adults with adult responsibilities and could not afford to give up their jobs to pursue their education. They sought programs of shorter length and attended school part time.

Nursing school enrollments are once again increasing after a steady decline in the 1980s. From 1987 to the fall of 1990, practical nursing program enrollments have experienced remarkable growth. This growth represents a 13% increase in enrollment. The enrollment levels continue to be lower than in previous years (*Nursing DataSource 1991,* p. 9). The continuing nursing shortage has helped make nursing an attractive career for many. Enrollments continue to rise, with some schools having waiting lists for admission. Nursing education programs have been successful in attracting older adult students, including college graduates. They are choosing nursing as a first or a second career because a job in nursing is guaranteed after graduation. This more mature type of student may lend more stability to health care institution work forces because these nurses generally tend to be less mobile and well established in the community. Nursing schools will continue to try to attract this type of student.

Reasons for a Continuing Nursing Shortage

Although an improvement has been seen, a shortage of nurses currently exists in most regions of the United States. Most hospitals continue recruitment efforts to attract nurses. The shortage is predicted through the year 2000. Why is the nursing shortage continuing despite increasing enrollments in nursing programs? The following offers an explanation for the continuation of the need for nurses:

1. Predecline enrollment numbers have not been realized.

2. New roles for nurses are continuously developed. All requests by employers for nurses cannot be filled from current supplies.

3. Schools of nursing cannot admit all qualified students that apply because of a lack of resources to enlarge existing programs. Lack of resources include money to expand present programs, facilities for clinical experience, and adequately prepared faculty.

4. Financial aid continues to decrease.

5. Women continue to choose from a wide variety of career opportunities, while the numbers of men enrolling in nursing programs are not large enough to offset this loss.

Impact on Jobs for Practical Nurses

Currently, some hospitals that previously laid off practical nurses are offering positions to these nurses. Some schools of practical nursing that were closed have been reopened. The help wanted section of newspapers display the continued need for registered and practical nurses.

The emphasis on quality assurance is being replaced with an emphasis on quality improvement. Quality assurance stressed the identification of care that needed to be given to patients and the evaluation of the results of that care. Quality improvement stresses the need to search continually for new ways to improve patient care. This makes approaches to nursing problems a never-ending quest (Hurley, 1991, p. 45).

A major way of ensuring quality of care in nursing has been the formulation of nursing care plans by the registered nurse, assisted by the practical nurse. The Joint Commission on Accreditation of Hospitals has removed the requirement for a separate nursing care plan for each patient (Hurley, 1991, p. 43). Whatever method might replace the nursing care plan, practical nurses will still have the responsibility of assisting the registered nurse with the task of planning care. They have proven themselves safe and effective in delivering patient care as planned by the registered nurse.

Increase of Health Care Costs

Perhaps the trend that is having the greatest impact on health care is the increasing cost of health care services. In 1960, $27 billion a year was spent on health care in the United States (Wolff, 1983, p. 46). In the 1990s, the cost of health care has climbed to over $500 billion a year (Anthony, 1991, p. 61). Reasons for this dramatic increase in the amount of money spent on health care include

1. The increased availability and demand of health care. The American consumer has come to expect health care services.

2. Development and use of costly technology for the diagnosis and treatment of disease.

3. Rising cost of salaries for persons working in health care careers.

Diagnosis-Related Groups (DRGs)

Since payment for health care was the fourth largest item in the federal budget and the federal deficit (less money on hand as compared with what is needed to run all programs) was consistently getting to be a larger amount, the federal government was the first group to try to stop the skyrocketing cost of health care. On

October 1, 1983, the Health Care Financing Administration adopted a system of paying hospitals a set fee for services by telling them in advance how much the hospitals would be reimbursed. Because the government announces to a hospital in advance what it will pay for health care costs, this system is called the prospective-payment system. Prior to 1983, hospitals submitted a bill to the government for total charges for Medicare and Medicaid patients and were reimbursed. Under the new DRG system, hospitals have an incentive to treat patients and discharge them as quickly as possible because they receive a flat fee for each patient regardless of length of stay. If the hospital keeps the patient longer than the government's fee will cover, the hospital has to make up the difference in costs.

Impact on Jobs for Practical Nurses

As Medicare patients are discharged sooner from hospitals than they were in the past (because of the DRG system of reimbursement), extended-care units are frequently used to continue convalescence. These units need more skilled health care workers, such as the practical nurse.

Rise of Alternative Systems of Delivery of and Payment for Health Care

The trend involving the rise of alternative systems of delivery of health care is a result, in part, of the dramatic increase in health care costs seen in recent years. Traditionally, the hospital was the major provider of health care. Today, the hospital is being used less and less, as the emphasis is on the more seriously ill patient and new delivery systems are being developed for health care. Ambulatory care centers for medical and surgical patients have dramatically reduced the need for overnight hospitalization. Home health agencies provide health care services in the home as an alternative to hospital admission. The popularity and effectiveness of these alternatives are displayed in the decreased number of inpatient hospitalizations. The new delivery systems also have made services more convenient and efficient for the consumer of health care.

Private Health Insurance

The government's DRG system has influenced private insurers for health care costs to adopt cost-cutting measures. Some employers offering health insurance are requiring second opinions for surgery, clearance for hospitalization, and are offering reduced premiums for selected wellness practices. Hospitalized patients with health insurance are finding themselves being discharged sooner than they expected.

Health Maintenance Organizations (HMOs)

In 1973, President Nixon passed the Health Maintenance Organization Act as a means of promoting private sector medicine through self-regulation, while giving incentives for containing health care costs. The law provided grants and loans to establish new HMOs. No new grants were awarded during the 1980s.

As a result of the above cost-cutting measures, the number of persons admitted to hospitals has decreased in the past few years. When patients are admitted, they are generally more acutely ill, requiring more skilled nursing care. On discharge, these same patients are leaving the hospital seemingly sicker than they were in the past on discharge. They really are not sicker, they are just leaving the hospital sooner. For this reason, a number of patients must go to extended-care facilities (long-term care) to complete their recuperation or have health care services in their home.

National Health Plan

Because of the number of persons who do not have access to Medicare, Medicaid, and private health insurance, nursing has suggested a National Health Plan. This plan emphasizes prevention, primary care, home care, and long-term care. It suggests that nurses are cost-saving key providers and coordinators of health care. This plan would provide universal access to health care for all persons in the United States.

Impact on Jobs for Practical Nurses

Practical nurses may obtain jobs in ambulatory-care settings, and acute care, but the home health care agencies are a frequent employer of practical nurses. Again, extended-care units are a source of employment for the practical nurse.

A decrease in health care agency admissions, especially for elective services, may be observed in some areas of the United States. This decrease may be accounted for by *inability to pay* for rising hospital costs, including *lack of insurance benefits* because of loss of jobs. As a result, regionally, some health care agencies have initiated a temporary hiring freeze for all levels of nursing. When hospital admissions increase, those agencies that initiated a temporary hiring freeze will resume standard hiring practices.

QUESTION: What could be three reasons for declining hospital admissions?

Summary

Health care services are delivered in the public and private sectors. Public health care agencies are classified as official and voluntary. Official health care agencies are supported by taxes, and voluntary health care agencies are supported by contributions. Private health care agencies are generally proprietary or for-profit. Public and private health care agencies are interested in the prevention of disease and promotion of wellness, but private agencies are more involved in providing direct care. Some public and private health agencies can potentially be places of employment for the practical nurse. The cost of health care has dramatically increased in past years, and method of payment is a major issue and concern for the consumer of health care. Insurance, both private and government-sponsored, are major third-party-payment systems today. Trends, or possible new directions of health care, can be identified and help the practical nurse become aware of potential employers.

REFERENCES

Anthony J. Anatomy of a hospital bill. Health, 1991; 5(2):60–62; 67–68.

Carty R, Bednash G. Insights from the past portray nurses of the future. Nurs Health Care 1985; 6:493–496.

Choate P, Linger JK. The shape of things to come. Voc Educ J 1986; 61(7):26–29.

Dire nursing shortage looms heavily over health industry horizon. Executive Director Wire (An NLN Publication). 1986; September/October:2.

Domers I. RUG-II, a case mix reimbursement systems for long term care. The Communique: Quarterly Publication of the Wisconsin League for Nursing 1986; 5(3):80–82.

Drew J. Health maintenance organization: history, evolution, and survival. Nurs Health Care 1990; 11:145–149.

Dugas B. *Introduction to Patient Care: A Comprehensive Approach to Nursing.* 4th ed. Philadelphia: WB Saunders, 1983: 3–9.

Fewer new nursing students may mean an RN shortage. RN 1986; 49(10):8.

Health United States 1989. Hyattsville, MD: Department of Health and Human Services. (DHHS publication no. (PHS) 90-1232.)

Hurley ML. What do the new JCAHO Standards mean for you? RN 1991; 54(6):42–46.

Kinney E. An LPN looks at the developing LPN role. Issues (A Publication of the National Council of State Boards of Nursing) 1986; 7(2):6—7.

League to prescribe Rx for recruitment and retention. Nurs Health Care 1985; 6(1):181.

Morrissey K. The nursing crunch is on. Nurs Health Care 1987; 8(3):198.

National Population Projections 1989. Special studies series P-23, No. 159, April 1989. Washington, DC: Department of Commerce.

Nook J. Trends forecast potential crises. The Communique: Quarterly Publication of the Wisconsin League for Nursing 1986; 5(2):49.

Nursing DataSource 1991. Vol. 2. Publication no. 19-2421. New York: National League for Nursing.

Nursing school enrollments up in 1988. Legislative Network for Nurses 1989; 6(1):1—8.

Ringold E. The crises in nursing. Working Mother 1985; October:36, 38, 40.

Rising nursing school enrollments are reason for optimism: NLN. Legislative Network for Nursing 1991; 8(1):1—6.

Rosenfeld P. Nursing education: statistics you can use. Nurs Health Care 1986; 7:327—329.

Rowland H. *The Nurse's Almanac.* 2nd ed. Rockville, MD: Aspen Systems, 1984.

Stanhope M, Lancaster J. *Community Health Nursing.* St Louis: CV Mosby, 1988.

Ten trends to watch. Nurs Health Care 1986; 7(1):17—19.

Wolff I. Fundamentals of Nursing, 7th ed. Philadelphia: JB Lippincott, 1983:43—54.

U.S. Lags in Child Health, Report Says. *Green Bay Press-Gazette.* Green-Bay, WI, March 26, 1992, Vol. 76, No. 273, p. A-4.

CHAPTER
17
Career Mobility and Vocational Organizations

Learning Objectives

Upon completing this chapter, you will
1. Identify areas of LPN employment available in your community at present.
2. State four types of progression programs available to practical nurses.
3. Discuss the purpose of
   a. NFLPN
   b. NAPNES
   c. HOSA
   d. NLN
   e. alumni associations
4. Name a journal written especially for practical nurses.

INTRODUCTION

Introductory courses in nursing are meant to excite you about the process of nursing education, the careers available in practical nursing, the vocational organization support groups, and how you can be a part of it all. The formal educational process opens up new doors of knowledge, skill, and responsibility for you. Many of the things you see and learn about will create a sense of awe and excitement for you. The careers in practical nursing are varied: some of you have already made decisions in advance, such as serving in the Peace Corps, working in a nursing home, or perhaps going into the military services. Both usual and atypical careers await you.

Many schools also introduce student practical nurses to the state affiliate of the National Federation of Licensed Practical Nurses (NFLPN) by having you attend the state association of Licensed Practical Nurses convention. Most state conventions include programming especially for student practical nurses. Some state and local associations offer a student membership rate as an inducement to joining prior to graduation. Keep in mind that practical nursing organizations and organizations that include practical nurses are your support groups. The members understand practical nursing—the joys and the challenges that you experience. Participation in your professional organization is encouraged to keep you up to date on issues that affect practical nursing. Remember—no voice, no vote!

CAREER MOBILITY
Employment Opportunities

Extended-Care Facilities

Chapter 16 discusses the growing number of persons age 65 and over which has a positive impact on the availability of jobs for practical nurses. The Omnibus Budget Reconciliation Act (OBRA) of 1987 mandates that as of October 1, 1990, "all Skilled Nursing Facilities (SNF) and Intermediate Care Facilities (ICF) provide 24-hour licensed practical nurse care 7 days a week, with at least one RN employed 7 days a week, 8 hours a day" (*Nursing DataSource 1991,* p. 4). Although this requirement can be waived if personnel are unavailable, if you enjoy longer-term contact with people, this employment option is certainly available and may be the area for you.

The nursing home population is made up of residents who are completing recovery from surgery or trauma and are too well for the hospital but not well enough to go home; elderly people who are unable to care for themselves because of medical or psychological impairment; mentally retarded people who are unable to live independently or in group homes; young to middle-aged victims of chronic debilitating disease or accidents; and young chronically mentally ill persons who need continuing supervision and are not candidates for independent living or halfway houses.

Special qualities needed for this kind of nursing include patience, ability to see below the surface, willingness to listen, maturity, ability to determine priorities, ability to set limits, interest in working with people with disabilities, willingness to work with other health care givers, communication skills, acute observation skills of physical change, and a sense of security regarding your value system. LPNs who work in nursing homes are challenged to assist in providing a homelike atmosphere, while dealing with immediate, long-term, and terminal health problems of the residents.

The level of responsibility is great, in that the LPN frequently works in a charge nurse role, and although supervision is available from a RN, at some periods of the day it may be general, meaning at the other end of the telephone. Consequently, a solid knowledge base is essential for knowing when to seek help and from whom.

The charge nurse role also means being responsible for managing care given by other LPNs, aides, and orderlies. It includes a willingness to assume responsibility for correlating assignments according to the skill of staff members, checking to see that care is given correctly and humanely, demonstrating appropriate care as needed, knowing the effect of medication dispensed, and always serving as a positive role model for care and treatment of the residents. Charge nurse responsibilities are usually not part of a basic curriculum. Prior to assuming that responsibility, you will need to take a "LPN charge nurse" continuing education course.

As the LPN in a nursing home facility, you frequently deal directly with the resident's response to being in the facility. It is not always the resident's wish to be there. Furthermore, you must be comfortable with your personal values in order to avoid judging the family members' reasons for admitting the resident. Family members need to be heard, as a prelude to gaining their cooperation in working with the resident. Much of your work ultimately relates to attaining or maintaining whatever the resident is capable of, in all areas of health. Residents who are recuperating from surgery or trauma realize their goal of discharge. For some residents, your role includes supporting them through the final step of the growth process—a dignified death.

Home Health Care

Because of shorter hospital stays, the home health care industry is flourishing. The actual care is under the supervision of a RN, who makes the initial assessment and the nursing diagnosis and develops the plan of care. The postdischarge (subacute) level of care fits in well with the LPN's basic education, thereby making the LPN invaluable in implementing the plan of care. The LPN's background adds to the continuing data collection and evaluation of the plan of care. Because of difficulty in receiving payment from nonprivate sources, some home health agencies use LPNs for private-pay patients only. Others employ LPNs as home health aides to avoid the restrictions. This is an unfortunate practice, since the pay is lower and you are always held to your highest license in legal situations.

Helpful qualities for home health nursing include: (1) flexibility—you will have to do an amount of improvising in the home and yet practice sound nursing principles; (2) communications skills—you will be working in the patient's domain; you have to both understand the patient's expression of needs and make sure that you express yourself clearly (and tactfully); (3) self-confidence—unlike the hospital area, an air of insecurity or uncertainty will be picked up by the patient, because the supervising person is not on the premises. This does not imply that you fake it. Rather it implies that you do what you know is accurate; do not ask for unnecessary reassurance when doing basic skills. Question what you do not know, but do it away from the patient unless an emergency exists; (4) sensitivity to physical and emotional changes—once the initial assessment is completed by the RN, it will be up to you to be alert to any changes of which the RN must be made aware. The RN must be able to depend on your observational skills for safety's sake; (5) ability to deal with emergencies—staying calm and following the agency protocol is essential; (6) nonjudgmental—a must, since you work right in the home. Remember at all times that you are providing a service. If you are comfortable with your own values, different values are no longer personally threatening.

Mental Health Nursing

Mental health nursing includes both community mental health centers and halfway houses for the recovering mentally ill. It is interesting to note that many community mental health centers are staffed primarily with LPNs and nursing assistants, with RNs in a supervisory role. Yet some practical nursing programs do not include a mental nursing component—theory or clinical experience.

In this area of work, LPNs are involved in doing treatments, dispensing medications, and tending to basic daily care needs such as bathing and supervision of eating. Furthermore, LPNs have a significant role in developing a therapeutic relationship with the client, and following through with appropriate interventions according to the patient-care plan.

Helpful qualities include (1) the ability to deal with stress; (2) empathic, rather than sympathetic approach to clients; (3) good communication skills; (4) nonjudgmental; (5) sound mental health; (6) alert to physical and emotional changes in clients; (7) ability to set client-centered limits; (8) ability to differentiate between personal and client goals; and (9) willingness to function as a team member.

Fortunately, some mental health facilities have an orientation and continuing inservice program. If this is an area of interest for you, the authors recommend Bauer and Hill's *Essentials of Mental Health Planning and Interventions*. This book is written for all psychiatric health care providers and is useful both as a textbook and as a continuing reference book.

Military Services

As a practical nurse, you will have to take basic training. Some branches of service are presently experiencing a nursing shortage at all levels. Consequently, they are willing to pay an immediate bonus upon signing up. There are also incentives involved for continuing education. If you are interested, contact recruiters for all branches of the military services. Compare the differences in order to determine which branch best fits your needs.

Desirable qualities include (1) interest in teamwork; (2) a strong ego; (3) ability to cope with changing situations; (4) emotional stability; (5) communication skills; and (6) self-direction. Certainly, a desire for continued education and the ability to adjust quickly to new situations are handy prerequisites for this kind of nursing.

Hospital Nursing

The major hospital experience in most practical nursing programs is on the medical and surgical units. Therefore, this is an immediate area of employment when available.

The NLN *Nursing DataSource 1991:* (p. 19) reports that although the number of LPNs employed in hospitals is declining, in 1989 LPNs were 18% of the hospital nursing staff. If you do consider speciality areas, they should be areas in which you have had both theory class and clinical experience. Areas with complex nursing duties mean that additional postgraduate education and experience are required.

Refer to the Nurse Practice Act for your state to see how the performance of nursing acts beyond basic nursing care is handled. These acts are referred to as the expanded role of the practical nurse or performance of acts in complex patient situations and will be discussed in Chapters 18 and 19.

Desirable qualities include (1)attention to detail in performing technical skills; (2) organizational skills; (3) observational skills; (4) strong ego; (5) ability to cope with stressful situations; (6) teamwork; (7) flexibility; and (8) ability to prioritize.

The anticipated pay scale is approximately two thirds of the RN pay scale. Other benefits vary according to agency policy.

Outpatient Clinics/Doctors' Offices

Jobs in outpatient clinics and doctors' offices continue to be jobs for many LPNs. For one thing, most clinics and offices are open Monday to Friday with weekends off. The day begins later and consequently runs a little later. Although the assigned work varies, it generally includes checking supplies, greeting the patient, taking vital signs, weighing the patient, a limited assessment regarding the purpose for being there, giving the patient directions on preparing for the examination, assisting the doctor with the examination, and performing any additional duties delegated by the physician. If you are working as a private nurse to a physician, you can also expect to accompany the physician on hospital rounds, assisting with examinations as needed. Because the clientele remains essentially the same, these nurses develop a rapport with the client—an asset to the client and to the doctor(s).

Desirable qualities include (1) communication skills; (2) attention to detail; (3) enjoying routine; and (4) organizational skills.

Other Job Opportunities

Some other job opportunities to consider are

- VISTA or the Peace Corps
- Industrial nursing—Some LPNs have found excellent support in this area and

work under the general supervision of a doctor.

- Veterans Administration hospitals and homes for retired veterans.
- Hospices—care of terminally ill patients in the institutional setting or in their homes.
- Insurance company—Companies will provide in-depth orientation for the work required.
- Veterinary clinic—an opportunity to combine your love of nursing with love of animals. In some states you may work as assistant to the veterinarian in the care and treatment of animals. Other states, such as California require a special training program and state test in order to assist veterinarians.
- Hospital equipment/supply salesperson— Some pharmacies, for example, select LPNs to staff this particular area. One such nurse, for example, has become the colostomy care expert in her city and gives seminars on the topic to agencies, patients, and health professionals. She enjoys the backing of the drug-store management and a pharmaceutical company.
- Coroner's nurse—A nurse doing the work commented, "I never saw myself as doing this, but it is so interesting. I've learned a lot about myself, people, pain, compassion. The doctor I work with is a born teacher."

Continuing Education

Historically, practical nurses have a reputation for being apathetic in pursuing continuing education classes. This is difficult to believe, since many LPNs have gone on to learn complex nursing skills after graduation. Continuing education classes are available in many formats and through many agencies. Often the agency you work for is willing to pick up part or all of the fee if the education benefits the agency. Some agency courses are free and are a part of contin-

uing service within the agency. Continuing education includes the following.

Orientation to the Facility

An opportunity to learn about variation in routine, plus review selected previously learned information and skills.

In-Service

Information chosen to meet specific needs within a facility. Attendance is required. Offer suggestions for content. Usually a specified amount of time is required, such as one hour per month or three times per year, according to agency policy.

Workshop

Presents information and an opportunity to practice what is being taught. Excellent opportunity to learn new skills. Length varies according to content.

Continuing Education Classes

Sometimes called *field services* in the vocational system. Classes are often on complex nursing skills such as intravenous therapy, physical assessment, LPN charge nurse, mental health concepts, nursing process for LPNs, and so on. Actually, many vocational schools and community colleges will provide any course you are interested in if you request it and have peers to help make up the required minimum enrollment. Many of these classes provide continuing education credits as opposed to course credit. You receive a certificate if you have attended faithfully and course work is satisfactory. One of the most valuable benefits of continuing education classes is the opportunity to get together with other working LPNs. You discover similarities in challenges and satisfactions. Ideas are shared on how to deal with difficult situations in the work setting. It would be a good idea to keep a running record of all in-service, seminars, and workshops, including dates, credits, and topics, for future reference. Ask for these records to be included in your file at your place of employment.

Moving Up

If you are a LPN who says "I want to be a LPN. I have no desire to be a RN," then good for you. You have obviously given careful consideration to your personal goals. Satisfaction in nursing both for you and the patients you care for is closely related to clear-cut goals. If you decided that you want to be a LPN, chances are that you will be satisfied with your choice and provide satisfactory care to your patients. If, however, someone else decided that you should be a nurse, chances are that you will never be entirely satisfied with the choice. This lack of satisfaction will be mirrored in the care you give to patients. The same process is true in regard to making a decision to become a RN. If you do not want to become a RN, avoid letting anyone push you into it. Only when a goal is truly your own will you be motivated to do your best both in the educational process and in the care of patients.

If, however, you want to go on into a RN program, it is important to know what is available educationally. A major problem in developing upward-mobility programs for LPNs is the belief held by some educators that a practical nursing course is terminal in nature; that state boards of nursing will not permit such programs, nor will credit be given by registered nursing programs. Although the same reasoning continues to be held in some parts of the country, it is exciting to note that other directors of nursing have negotiated with boards of nursing successfully in order to develop progressive LPN-to-RN programs.

Career Ladder

Ahl (1975, p. 143) states "I believe that historically the Helene Fuld School of Nursing at the Hospital of Joint Diseases and Medical Center (New York City) is the first program to demonstrate the belief that practical nursing is indeed a part of the nursing profession, and that a curriculum can be constructed that effectively articulates with one that prepares for registered nurse licensure with minimal repetition." The program, initially a 15-month course trimmed down to 47 weeks, was initiated in 1964. Jus-

tine Hannan, hospital Director of Nursing, worked with the Board of Nursing within New York State's Education Department, and by 1968, the department granted full registration to the program. By 1970, it was accredited by the National League of Nursing (NLN). "The school has had an impact on the quality of nursing in its home hospital, and has sent graduates into dozens of other health care facilities throughout New York and fifteen other states. It has willingly shared its experience with educators who have made inquiries about its work, and has demonstrated that career ladder education is both valid and appropriate for a large number of persons who have the aptitude and commitment to such a goal" (Ahl, 1975, p. 150).

Career-ladder programs are carefully planned to avoid duplication of content. "The curriculum is not a Practical Nursing curriculum for the first year and an Associate Degree Nursing curriculum for the second. It is a totally new curriculum designed in terms of essential learnings for beginning nursing competencies. It allows the student to be a competent Practical Nurse practitioner at the end of one year of study and a competent Registered Nurse practitioner at the end of an additional year" (Story, 1974, p. 2).

The career-ladder concept is also being used successfully in vocational systems. One of the best-known vocational–technical career ladders is the open curriculum program developed at Iowa's Area One Vocational-Technical School of Nursing in 1969, under the guidance of Donna K. Story. In this program, all students are admitted as nursing students with no effort being made to differentiate between practical nursing and registered nursing students. All students take the same courses during the first three quarters. Tests during the third quarter assist the student in making a decision whether to continue on into the associate-degree level or to exit at the first level to become a LPN. The fourth quarter varies depending on this decision. All students, regardless of their decision to exit or continue, take the practical-nurse licensing examination. It gives the student practice in taking a licensing examination, and provides her with the opportunity to work as a LPN, either as a career or to help support the remainder of her schooling. This school has taken an additional step of working with a private college so that students can obtain their BSN (Bachelor of Science in Nursing) in an additional two years, that is, $2 + 2 =$ a BSN. Once again, it was through articulation with the state board of nursing that this innovative program came into being.

Similar programs exist in other areas of the country. Your board of nursing is an excellent resource.

Accelerated AD (Associate Degree) Nursing Program An innovative one-year ADN completion program was initiated in 1980 by MANEC (Metro Area Nursing Education Consortium of Minnesota). The faculty of three area vocational–technical institutes and two community colleges completed detailed curriculum comparisons and identified the common core of theoretical and technical skills taught in the PN and AD nursing programs. Based on this preliminary work, LPNs who have graduated from January 1978 on and are admitted to the AD nursing program, are awarded 21 quarter credits in nursing, 4 credits in anatomy, 3 credits in nutrition, and 3 credits in psychology. Licensure as a LPN is required. No work experience is required if the LPN has graduated within the past three years. If the period of employment is more than three years, then six months of work experience is needed. LPNs are required to take 15 credits of general education, maintaining a 2.5 grade-point average prior to admission to the AD program. The program has received NLN accreditation.

Progression Program Some educators continue to believe that it is necessary for an LPN to prove a certain level of knowledge in order to attain advanced standing in an ADN program. The Northeast Wisconsin Technical College Nursing Program (Green Bay) developed an LPN progression into an ADN program in 1985. LPNs were expected to have at least one full year of work experience within the past three years to be eligible for the program. LPNs meet the same criteria for admission as students to the general ADN program; the minimum length of the program is two years because the nursing process courses must be taken in proper numerical sequence. The program may be completed on a part-time or full-time basis. The LPNs receive advanced-standing partial credit through a series of tests intended to determine competency in each of the first four nursing-process steps (the curriculum is based on a five-step nursing-process sequence). To receive the total number of credits required, a student who successfully passes the test must take the appropriate bridge class. The bridge class content is intended to be different from the full-credit process class taken by general students, and eliminates the need to repeat some of the skills the LPN has already learned. Only LPNs who pass the bridge class will receive credit for the passed challenge test.

No-Credit RN Programs There continue to be RN programs that do not recognize the worth of LPN education. These programs insist that LPNs start from the beginning, and repeat all previously covered information, including basic nursing skills. The bottom line is that there are a number of programs throughout the country that the LPN can use to become a RN— if that is what is right for you. Contact your board of nursing. They are an excellent resource in regard to programs in your state. Contact boards of nursing in other states to inquire about educational opportunities, especially if you have the advantage of personal mobility. The addresses for boards of nursing are available in Appendix A.

NURSING ORGANIZATIONS

If you want a voice in nursing—your vocation— join your vocational organization(s). The narrative below will be limited to discussion of organizations that are made up of, or include LPN members. Additional information can be obtained by writing to the organization headquarters.

NFLPN
3948 Browning Pl.
Suite 205
P.O. Box 18088
Raleigh, NC 27619

The NFLPN (National Federation of Licensed Practical Nurses, Inc.) is the policy-making body for LPNs. Made up entirely of LPNs and student practical nurses, it was formed by LPNs in order to have an organization to work for and speak on behalf of them. Membership includes a newsletter. The organization keeps its members involved with matters of interest to practical nursing, makes health, accident, malpractice, and personal liability insurance plans available to its members, works for LPN representation on boards of nursing, provides a voice in nursing legislation on a national level, encourages agencies to provide continuing education, provides a statement of functions and qualifications of LPNs, and works with other health organizations for quality patient care.

NAPNES
1400 Spring St.
Suite 310
Silver Spring, MD 20910

NAPNES (National Association for Practical Nurse Education and Service) is a multidisciplinary organization that is involved with practical nursing, both on a student and graduate level. It was the first organization formed for promotion of practical nursing schools and continuing education for LPNs. The membership fee includes a subscription to *The Journal of Practical Nursing*, the official magazine of NAPNES. Membership is open to anyone concerned with the advancement of practical nursing.

HOSA
6309 N. O'Connor St.
Suite 215 LB117
Irving, Texas 75039

HOSA (Health Occupations Students of America) is a national vocational organization for students of health occupations. The national motto, "The Hands of Youth Hold the Health of Tomorrow," reflects the purpose of the organization: better understanding of health-related issues, cooperation with other students of health occupations, and strengthening of leadership and citizenship abilities in preparing for health care of tomorrow.

NLN
350 Hudson St.
New York, NY 10014

The NLN (National League for Nursing) is an organization involved with all types of nursing: consultation; accreditation of nursing education programs; professional testing services; surveys on admissions, enrollments, graduation, studies on nursing education, and service; information source on trends in nursing; and conventions, meetings, workshops, and continuing education. NLN membership is open to all nurses and others concerned with health care. The membership fee includes a subscription to its journal *Nursing and Health Care*.

Alumni Association
Your school

Practical nursing alumni associations provides a familiar, proud connection for classes past and those to come—you share a common bond. Activities vary from social gatherings to welcoming a new class or celebrating graduation, to those with educational intent and content. If your school does not have an alumni association, consider getting together with peers to start one. Seek help from your faculty.

Summary

Career opportunities, to a large extent, depend on where you live, the current trends in nursing and your ability and/or willingness to go after the job you want. Career mobility on the other hand, depends on your personal goal in regard to nursing. If additional education is a goal, continuing education classes in various forms are available to you. RN completion programs vary considerably in regard to admission requirements, prerequisites, and length of program. Inquiries can be made directly to your state board of nursing to assist you in locating a suitable program.

Valuable support groups exist for you in the form of nursing organizations. Student membership is available in the NFLPN and state conventions frequently sponsor a student day. NAPNES continues to fight for the rights of practical nurses, and supports continuation of the vocation. HOSA is a Health Occupations Student Organization that provides a balance of social and educational activity. The NLN focuses on nursing needs at all levels of nursing, and provides broad services for nursing in all areas. Your alumni association will always be a touch of "home."

REFERENCES

Ahl ME. In: Lenburg C, ed. *Open Learning and Career Mobility in Nursing.* St Louis: CV Mosby, 1975.

Anastas L. *Your Career in Nursing.* New York: National League for Nursing, 1984.

Bauer B, Hill S. *Essentials of Mental Health Planning and Interventions.* Philadelphia: WB Saunders, 1985.

Downs F, Brooten D. *New Careers in Nursing.* New York: ARCO Publishing, 1983.

Northeast Wisconsin Technical College, Green Bay. Application for Advanced Standing, ADN Fall, 1985.

Nursing DataSource 1991. Vol. 2. New York: National League for Nursing.

Robertson S on MANEC (Metro Area Nursing Education Consortium) Project, 1991.

Story D. *Career Mobility.* St Louis: CV Mosby, 1974.

CHAPTER
18

Leadership Skills for the Practical Nurse

Learning Objectives

Upon completing this chapter, you will
1. Describe the expanded role of the practical nurse as described in your state's Nurse Practice Act.
2. Identify your personal leadership style.
3. In your own words, explain the following leadership styles
   a. autocratic
   b. democratic
   c. laissez-faire
4. Identify ways to obtain competence in the three general areas in which knowledge is needed to be an effective leader:
   a. occupational skills
   b. organizational skills
   c. human relationship skills
5. Describe how Maslow's Hierarchy of Needs acts as a motivator of human behavior.
6. Describe how The Howlett Hierarchy of Work Motivators can help the practical nurse leader motivate subordinates.
7. Discuss leadership strategies for handling the following common workplace problems:
   a. chronic lateness
   b. difficulty completing work assignment

INTRODUCTION

Polly Practical, LPN, Charge Nurse days, comes on duty for the day shift in a frenzy. The staff shudders as she rearranges her uniform and papers. They murmur to each other, "Another day with Attila the Hun." Polly barks out the assignments after report. She reminds the staff (1) not to dawdle in their cares, (2) to have everything done by 10 A.M., (3) to stay out of her way when she gives her meds, and (4) to have a thorough end-of-shift report, as Polly has a headache and will be unable personally to check up on the patients that day.

Ann Assistant, NA, asks why everything has to be done by 10 A.M. Polly takes off in a whirlwind of prose and assorted dramatics. Polly, PN, never answers Ann's question, which is unfortunate. The reason for getting cares done by 10 A.M. that particular day is because of a visit to the nursing home by Doc Severinsen and his entire orchestra. Had Ann and the other nursing assistants known the reason for the command, they would have worked twice as hard to complete care in time for the residents' favorite entertainers.

Briefly stated, the purpose of this chapter is to help you get started in developing more skill and tact to lead than is displayed by Polly Practical.

THE PRACTICAL NURSE AS FIRST-LINE LEADER

Have you ever experienced an employment situation similar to the one with Polly Practical? Perhaps you received directions as a nursing assistant or in another job capacity and did not like the way in which you were approached by your supervisor. In the 1990s, in many states, the licensed practical nurse is used as a first-line leader in selected health care settings. This means you will be the person filling Polly Practical's shoes. Practical nurses need to develop leadership skills so they can direct and supervise others in a manner that will effectively meet the goals of the employing agency.

The Organizational Chart

The organizational chart is a picture of responsibility in an employment situation. Individuals lower on the organizational chart report to the person directly above them on the chart. See Figure 18-1 to visualize where the practical nurse fits into the organizational chart as a first line leader. In Figure 18-1, the practical nurse reports to the nurse manager who is a registered nurse. Nursing assistants report to the practical nurse. To whom does the director of nursing (DON) report? Organizational charts may differ by regions of the United States. Refer to the organizational chart of specific agencies of your interest for clarification of specific levels of responsibility in your area.

The Expanded Role of Practical Nursing

It is important for you to review the Nurse Practice Act of your state as it legally defines the exact role and boundaries for practical nurses. Also, review the National Federation of Licensed Practical Nurses (NFLPN) Specialized Nursing Practice Standards found in Chapter 19 (Table 19-3) for more guidelines for the expanded role of the practical nurse.

An example of the expanded role of the practical nurse is the Charge Nurse position. In Charge Nurse situations, the practical nurse has the responsibility for the care given by nursing assistants. The practical nurse will direct, guide, and supervise these health care workers as they attempt to meet the goals of the agency of employment. A common site for utilization of the practical nurse in the expanded role as Charge Nurse is the nursing home and long-term–care unit. To carry out the Charge Nurse role, you will need the abilities found in a leader.

How You Are Already Preparing for a Leadership Role

The topic of leadership and the practical nurse is a vast one. The references and annotated bib-

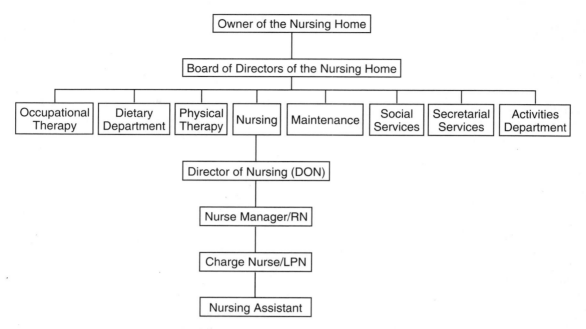

FIGURE 18-1   Sample Organizational Chart for the Role of the Practical Nurse in the Nursing Home/Long-Term Care Setting

liography (a bibliography that tells you the main points of the books listed and how the books may benefit you) at the end of this chapter provide valuable references.

All practical nurses are leaders in the sense that they consistently need to direct, handle, and organize care for assigned patients. It is worthwhile for you to review the ways in which your one-year program helps to prepare you for a leadership position.

The one-year practical nursing program encourages development of the following skills necessary for functioning successfully as a charge nurse:

1. Basic nursing skills, including the nursing process

2. Time management techniques for home and clinical time

3. How to learn new information, including use of resources for learning

4. The power of positive self-talk and thinking

5. Rules for assertiveness

6. Communication skills

7. Legal and ethical aspects of health care

8. Problem solving and critical thinking

9. Stress management

You have received frequent verbal and written evaluation of your behaviors both in class and the clinical area. This experience with evaluation will help prepare you for the need to evaluate others in your job as charge nurse.

"Learning leadership," as you can see, is much more than taking one course that turns you into a leader. Learning leadership is a process (continual development) that includes many skills and is something that evolves over time. This chapter will focus on leadership in practical nursing and help you to think specifically of a leadership role.

WHAT KIND OF A LEADER ARE YOU?

There are several different ways to lead. What is your predominant leadership style? Each of the following statements of "A Short Test of Leadership Style" is an extreme. The responses are not positive or negative. They have no value over one another. They just are. Make a check next to the statement that *best* describes the way you *might be* at work, not how you want to be.*

A Short Test of Leadership Style

1. My primary goal at work is to
   a. get the job done
   b. get along with the people with whom I work
   c. do the job correctly
   d. hope the work I do is noticed

2. My clinical coworkers would say I am
   a. domineering in my relationships
   b. friendly and personable in my relationships
   c. likely to attend to details of the patient care plan
   d. creative and energetic in giving care

3. At work, I feel like I have to be
   a. in control of the patient situation
   b. liked by my coworkers
   c. correct in giving care
   d. recognized and praised for my care

4. When I communicate on the nursing unit:
   a. I am usually direct and to the point.
   b. I am more considerate of the person to whom I am talking rather than strongly getting my point across.
   c. I usually give detailed information.
   d. I usually elaborate on the point at hand.

5. My coworkers would say I am a person who
   a. gets the job done regardless of what shift I work
   b. is very likable and patient
   c. is precise and accurate in giving nursing care
   d. is optimistic and has good verbal skills

---

*Idea adapted from the Career Track Seminar entitled "How to Get Along with Difficult People" given by Dr. Rick Brinkman, April 1989 in Green Bay, Wisconsin.

6. Select the behavior your charge nurse might attribute to you while on your shift.
   a. *Sometimes* I alienate people.
   b. *Sometimes* I waste time and fall for excuses others may give.
   c. *Sometimes* I can be stubborn with coworkers.
   d. *Sometimes* I appear like a flake to my coworkers.

7. How do you react to a stressful incident on the nursing unit?
   a. By being arrogant, blaming other departments, yelling at coworkers.
   b. By being accommodating to the person in charge and passive in behavior.
   c. By becoming silent and withdrawing from the situation.
   d. By talking faster and louder.

8. When I deal with my coworkers on the nursing unit regarding patient matters, I like them to
   a. get to the point and be businesslike in their behavior
   b. be casual and sincere in their behavior
   c. use the facts of the matter and go step-by-step when explaining a patient-care situation
   d. be enthusiastic about the situation and use demonstrations to explain their points

Count up your A and C answers. These answers are more characteristic of a task-oriented person. This person in leadership terms is called an *autocratic* leader. Add up your B and D responses. These are more characteristic of a people-oriented person. In leadership terms, this person is called a *laissez-faire* leader. Your score can give you a rough estimate of the tendency of your leadership style.

LEADERSHIP STYLES

The literature abounds with examples of leadership styles. Figure 18-2 illustrates a continuum (a line with extreme opposites at each end) of leadership styles and Table 18-1 compares and contrasts the leadership styles found on this continuum.

Table 18–1 Comparing Autocratic, Democratic, and Laissez-faire styles of Leadership

	AUTOCRATIC	DEMOCRATIC	LAISSEZ-FAIRE
GENERAL DESCRIPTION	Does not share responsibility and authority with employees	Shares responsibility and authority with employees	Gives away responsibility and authority to employees
IMPORTANCE OF AGENCIES' POLICIES	Emphasis on policies	Enforces policies but with concern for employees	Puts employees before policies
HOW LEADER GETS THE JOB DONE	Tells employees what tasks to do. Does not seek input from employees	Seeks input from employees and encourages problem solving.	Tries to please everyone
WHAT GETS DONE	May reach goals	Because of involvement of employees, goals may be achieved with positive staff feelings	Maybe nothing
WHEN STYLE CAN BE USED	Crisis situations Code situations Emergencies	Daily nursing care situations Meetings Committees Review of care plans	When agency goals/policies are not a consideration

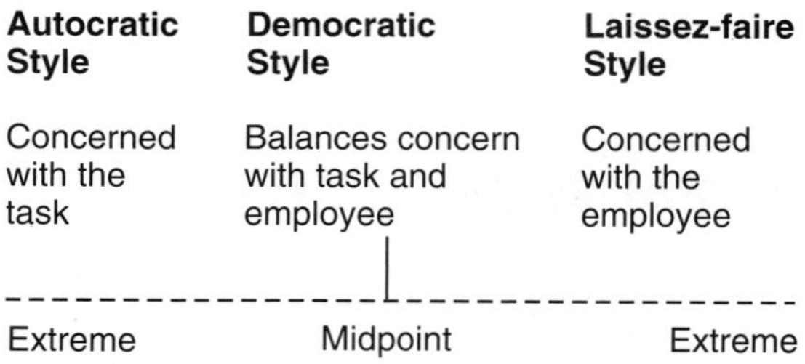

Autocratic Style	Democratic Style	Laissez-faire Style
Concerned with the task	Balances concern with task and employee	Concerned with the employee
Extreme	Midpoint	Extreme

FIGURE 18-2 Extremes of Leadership Styles on a Continuum

BENEFITS AND DISADVANTAGES OF LEADERSHIP STYLES

To adopt one of the extreme columns in Table 18-1 (autocratic or laissez-faire) to be used consistently as a leadership style is unrealistic and could be disastrous. As you can see, there is room for an autocratic leadership style, for example, in times of emergency. A purely task-centered leadership style (autocratic style) thrives on power. It involves telling someone what to do with little regard for the employee as a person who may have ideas as how to reach agency goals. List below two additional examples of situations that might require the autocratic style of leadership.

1.
2.

A purely people-oriented style (laissez-faire) focuses on people's feelings but ignores the task at hand and allows employees to act without any direction. The goals of the organization will be compromised when the laissez-faire leadership style is used. At times, persons in leadership roles may feel the need to be liked by all subordinates and use this leadership style, but the task of accomplishing goals will be seriously compromised.

SITUATIONAL LEADERSHIP

A popular system of leadership is called *situational leadership*. Situational leadership involves varying your leadership style to meet the demands of the situation in the work environment. According to this system, the practical nurse needs to pick a leadership style that fits the work situation at hand.

Using the Leadership Continuum as a Guide

The value of a continuum, as shown in Figure 18-2, is that as you move along the continuum from each extreme toward the center or midpoint, the two extremes begin to blend together. You have some of each style, depending on where you are on the continuum. A blend of the two extremes to some degree in the appropriate work situation would be the leadership style needed at the moment.

The leadership model presented by Hersey and Weaver (1989, pp. 9–10) illustrates the use of the concept of situational leadership. These authors identify four main leadership styles as

1. Sell
2. Tell
3. Participate
4. Delegate

Referring to Figure 18-2, *tell* would be the direct, power approach used when the situation, such as an emergency, demands the autocratic style of leadership. *Delegate* would allow subordinates who are self-directed and have proved their responsibility to function on their own to meet organizational goals once the goals are made clear. *Delegate* comes between autocratic and democratic styles. *Sell* offers ideas and suggestions to subordinates (workers for whom you have responsibility) of the positive benefits of organizational goals. The intention of *sell* is to persuade workers of the value of carrying out the goals. The staff then adopts the desirability of meeting the goals and will work hard to achieve them. *Sell* comes between the autocratic and the laissez-faire styles of leadership. *Participate* involves staff and leader working together on identified goals. The leader offers various degrees of support or direction, as needed by subordinates. This is an example of the democratic style of leadership.

My Leadership Style Score

How did you score on the test of leadership style? Place an X on the continuum in Figure 18-2 to indicate where you are at this point in general leadership style tendencies. Remember, this score is your tendency. If your X is far to the left or right, it may benefit you to be aware of this tendency and to avoid using this style consistently. Remember the continuum and the need to be flexible in your style. Balance task- and people-orientation as needed. Knowing what your predominant style of leadership is will be helpful in your evaluation of work situations and the style needed at that time. Some situations require a supportive style while others require a more directive approach.

LEARNING ACTIVITY

Using "A Short Test of Leadership Style" as a guide, have students in class identify their general personal leadership style tendencies. Total up the number of autocratic styles as compared with laissez-faire styles. If students will share their results, have peers offer feedback as to what style they see each class member as having.

SPECIFIC SKILLS NEEDED FOR LEADERSHIP

In order to function well in your expanded role, you must be a good leader. The scenario at the beginning of this chapter is an example of what not to do as a nurse leader. It may be the sad fact that you can relate to the scenario by having experienced Polly's style in your work environment. Much research in learning about the business of leading others and the theories that go with leading are evident in the literature. To lead, research points out the need to have knowledge in three general areas:

1. Occupational skills
2. Organizational skills
3. Human relationship skills

The focus of your role as leader will be tasks and people in an organization. Does the continuum of leadership styles come to mind? Developing the needed skills for your job is a responsibility you share with your employer.

Occupational Skills for First-Line Practical Nursing Leaders

Solid nursing skills are necessary to be a good nursing leader. Visible expertise in nursing skills is a plus with your coworkers. This means the desire to see the patient situation for yourself, assist in providing care, and demonstrate nursing skills to peers as needed. Your practical nursing program has started your skill development in this area. This is an area you will need to keep current and fresh.

Organizational Skills for First-Line Practical Nursing Leaders

Survival skills and personal growth are essential ingredients for leaders. The emphasis on the personal and vocational issues/concepts course in your practical nursing program has given you the opportunity to learn and apply principles of assertiveness (Chapter 11), time management (Chapter 5), and methods of stress control (Chapter 10). These skills are necessary ingredients for the development of any nursing leader.

Human Relationship Skills for First-Line Practical Nursing Leaders

Although nursing and specific organizational skills are important, human relationship skills are necessary in your leadership role. Polly Practical *might* get the job done. Leaders with human relationship skills will get the job done with finesse, style, and tact. Subordinates will like their leader's style a whole lot more and be more effective in reaching the goals of the nursing unit. One of the nursing leader's most productive tools is the effective use of verbal and nonverbal communication. A review of principles of communication in "Job-Related Communication" (Chapter 13) will benefit you.

Additional Resources for Developing Organizational, Occupational, and Human Relationship Skills

There are various ways of obtaining other occupational, organizational, and human relationship skills for survival. See "Suggested References" at the end of this chapter for an annotated bibliography of resources for this area. Many of the following suggestions for additional learning offer continuing education credits.

1. Check with your local vocational/technical school for a practical nursing leadership course.

2. Ask your boss to consider in-services on leadership techniques as well as updates on nursing skills. Consider cosponsoring such in-services with the local technical college and making them available to a wide geographic area.

3. Form a network with other persons who fill first-line leadership positions. Be sure to go outside your institution as well as the discipline of nursing. You will find that the problems leaders have are very similar regardless of the discipline.

4. Attend seminars relating to leadership topics as well as nursing topics. Career Track is one example of companies that offer informative, interesting, fun, and affordable one-day seminars that could be of benefit to the first-line leader in nursing.

5. Read books and articles that offer hints for leaders. Be sure your nursing library is up to date. The annotated bibliography at the end of this chapter can help in this area. Some sources are new and some have stood the test of time.

UNDERSTANDING HUMAN NEEDS

As a leader, you will have the task of getting your subordinates to meet goals set by your employer. Getting persons to do what needs to be done is a complex task. Understanding human needs will help you get started.

All persons have needs that must be filled in order to meet goals. Individuals engage in various activities in order to fill needs. The activity is called behavior and can be observed. Abraham Maslow, a psychologist, presented a pyramid of human needs that can assist the learner in understanding the ranking of human needs (Figure 18-3). Meeting each level of needs on the pyramid acts as a motivator for meeting higher levels of needs. For example, before individuals can meet Safety and Security needs, they must have met Physiologic needs.

Adapting Maslow's Hierarchy

Maslow's Hierarchy of Needs can be adapted to help the first-line practical nursing leader understand motivation of subordinates in a health care setting (see Figure 18-4).

The lower three levels of the pyramid in Figure 18-4, the Howlett Hierarchy of Work Moti-

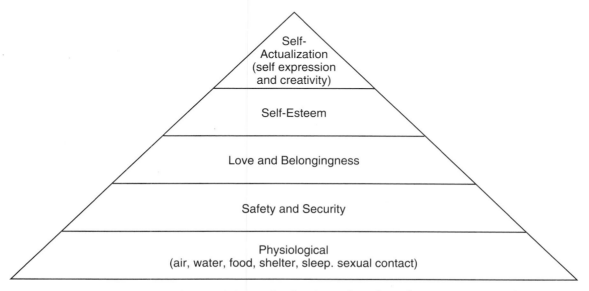

FIGURE 18-3 Maslow's Hierarchy of Needs.

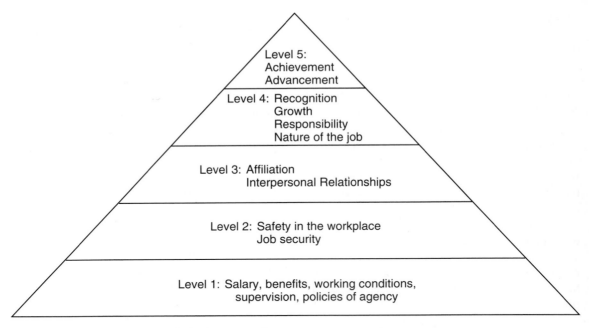

FIGURE 18-4 Howlett Hierarchy of Work Motivators

vators, are considered to be externally moti-vated needs. These motivators exist outside a person. They depend on the employer or any-one else outside of self. If these needs are met, the person can proceed to the next higher level of the pyramid. If these needs are not met, a person will become dissatisfied with the work situation.

The upper two levels of the pyramid in Fig-ure 18-4 represent internal motivators in the work environment. Internal motivators come from inside the individual. They result in indi-viduals motivating themselves to reach goals.

Meeting needs on the Howlett Hierarchy can motivate employees to behave in certain ways. It is a challenge for the leader to channel the motives of subordinates to meet the goals of the employer. As you go up the Howlett Hierarchy in Figure 18-4, begin identifying behaviors that could be done to encourage meeting needs at each level. Also, identify if the employer needs to initiate the behavior or if behavior could be initiated by the first-line practical nursing leader. As needs are met on one level, move-ment can then be encouraged to the next level of the Howlett Hierarchy.

Using the Howlett Hierarchy in Leadership Situations

The following activity gives you an opportunity to assume responsibility as a practical nursing leader. Examples of behaviors to encourage meeting needs at each level of the hierarchy are given. The person responsible for the behavior is listed in parentheses. Space is provided for you to fill in additional suggestions of behaviors for each level to show how you can encourage meeting subordinates' needs at each level.

Level 1: **Salary, benefits, working condi-tions, supervision, policies of agency**
Examples:
Explanation of policies that affect employees. (first-line PN leader)
Cafeteria-style benefits—pick and choose benefits (employer)

_____

_____

Level 2: **Safety in the workplace, job secu-rity**

Provision of adequate equipment to carry out universal precautions (employer and first-line PN leader)

Policy for hostile patients (employer and first-line PN leader)

_____

_____

Level 3:   Affiliation, interpersonal relationships

Plan monthly potluck dinners, pizza lunches, get-togethers (first-line PN leader)

_____

_____

Level 4:   Recognition, growth, responsibility, nature of the job

Encourage attendance at continuing education seminars, in-service, etc. (employer and first-line PN leader)

Recognition for working short-staffed (employer and first-line PN leader)

_____

_____

Level 5:   Achievement, advancement

Recognition of successful completion of class, seminar (employer and first-line PN leader)

_____

_____

Appendix D: The Howlett Style of Nursing Leadership contains additional suggestions.

*L*EARNING EXERCISE

Share with your peers the behaviors you have listed to meet needs at the five levels of the Howlett Hierarchy. Then, give objective examples of how you can implement each of your suggested behaviors. For example, Level 5: recognizing successful completion of classes and seminars could be implemented by:

1. A written account in the institution's newsletter
2. Announcement on special section of bulletin board
3. Recognition by note from the charge nurse

This learning activity can be fun. It allows the nurse to be creative in finding ways to give recognition.

*D*EALING WITH COMMON PRACTICAL NURSING LEADER PROBLEMS

You have learned about the problem-solving method of nursing, the nursing process (Chapter 2), and its benefit in planning care for patients. This same problem-solving process can be used by the first-line practical nursing leader to deal with problems that present on the clinical area. Common problem areas are absenteeism, tardiness, poor appearance, and not completing assigned work in a timely and/or quality manner. Each leadership problem will differ. Problems need to be approached individually. Use the nursing process and elements of Appendix D: The Howlett Style of Nursing Leadership as guidelines.

The following scenario may be used as a model. Actual times for observing behavior may differ depending on the specific employee. The following sequence of discipline was suggested in an article by Janet Wilson (1987, pp. 121–123). It represents a legally sound way of handling an employee problem. Be sure to follow the recommended procedure for discipline as found in your institution.

Scenario: Late for Assigned Shift

Penny, a nursing assistant, is assigned to the day shift in a nursing home. Her shift begins at 0645 with a verbal report from the night nurse.

Assessment

On May 8, 10, 15, 16, 23, and 24 Penny came to work either during the night report or after report was finished. When questioned about this behavior, she states she has problems getting her teenagers up and started for school.

Problem

A record of Penny's tardiness indicates this is a recurring problem and not an isolated incident. A pattern has been established.

Interventions

As the first-line practical nursing leader, it is your responsibility to talk to Penny about this tardiness. This includes the times and days of her tardiness. Select a private spot for your discussion. Encourage Penny to determine why this behavior is inconvenient for the staff and residents. Review the institution's policy on punctuality. Encourage Penny to come up with ideas for improving her home situation so she can be on time. Set limits with Penny. Identify that she needs to be on time for her assigned shifts. Plan to meet with her in one month to discuss her improved performance. At that time, if she has not improved her performance, a written reprimand will be given and included in her personal file. At the end of the meeting, compliment Penny on an area of her work that has been going well.

Evaluation

During the next month, continue to document Penny's arrival for her assigned shifts. If she complies, note and praise her change in performance. If she continues to be late for her shift, issue a written reprimand. Place a copy in her file. Give a copy to your supervisor. Keep a copy in your file. Be sure the warning contains objective information containing:

1. Days and times late for shift
2. Date of oral warning
3. Seriousness of situation
4. The consequences

Be sure to discuss the written reprimand privately with Penny. At this time another interval might be set. If performance has not improved, disciplinary action may be carried out.

Using the nursing process and principles found in Appendix D, develop a plan of action to handle the following employee problems. Suggested, but not definite, ways of handling these problems can be found in Appendix E.

Scenario 1

Wayne, a nursing assistant, is a full-time employee of the evening shift of his local nursing home. He has missed 5 of 20 scheduled shifts this month. When questioned about his absences, Wayne states he has personal problems. Frequent absences have been a problem since Wayne was first employed.

Scenario 2

Ceil completed her nursing assistant training four months ago. She has been employed at a nursing home since she became certified. Since completing her orientation to the nursing home, she has had continuing problems getting her assignment completed in an acceptable time frame. Ceil claims her patient load is always too heavy and is impossible to complete. The other nursing assistants have helped Ceil with her patients but they tell you they are tired of carrying her load because frequently she can be seen sitting at the nurse's desk talking on the telephone.

Summary

When the state Nurse Practice Act allows, practical nurses are used as first-line leaders, especially in the nursing home. The practical nursing program itself offers students the opportunity to develop skills in nursing procedures, time management, assertiveness, and stress control. These are skills needed for everyday practice as well as leadership positions. Development of a leadership style is important in guiding staff to meet the goals of the health care organization.

Established leadership styles range from the extreme of autocratic, with a pure emphasis on the task, to laissez-faire, which solely emphasizes concern with the employee. Situational leadership adapts a leadership style to the environment and situation at hand. It is the suggested way of leading in the 1990s. Specific skill areas for nursing leadership include (1) occupational skills (2) organizational skills, and (3) human relationship skills.

No one chapter can teach you how to become a leader. In addition to training given by the institution, first-line practical nursing leaders need continually to educate and update themselves in the three specific skill areas noted. The references listed in the annotated bibliography at the end of this chapter can help you in your development as a first-line leader in nursing.

REFERENCES

Barker A. An emerging leadership paradigm. Nurs Health Care 1991; 12:204–207.

Bauer B, Hill S. *Essentials of Mental Health Care: Planning and Interventions.* Philadelphia: WB Saunders, 1986.

Blanchard K, Lorber R. *Putting the One Minute Manager to Work.* New York: Berkley Publishing, 1984.

Blanchard K, Johnson S. *The One Minute Manager.* New York: Berkley Publishing, 1981.

Blanchard K, Orcken W, Burrows H. *The One Minute Manager Meets the Monkey.* New York: William Morrow, 1989.

Gable FG. *The Third Force: Abraham Maslow.* New York: Pocket Books, 1976.

Henry B. New organization theories for future nursing administration research. Nurs Admin Q 1986; 11(1):73–80.

Hersey P, Weaver B. *Situational Leadership in Nursing.* Norwalk, CT: Appleton & Lange, 1989.

Herzberg F. *The Managerial Choice.* Homewood, IL: Dow Jones-Irwin, 1976.

Howlett H. *The Howlett Theory of Management for Nursing Instructors* (unpublished paper), November 1989.

Keenan M, Hoover P, Hoover R. Leadership theory lets clinical instructors guide students towards autonomy. Nurs Health Care 1988; 9:83–86.

Lilley L, Davis L. Building a management library. Nurs Health Care 1991; 12:130–134, 149–50.

Nowlin W. Supervisory leadership characteristics: a health care agency profile. Nurs Health Care 1986; 7(Fall): 9–14.

Smoyak S. High tech high touch. Nurs Success Today 3(11):9–16.

Wilson J. Have a problem employee? Use this plan. Nursing 87 1987; April:121–123.

Annotated Bibliography

Suggested References for Occupational Skills

Berenson A, ed. *Control of Communicable Diseases in Man.* 15th ed. Washington, DC: American Public Health Association, 1990.

This publication is a handy reference containing basic information on how to recognize a specific communicable disease and how to treat patients so disease does not spread. It provides guidance on how to prevent the spread of specific communicable diseases. Diseases are listed alphabetically.

Burnside I. *Nursing and the Aged: A Self-Care Approach.* 3rd ed. New York: McGraw-Hill, 1988.

Burnside's approach to nursing care of the elderly patient focuses on this patient's responses to aging and nursing interventions directed to those responses. This book is readable and filled with excellent tables and figures, which are used to summarize useful information.

Johnson B. *Psychiatric Mental Health Nursing.* Philadelphia: JB Lippincott, 1989.

The nursing process is used to present mental health concepts in a concise, clear, interesting, and easy-to-understand manner. Besides strategies to use to intervene in developmental and situational crises, a chapter is included on the topic of "Mental Health of the Aging."

Murray R, Zentner J. *Nursing Assessment and Health Promotion Strategies Through the Lifespan.* 4th ed. Norwalk, CT: Appleton & Lange, 1989.

Murray and Zentner present a usable text that discusses the total person (physical, mental, emotional, sociologic, cultural, and spiritual aspects). Emphasis is on assessment and health promotion through the entire lifespan, with the chapters on the person in later maturity and death as the final developmental stage, particularly useful for the long-term–care setting.

Abramson B, Groom M. *Senior Citizens and the Law.* Madison, WI: Center for Public Representation, 1989.

Discusses various laws that affect the elderly, especially Medicare and Medicaid.

Ignatavicius D, Varner Bayne M. *Medical-Surgical Nursing: A Nursing Process Approach.* Philadelphia: WB Saunders, 1991.

By means of a nursing process approach, this book emphasizes care of the seriously ill elderly patient throughout the text. Common assessment findings in elderly patients are highlighted. Each assessment chapter contains a "Focus on the Elderly" table that summarizes useful information.

Ringsven M, Bond D. *Gerontology and Leadership Skills for Nurses.* Albany, NY: Delmar, 1991.

This text is of value to the student and graduate practical nurse. Using a nursing process focus, active and dependent elderly populations are discussed. In addition to discussion of physical and psychological conditions, community services and approaches to patient teaching are included. *See listing in references for organizational skills.*

Additional Suggested References For Organizational Skills

(*Note:* All books listing Blanchard as an author are easy and fun to read and can be completed in a few hours time, at the most. They offer excellent suggestions for leaders.)

Blanchard K, Peale NV. *The Power of Ethical Management.* New York: William Morrow, 1988.

These authors bring integrity back to the workplace with their practical ethical strategies that build productivity in the workplace. A three-step ethics check to evaluate a leader's actions/decisions is offered.

Blanchard K, Carew D, Parisi-Carew C. *The One Minute Manager Builds High Performing Teams.* New York: William Morrow, 1990.

The teamwork emphasis of this book will help increase any working group's productivity and satisfaction. Four stages that groups move through on their way to becoming high-performance teams is discussed as well as ideas on how to make groups more effective sooner while experiencing less stress.

Blanchard K, Zigarmi P, Zigarmi D. *Leadership and the One Minute Manager.* New York: William Morrow, 1985.

Situational leadership is described and the hints given can help you become a flexible and successful leader. Suggestions given to help you diagnose the work situation can help you determine when to delegate, support, or direct subordinates.

Blanchard K, Oncken W, Burrows H. *The One Minute Manager Meets the Monkey.* New York: William Morrow, 1989.

Do you have the time at work to do all the things you want and/or need to do? If not, this book will help you decide if you are taking on problems at work that really belong to other people. The scenarios are funny, especially the manager who is loaded down by monkeys that have jumped from their owners' (the workers) backs to the manager's back. Oncken's Rules of Monkey Management will help you get the worker's monkeys off your back and become a more effective leader.

Fisher R, Ury W. *Getting to Yes: Negotiating Agreement without Giving In.* New York: Penguin Books, 1981.

This book discusses conflict and gives a "how-to" on reaching mutually acceptable agreement between opposing parties. Specific "how-to" advice is given for (1) separating people from the problem, (2) focusing on interests and not position, (3) creating options that are agreeable to all, (4) and negotiating with persons who do not play fair or by the rules. This book can be helpful at home as well as at work.

Peters T. *In Search of Excellence.* New York: Harper & Row, 1982.

This highly successful and readable book presents eight basic practices that are characteristic of successfully managed companies.

Ringsven M, Bond D. *Gerontology and Leadership Skills for Nurses.* Albany, NY: Delmar, 1991.

Includes a thorough, easy-to-read section on specific leadership skills for the first-line nurse manager. Very helpful for the practical/vocational nurse in a leadership position. *See listing in references for occupational skills.*

Sullivan E, Decker P. *Effective Management in Nursing.* Menlo Park, CA: Addison-Wesley, 1988.

Although not published as a practical nursing book, this book can provide the first-line nurse manager with a discussion of organizational structure of health care agencies, managing and initiating change, managing the chemically dependent nurse, improving communication skills, motivating staff, developing leadership skills, managing time, problem solving, decision making, staffing, performance appraisal, managing absenteeism, dealing with conflict, stress management, and working with higher management. You probably will find some helpful information in this book if you are a first-line manager.

SUGGESTED REFERENCES FOR HUMAN RELATIONSHIP SKILL DEVELOPMENT, INCLUDING PERSONAL GROWTH

Satir V. *The New People Making.* Mountain View, CA: Science and Behavior Books, 1988.

The editor's note to this book states that the author's "writings are like homemade bread. They are yeasty, hearty, and nourishing." This readable book by a family therapist offers suggestions for improving communication, increasing self-esteem, and getting along with others. Another book that benefits one's personal as well as career self. Just reading this book makes one feel good!

von Oech R. *A Whack on the Side of the Head.* New York: Warner Books, 1990.

Activities in the form of puzzles, games, exercises, and stories are presented to help break through mental blocks and unlock one's mind for creative thinking. Activities may be useful to help committees, the nursing team, etc. to develop problem-solving abilities by awakening the right side of the brain. This author also published *Creative Whack Pack* (Stamford, CT: U.S. Systems Games, 1988), which offers the above activities on individual game cards.

Zigler Z. *See Yourself at the Top.* Gretna, LA: Pelican Publishing, 1975 (original); 1990—48th ed.

This book is funny and has a conversational style. The value of a healthy self image and how to build one for yourself (or help others to do so) is stressed. The power of thinking positively is also stressed, and a step-by-step plan is given to change motivation and performance by changing the way one think's about oneself and the environment. The author describes the book as the "How-to" book that gives you a "Check-up" from the "Neck up" to eliminate "Stinkin' Thinkin'" and avoid "Hardening of the Attitudes."

part VI
HOW TO GET THERE

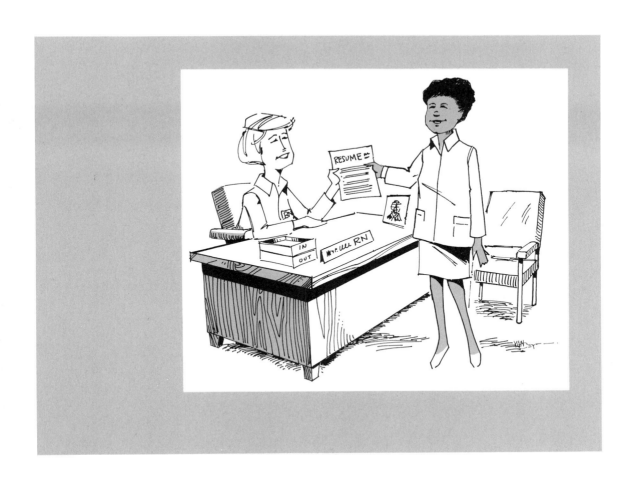

CHAPTER
19
Legal Aspects and Nursing Ethics

Learning Objectives

Upon completing this chapter, you will
1. Explain the relationship between legal aspects and nursing ethics.
2. Discuss what is meant by the patient's bill of rights.
3. Differentiate between civil action and criminal action.
4. List the five steps of the legal process, using the correct terms.
5. Explain the purpose of the Nurse Practice Act, an example of statutory law.
6. Define terms commonly used in Nurse Practice Acts:
   a. basic nursing care
   b. basic nursing situation
   c. complex nursing situation
   d. delegated medical act
   e. delegated nursing act
   f. direct supervision
   g. general supervision
7. Differentiate between mandatory and permissive licensure.
8. Describe how the nursing standard of care has come into being.
9. Review the four elements necessary to prove negligence.
10. Describe three intentional torts.
11. List six common causes of recurring liability for nurses.
12. Discuss how to document in a legally correct way.
13. Explain liability as it applies to the student nurse and instructor.
14. Differentiate between personal values and nursing ethics.
15. Give an example of how the patient's religious preference may relate to acceptance of treatment.

GENERAL LEGAL ASPECTS

Relationship of Legal Aspects to Ethics

Legal aspects of nursing refer to rules and regulations developed by society that help to control the practice of nursing. Ethics are not unlike the law in that each deals with rules of conduct that reflect underlying principles of right and wrong and codes of morality. Ethics are designed to protect the rights of human beings (Kozier et al., 1991, p. 132).

Importance of Legal Aspects

As practical nursing responsibility for involvement in the nursing process and accountability for providing quality nursing care increases, it becomes important for you to understand basic concepts of the laws that govern your nursing performance. This knowledge base will be of value to you in making decisions, and will help you to protect yourself from acts and decisions that could involve you in lawsuits and criminal prosecution.

Rights of Patients

It is recognized that a personal relationship between the physician and the patient is essential for the provision of proper medical care. The traditional physician–patient relationship takes on a new dimension when care is rendered within an organizational structure. Legal precedent has established that the institution itself also has a responsibility to the patient. It is in recognition of these factors that these rights are affirmed.

Patients have become increasingly concerned and vocal about the level of care they expect to receive. Several agencies have issued "Patient's Rights" statements. One of the most widely circulated statements is called the Patient's Bill of Rights and was issued by the American Hospital Association. It reads as follows:

1. The patient has the right to considerate and respectful care.

2. The patient has the right to obtain from his or her physician complete current information concerning his or her diagnosis, treatment, and prognosis in terms the patient can be reasonably be expected to understand. When it is not medically advisable to give such information to the patient, the information should be made available to an appropriate person in his or her behalf. He or she has the right to know, by name, the physician responsible for coordinating his or her care.

3. The patient has the right to receive from his or her physician information necessary to give informed consent prior to the start of any procedure and/or treatment. Except in emergencies, such information for informed consent should include but not necessarily be limited to the specific procedure and/or treatment, the medically significant risks involved, and the probable duration of incapacitation. Where medically significant alternatives for care or treatment exist or when the patient requests information concerning medical alternatives, the patient has the right to such information. The patient also has the right to know the name of the person responsible for the procedures and/or treatment. The patient receives this information from the physician prior to deciding whether or not to sign the consent form.

4. The patient has the right to refuse treatment to the extent permitted by law, and to be informed of the medical consequences of his or her action.

5. The patient has the right to every consideration of his or her privacy concerning his or her own medical care program. Case discussion, consultation, examination, and treatment are confidential and should be conducted discreetly. Those not directly involved in the patient's care must have the permission of the patient to be present.

6. The patient has the right to expect that all communications and records pertaining to his or her care should be treated as confidential.

7. The patient has the right to expect that, within its capacity, a hospital must make reasonable response to the request of a patient for services. The hospital must provide evaluation, service, and/or referral as indicated by the urgency of the case. When medically permissible a patient may be transferred to another facility only after he or she has received complete information and explanation concerning the needs for and alternatives to such a transfer. The institution to which the patient is to be transferred must first have accepted the patient for transfer.

8. The patient has the right to obtain information as to any relationship of his hospital to other health care and educational institutions insofar as his or her care is concerned. The patient has the right to obtain information as to the existence of any professional relationships among individuals (by name) who are treating him or her.

9. The patient has the right to be advised if the hospital proposes to engage in or perform human experimentation affecting his or her care or treatment. The patient has the right to refuse to participate in such research projects.

10. The patient has the right to expect reasonable continuity of care. He or she has the right to know in advance what appointment times and physicians are available and where. The patient has the right to expect that the hospital will provide a mechanism whereby he or she is informed by his or her physician or a delegate of the physician of the patient's continuing health care requirements following discharge.

11. The patient has the right to examine and receive an explanation of his or her bill, regardless of source of payment.

12. The patient has the right to know what hospital rules and regulations apply to his or her conduct as a patient.

Legal Aspects of Nursing and the Legal System

In order to understand the connection between legal aspects of nursing and the legal system found in the United States and Canada, a brief review of the legal system is in order. Both countries have their origins in the English Common Law System, hence the similarity. Common Law, sometimes called Judge-made Law, since it has its origin in the courts, is one way of establishing standards of legal conduct. It is useful in settling disputes, because once the judge has made a decision, this decision sets the precedent for a ruling on a case with similar facts in the future.

The legislative branch of the state and the federal government enact statutory laws. The Nurse Practice Act, which governs the practice of nursing, is an example of statutory law. Each state has its own nurse practice act; the states can do this as long as items in their law do not conflict with any federal statutes.

Types of Legal Action

The two classifications of legal action are civil action and criminal action. A civil action is related to individual rights, that is, to relationships between people. For example, if you cause harm by administering incorrect medication, the patient can bring a civil action suit against you. A criminal action involves persons and society as a whole. If nurses take it upon themselves to remove life-sustaining devices and the patient dies, this is considered murder, and a criminal action suit will be filed against the nurse.

Steps in Reaching Legal Decisions

Legal decisions are based on an orderly process generally consisting of five steps.

1. The plaintiff (who claims to have had his or her legal rights violated), files a complaint (document stating the grievance), and this is served to the defendant (individual the plaintiff claims is at fault).

2. The defendant responds with an answer (written response).

3. The plaintiff and defendant attempt to get all the facts during the discovery period (pretrial activities).

4. All important facts are presented to the judge and/or jury at the trial and a verdict (decision) is reached. The plaintiff bears the burden of proof (evidence of wrongdoing) during the trial.

5. An appeal (request for another trial), can be made if the judge's or jury's decision is not considered acceptable by either the plaintiff or the defendant.

(Adapted from Kozier and Erb, 1979, p. 84).

SPECIFIC LEGAL ASPECTS
Nurse Practice Acts

The duties and functions that nurses can perform are dictated on the state level by Nurse Practice Acts. The nurse practice act of each state defines what nursing is, what it is not, and under what circumstances it can be practiced for compensation.

The definitions of practical nursing found in state licensure laws clarify the type of nursing practical nurses will do as well as the leadership they will need. It is necessary for practical nurses to understand that they must limit their work to the area of authorized practical nursing. Practical nurses must realize, too, that no physician or registered professional nurse can give them a right to do more than what legally may be done.

In 1981 a practical nursing organization, NAPNES (National Association of Practical Nurse Education and Service), issued the following statement of responsibilities required for practice as a practical/vocational nurse:

- Recognizes the LPN/LVN's role in the health care delivery system and articulates that role with those of other health care team members

- Maintains accountability for one's own nursing practice within the ethical and legal framework

- Serves as a patient advocate

- Accepts a role in maintaining developing standards of practice in providing health care

- Seeks further growth through educational opportunities

Statements from official nursing organizations do not carry the weight of law. They are useful as a guide for behavior and may be used in a court of law as a point of reference. *The Nurse Practice Act of your state is your final authority.*

Terms Used in Nurse Practice Acts

Terminology remains standard in many states. As you study the standards of practice for licensed trained practical nurses in your state, knowledge of the following terms may be helpful.

Basic Nursing Care Nursing care that can be performed safely by the LPN, based on knowledge and skills gained during the educational program. Modifications of care are unnecessary and patient response is predictable.

Basic Patient Situation Situation as determined by the RN. Patient's clinical condition is predictable. Medical and nursing orders are not changing continuously and do not contain complex modifications. The patient's clinical condition requires only basic nursing care.

Complex Nursing Situation Situation as assessed by an RN. Patient's clinical condition is not predictable. Medical or nursing orders are likely to involve continuous change or complex modifications. Nursing care expectations are beyond that learned by the LPN during the educational program.

Delegated Medical Act Doctor's orders given to a RN or LPN by a physician, dentist, or podiatrist.

Delegated Nursing Act Nursing orders given to an RN or LPN by a RN.

Direct Supervision Supervisor is continuously present to coordinate, direct, or inspect nursing care.

General Supervision Supervisor regularly coordinates, directs, or inspects nursing care and is within reach either in the building or by telephone.

Licensure

Upon completion of a state-approved LPN/LVN nursing education program, a graduate is eligible to apply to take a national licensing examination (NCLEX-PN). Each state has established its own criteria for passing the examination.

States also have arrangements for interstate endorsement (reciprocity) for nurses who choose to work in other states. This means that it is possible to work in another state without repeating the NCLEX-PN if you have met that state's criteria for passing. Check Appendix A for the location of your state licensing board. All nurse practice acts address nursing licensure. Depending on the state in which you work, licensure will be mandatory or permissive.

Mandatory licensure protects, by law, the role of the nurse. This means that anyone who practices nursing must be licensed. Permissive licensure protects the title of the nurse. This means that the practical nurse may practice nursing without a license, but cannot use the title LPN or LVN.

> QUESTION: Which kind of license is required in your state?

The practice of licensing was instituted by nurses themselves. Nurses were concerned about the nursing care that they delivered and the safety of their patients.

All states and provinces have examining councils, which provide nursing examinations for licensure, and review complaints that can lead to revocation of a license. Because of the sheer numbers of complaints involved and the small number of board members, it is difficult to review all complaints. (Some states employ a compliance officer, who investigates suspected cases of drug/alcohol abuse.) It is interesting to note that the highest number of revocations are related to drug addiction, an illness, and rarely to incompetency in nursing practice or failure

to update nursing skills. This is something to think about, since a significant criteria for licensure is the need to protect the public's safety or welfare.

> QUESTION: What happens to the LPN whose license is revoked for drug addiction, and who remains untreated?

There is a phrase used in nursing that has important legal implications: "You are held to the nursing standard of care." "The standard of care is established when an ordinary, prudent nurse would have performed in the same or similar manner" (Calloway, 1986, p. 8). Resources for nursing standard of care are

- Nurse practice act—identifies the minimum competency necessary for you to function as a LPN in your state.

- Nursing licensure examination—written tests for minimum competency.

- Practical nursing programs—based on guidelines provided by the board of nursing, to guarantee a minimum knowledge base and clinical practice necessary to give safe nursing care. Curricula, textbooks, and instructors are resources for standard of care.

- Written policies and procedure—the agency for which you work provides a standard of nursing care for you to follow. This is the reason it is so important for you to read the policies of the agency in order to find out if verbal directions are supported by written policies. If ever a question regarding care comes up in court, a lawyer will use the hospital policy and procedure manual as one guide to expected behavior. Remember that policies and procedures do not overrule your state's Nurse Practice Act and educational preparation.

- Custom—an unwritten, usually acceptable way of giving nursing care.

- Law—Decisions that have been arrived at in similar cases brought up before a court.

- Statements from the NFLPN and NAPNES.

Nursing Negligence

The terms **negligence** and **malpractice** are often used interchangeably in nursing, since malpractice is the part of the negligence law that relates to lack of skill or misconduct by professional persons. Some states, however, differ on the issue of whether nurses are professional and can commit malpractice. "Negligence is conduct which falls below the standard of care established by law for the protection of others, and thus, involves an unreasonable risk of harm to the patient" (Calloway, 1986, p. 11). It relates to the action or lack of action, not to what you intended to do. Good intentions do not enter in. As a nurse you are held responsible for your conduct. Students are held to a level of graduate performance.

Elements Necessary for Negligence

Duty, breach of duty, proximate cause, and damages are the four elements that must be present to cause an action for negligence against the nurse. Each of the four must be proven by the patient in order to receive compensation. *Duty* refers to the nurse's responsibility to provide care and to do so in an acceptable way. For example, the nurse has a duty based on education as well as the expectations and standards of his or her place of employment. *Breach of duty* means that the nurse did not adhere to the nursing standard of care, that is, what was expected of the nurse was not done or was not done correctly. *Proximate cause* means that a reasonable cause-and-effect relationship can be shown between the omission or commission of the nursing act and the harm to the patient, that is, did the nurse's negligent act cause the injury in question? *Damages* means that the patient must be able to show that the nurse's negligent act injured him or her in some way—he or she must prove actual damage.

Torts

A **tort** is a wrong or injury done to someone that violates his or her rights. Negligence fits into the category of unintentional torts, since the nurse's conduct, not state of mind, is the issue. Intentional torts require a specific state of mind, that is, that the nurse involved intended to do the wrongful act. Significantly, not all insurance companies cover intentional torts in the malpractice insurance policy. Check your policy. Examples of intentional torts include

- **Assault** and **Battery**—**Assault** is an unjustified attempt or threat to touch someone. **Battery** is actual physical harm to someone. Remember this when a patient refuses a treatment or medication. The patient gives implied consent (permission) by entering the institution for certain routine treatments, but retains the right verbally to refuse any treatment, and may leave the institution when he or she chooses unless he or she is there for court-ordered treatment. Nurses can protect themselves from assaultive patients, but can use only as much force as is considered reasonable to protect themselves.

- **False imprisonment** and use of restraints—False imprisonment is keeping someone detained against their will and can include use of restraints, or secluding a patient in a room without cause and without a doctor's order. Restraining by verbal threats of physical harm, is also included in this category.

QUESTION: How does the Patients' Bill of Rights relate to the care of an elderly confused patient?

- **Defamation**—Defamation means damage to someone's reputation through false or unprivileged communication. **Libel** is defamation through written communication or pictures. **Slander** is defamation by verbalizing untrue or private information (gossip) to a third party. Each patient has the right to expect that you will share information about him or her only with health providers who are actively involved in promoting his or her health. This is called **confidentiality.** He or she further has the right to expect you to speak the truth. Additional unnecessary conversation with coworkers and those outside of the agency can result in a charge of defamation. The same is true with all documented information or invading his or her privacy by taking unwanted photographs or showing his or her affliction to others, students included, without permission. Patient privacy is protected by law. Remember: Loose lips may sink your ship

Consider also, that you and other health care providers have the same right to privacy. You often are privy to information about personal lives of nurses, physicians and other coworkers. While the desire to repeat the information you hear may be tempting, it is best left unsaid.

COMMON CAUSES OF NURSING LIABILITY

Many of the errors leading to common nursing liabilities can be avoided by following the guidelines that you learn in nursing school.

QUESTION: In what major areas are you evaluated during each clinical rotation?

Areas of liability involved can be categorized as safety, knowledge, skill, observation and reporting, documentation, accepting responsibility for nursing actions, and delegation of tasks—all part of the usual clinical evaluation. The most common errors are drug errors, most of which can be avoided if you follow the guidelines you learn in basic nursing and practice in the clinical areas. Other recurring liabilities include falls, burns, failure to note and report changes in condition, error in patient identity, infection or cross-infection resulting from lack of aseptic technique, inability to recognize and to refuse to follow improper doctor's orders, and failure to note patient allergies (Calloway, 1986, p. 35). One of the best defenses against malpractice is developing rapport with the patient. The very best defense is to not err in the first place.

Charting

Proper documentation is basic nursing no matter which institution you visit. The forms may be different, but the basics remain the same. The chart is a legal document and can be used in court. Be sure to review the charting procedure for your specific institution and adhere to it. Proper charting is also an opportunity for you to show that you have a legitimate knowledge base, and it gives credibility to practical nursing as a vocation. As recommended in Chapter 2, use the patient-care plan as the format for charting.

General Guidelines for Legal Documentation

Regardless of the method of charting used by an institution, the following guidelines will apply.

1. Each entry should be accurate, factual, and objective. Nurses must consistently remind themselves to avoid subjective comments when charting. Eliminate the word "appears" except for sleeping.

2. Each entry should be legible and spelled correctly. Print, if this is an agency policy or if your handwriting is hard to read. Use correct punctuation, as the meaning of a sentence can change based on punctuation.

3. Charting entries are generally written in chronologic order, indicating when the event happened in the time column. If someone else writes on the chart before you are able to record an entry or you have forgotten an entry, a late entry may be used. Put actual charting time in the time column for the late entry and include actual times events occurred in nurses' notes. Strive to place entries on the chart as soon as possible after they occur. Check the policy manual to clarify if the time column indicates the time the event happened or the time that the charting took place.

4. Use permanent ink (no erasable pens) in a color identified in the institution's procedure manual.

5. Do not leave blank lines or spaces in your charting. If an item on a flow sheet does not apply, write in N/A (not applicable). If other staff persons need to make an entry, do not save lines, as they can make a late entry. Write your signature immediately after the period.

6. Ditto marks are never used.

7. *Use only approved abbreviations as found in the institution's policy and procedure manual.*

8. Document medical and nursing treatments performed and the patient's response to these treatments. If the patient refuses these treatments, document the refusal.

9. Chart communication with the doctor, especially phone conversations. Avoid writing, "Doctor called; no orders received." Document communication with supervisors by name and content of conversation.

10. As a LPN, do not cosign for nursing students. If you must sign off a patient chart that is not for one of your patients, write "I'm signing this to complete the record; I have no knowledge of the patient."

11. Do not add notes once charting is complete unless using a *late entry format.*.

12. Do not delete notes or correct errors with "white out."

13. Chart all abnormal observations, including change in patient's condition and to whom these observations are reported.

14. Record care actually given, not care that will be given in the future.

15. Each timed entry should be signed using your full, legal title as determined by your state.

ADDITIONAL LEGAL CONCERNS
Employer Liability

The employer may be held responsible for acts performed by the nurse within the scope of employment. However, the employer may sue the nurse to recover fees and other monies involved while defending him or her.

Verbal Orders

Should not be accepted except in emergency situations. Written order by the physician protects the doctor, the patient, and the nurse. It is difficult to explain to the court why the physician, who has access to the chart, did not write the order. *Verbal orders should be repeated for accuracy.*

Telephone Orders

When used, should be given directly to the nurse, who checks it out with the doctor, including spelling if necessary, since so many medications sound alike these days and doses can be confusing. If it is a sensitive order, meaning one that carries special risk, have two people listen to the order.

Be sure to check the policy of your employer as to the appropriateness of an LPN accepting phone orders.

Telephone Logs

These can be used routinely to document the time, problem, and the advice received or given. Also log attempted calls.

Discharge Instruction/Patient Education

This is the domain of the nurse, in which LPNs play a supportive role, once the instruction or education is started by the RN. This needs to be done verbally and in writing, with the patient signing a form indicating he or she understands the information. Preprinted information is valuable and available in many agencies.

Incident Reports

Intended for in-house improvement in care. They should, however, be written with the thought that they may be viewed by attorneys on the "other side." Should be written immediately by the health provider(s) who witnessed the incident. Include the patient's description of what happened. The report needs to be legible, factual, objective, in permanent ink and should not be worded to accept or place blame. Avoid drawing conclusions. While the incident itself is also recorded on the patient's chart, avoid writing "Incident Report Filed" here.

General Consent

Obtained for treating a patient upon admission. May be obtained by the nurse. The fact that a person has voluntarily sought admission and willingly signs a general admission form is an example of general consent. A patient may revoke this permission verbally.

Informed Consent

Informed consent must be obtained for invasive procedures for therapeutic or diagnostic purposes (for example, surgery). This means that the patient is told in nontechnical language

- What the treatment is
- What the risks are
- Alternative treatments
- Who will do the treatment
- If the treatment is really necessary

The patient must also indicate understanding of the above information.

Parents cannot give informed consent for the treatment of their children. What they can do is authorize treatment for their children up to a certain age.

In most states, informed consent is the responsibility of the doctor, since he or she must explain the implications and complications of the procedure to the patient before obtaining written permission. The patient may revoke this permission verbally.

Access to Medical Records

The medical record belongs to the hospital, but the patient has the right to see the record. The

practical nurse, however, does not have the authority to give the record to the patient. Refer patient requests to view the medical record to your supervisor and the doctor.

Abandonment

You may not leave your place of employment until you can transfer care of patients to your replacement. Notify your supervisor if you are short staffed. Follow with a memo, since a memo is more effective than verbal notification alone. Keep a copy for yourself.

Duty to Refuse to Carry Out Improper Orders

A doctor's written or verbal order is a legal order for the nurse to carry out. However, the nurse has the responsibility to recognize an order that may harm the patient and refuse to carry it out. Deal directly with the doctor first. If this is unsuccessful, use the nursing chain of command, beginning with your immediate supervisor. However, if it is not resolved through nursing, it must reach the physician chain of command quickly, in order to avoid harm to the patient. Document in the nursing notes and prepare an incident report identifying "inappropriate MD behavior." *Remember:* Always check out any order a patient questions before carrying it out.

Standing Orders

Some states do not allow standing orders except in intensive and coronary care units. Since standing orders call for making judgments, the practical nurse must always check first with the RN before carrying them out.

No-Code Orders

These are legal orders written by the physician and do not have to be updated, unless the patient changes his mind. "If no written order exists and the nurse does not code the patient, he/she is in effect making a medical decision. This amounts to practicing medicine without a license" (Calloway, 1986, p. 99). There is no such thing as a partial or slow code. All care givers must know when a written no-code order exists. Check your state and agency policy regarding no-code orders.

Signing a Will

Nurses may usually witness the signing of a will if they do not stand to gain personally from the will. Check your agency policy before doing so.

As a student, check with your instructor before agreeing to witness the signing of a will. If the instructor gives approval, you must document in the patient's record that you witnessed signing of a will.

Removal of Life Support Systems

The doctor must pronounce the patient dead and document same *before* the nurse turns off the ventilator.

Malpractice Insurance for Nurses

These days, more and more nurses are being sued. Nurses are responsible for their own acts. While the agency may assume responsibility for you during a suit, they can turn around and sue you. Did you know that you can also be held responsible for "neighborhood advice"; for example, telling a neighbor how to care for her sick child?

Each nurse must carefully consider if it is necessary to purchase a malpractice insurance policy. Look very carefully at the circumstances that are a part of the agency of which you are an employee. See Table 19-1.

Liability of Student Nurses and Instructors

Student nurses are held accountable for their nursing care. You are held to the standards of a graduate; this emphasizes the necessity of

1. preparation for working in the clinical area. The instructor is held responsible for making

Table 19-1 Malpractice

Reasons for your own malpractice insurance coverage.

1. The jury's award could exceed the limits of your hospital's coverage.
2. Your employing hospital could pay out an award to a plaintiff and then countersue you.
3. You acted outside the scope of employment and the hospital argues it is not liable.
4. Your employer's policy covers you only on the job.
5. A hospital might carry a policy that covers you only while you are employed by that institution and a suit may come up years after you have stopped working for an employer. It is suggested that nurses purchase *occurrence* coverage and not *claims coverage*. For this reason, occurrence coverage protects the nurse for each incident regardless of present employer.
6. Hospital may decide to settle out of court. Plaintiff could pursue a case against the nurse.
7. Has your employer paid the insurance premium?
8. After a settlement, insurers could turn around and sue the nurse.
9. With your own coverage, you will have your own lawyers, not the lawyers also defending the hospital.

sure that the student assigned to a patient has the necessary knowledge base and skill to give safe nursing care. The instructor is also expected to provide reasonable supervision for the care given by a student.

2. requesting additional help or supervision if needed

3. complying with agency and school of nursing policies.

Floating

"Floating" is working in an area that is not your usual work area. In 1991, the Joint Commission on Accreditation of Health-Care Organizations (JCAHO) revised its nursing care standards that are used as a basis for accreditation decisions. One of the standards states that nursing staff are competent to fulfill their assigned responsibilities. Directives from the Joint Commission include the need for timely and adequate orientation and cross-training, so it is hoped that practical nurses will have adequate orientation and cross-training for float areas. You will have the responsibility for informing supervisors if you do not feel competent working in any assigned area.

Reporting Incompetence of Other Health Providers

A drug- or alcohol-abusing nurse should be reported. Document incidents to support your report; this is a moral, ethical, and legal responsibility. A nurse must determine at the beginning of a nursing career, who is the priority. Hopefully the answer is "the patient."

Money and Gifts

Nurses may not accept money or gifts from patients. Some cultures feel it is an insult to turn down their offer of a gift. The nurse might tactfully suggest a gift be given to the facility instead.

Good Samaritan Acts

Good Samaritan Acts govern how a person who renders emergency care at the scene of an accident, in good faith, will be immune from civil liability for their actions while providing the care. The state statutes are of special concern to nurses and physicians who provide emergency care outside of the agency that employs them.

QUESTION: What does your state's Good Samaritan Act say?

Physical and Emotional Abuse

In the course of your career in practical nursing, you will probably suspect or actually see the results of some type of abuse. As a practical nurse, you have a special legal responsibility to report your suspicions/observations of abuse to your supervisor immediately. Refer to your state's abuse laws for specific rules that govern your responsibility for reporting abuse.

It is especially important to be empathetic (as opposed to sympathetic) so that your observations/reporting will be as objective as possible. Becoming a part of the patient's emotions may lead you to jump to conclusions or accept a particularly convincing, but untrue, explanation. Remember that whether this is a child, woman, man, or elder, reputations are at stake. Once accusations are made, it is difficult to be truly free, even when not guilty.

Report your suspicions to your supervisor right away. Offer concrete, specific observations. Quote statements made and avoid offering a personal interpretation. Let the facts speak for themselves.

Euthanasia

Euthanasia is often referred to as mercy killing, that is, assisting with a killing or permitting the death of a person who is terminally ill.

Euthanasia is not the same as a no-code order written by a physician based on a decision between the physician and the patient and/or family. Active euthanasia is illegal and considered a crime in the United States. You are to avoid participation in euthanasia.

Organ Donation

Organ donations are voluntary; they cannot be bought or sold. Many patients and families give permission for organ donation after death. In fact, you may have been asked to agree to personal organ donation at the time you got your driver's license. Many states participate in this effort.

Body tissue that can be donated include skin, cornea, bone, and heart valves. Body organs include the heart, liver, kidneys, lungs, and pancreas.

Nursing Ethics

A code of ethics is basic to all cultures, groups, and professions. Ethics provide guidelines for living and/or performing, and the basis for difficult decisions. "In nursing, ethics provide professional standards for nursing activities, which protect the nurse and the patient" (Kozier et al., 1991, p. 132).

As a student nurse, your initial functioning is based on your personal values, the beliefs that you have gained primarily from your family and significant others. It is helpful if these values correlate with the nursing code of ethics. This is an important reason for having you learn nursing ethics and for asking you to evaluate your personal value system. As a practical nurse, you inherit the responsibility of carrying out ethical nursing actions and behaving in an ethical manner.

The International Council of Nurses (ICN) first adopted a code of ethics for nurses in 1965. The National Association for Practical Nurse Educators and Service (NAPNES) adopted a code of ethics for the LPN in 1941. NAPNES currently has 19 state correspondents of the organization. It keeps practical nurses apprised

of updates and changes through *The Journal of Practical Nursing.*

The National Federation of Licensed Practical Nurses (NFLPN) has 26 state affiliates. Many state affiliates continue to encourage student nurses to participate in the organization after graduation. NFLPN encourages student participation at the state convention and plans a portion of the program around student needs. In order to understand this effort, it is helpful to explore the NFLPN code of ethics for practical nurses before attending the convention.

The National Federation of Licensed Practical Nurses (NFLPN) has developed a code for licensed practical/vocational nurses. Table 19-2 presents the code on the left, with space on the right for you to write a statement about your personal value system as it applies to the code. Evaluate your value system as it is today.

When you have completed writing in your personal values regarding the code, go back to the beginning and decide if a value adjustment is needed. Remember that values are learned; therefore, they can be unlearned. New values can be practiced until they become a part of you and meld with the NFLPN code for nurses.

Examples of Ethical Issues in Nursing

There are numerous life-and-death issues that are directly related to personal values and nursing ethics. These include such issues as the acquired immunodeficiency syndrome (AIDS), confidentiality, abortion, prolonging life through artificial means, organ transplants, withdrawing or withholding nourishment, and withholding a blood transfusion because it conflicts with the patient's beliefs/values.

The following examples may help you to put the NFLPN code to work for you.

AIDS and Other Communicable or Infectious Diseases

NFLPN code #3 directs you to provide health care to all patients regardless of race, creed, cultural background, or lifestyle. In essence, the

Table 19-2 Nursing Ethics versus Personal Values

NFLPN CODE FOR LICENSED PRACTICAL/ VOCATIONAL NURSES	A STATEMENT OF MY PERSONAL VALUE SYSTEM	ADJUSTMENT NEEDED
Know the scope of maximum utilization of the LP/VN as specified by the nursing practice act and function within this scope		
Safeguard the confidential information acquired from any source about the patient		
Provide health care to all patients regardless of race, creed, cultural background, disease, or lifestyle		
Refuse to give endorsement to the sale and promotion of commercial products or services		
Uphold the highest standards in personal appearance, language, dress and demeanor		
Stay informed about issues affecting the practice of nursing and delivery of health care and, where appropriate, participate in government and policy decisions		
Accept the responsibility for safe nursing practice by keeping oneself mentally and physically fit and educationally prepared to practice		

Table continued on the following page.

Accept the responsibility for membership in NFLPN and participate in its efforts to maintain the established standards of nursing practice and employment policies that lead to quality patient care

From Nursing Practice Standards booklet. Raleigh, NC: National Federation of Licensed Practical Nurses (NFLPN).

nurse's moral values do not cancel out the nurse's moral responsibility to care for patients.

Confidentiality

NFLPN code #2 directs you to safeguard the confidential information acquired from any source about patients. Translated, this means that you do not share patient information with anyone not directly related to patient care. However, you must let patients know from the beginning that you will be sharing information pertinent to their care and well-being with others involved in their care. In this way, you will not be trapped into promising to keep a secret only to discover that the secret is directly related to the patient's current hospitalization and treatment.

Abortion

NFLPN code #6 directs you to stay informed about issues affecting the practice of nursing and the delivery of health care. Most states/provinces have a "conscience clause," which permits nurses to refuse to assist in doing an abortion if doing so violates their religious or moral principles. Refusal can occur without fear of reprisal. Equally important are patients' rights to their personal values. You do not have the right to attempt to impose your values on them.

Withdrawing and Withholding Food

NFLPN code #1 directs you to know the scope of maximum utilization of LPNs as specified by the Nurse Practice Act of the state and function within this scope. This means that withholding or withdrawing food is *not* a practical nursing decision.

A recent ethical and legal issue that has surfaced is the replacement of the Living Will with a document called the Durable Power of Attorney-Health (DPOA-Health). The Living Will listed patient preferences to the doctor. The DPOA-Health allows individuals, while lucid, to appoint an individual to speak on their behalf when they are unable to make decisions. The document informs their spokesperson of the decisions they wish to have made regarding their health care.

These are serious issues for you to think about, right now, at the beginning of this personally demanding vocation.

Accountability in Nursing

You have already learned that nursing demands that you be responsible, that is, reliable and trustworthy. At no time can you expect a peer or supervisor or patient to say to you, "It's OK that you didn't come to work today because your car isn't functioning properly," or "It's OK if we talk about your interests and problems today" (rather than those of the patients), or "It's OK that you didn't do the work you were assigned because it is an 'off' day for you." Nursing says, "I'm sorry that you have problems to cope with that are heavy, but it's up to you to deal with them because your priority, in this vocation, is the patient."

The word "accountability" means that you are answerable. As a nursing student you are answerable to yourself, to your assigned patient, to the team leader, to the physician, and certainly to your instructor, who constantly evaluates your work. As a LPN, accountability to the instructor is replaced by accountability to the employing agency. You are held accountable for all of the nursing actions that you perform or are assigned to perform. The measures of accountability are the nursing standards of practice. (See Tables 19-3 and 19-4.) Through theory class, and by providing nursing care to patients using this knowledge, many of the issues of both responsibility and accountability become an integral part of you.

Table 19-3 NFLPN Nursing Practice Standards

INTRODUCTORY STATEMENT

DEFINITION

Practical/Vocational nursing means the performance for compensation of authorized acts of nursing that utilize specialized knowledge and skills and that meet the health needs of people in a variety of settings under the direction of qualified health professionals.

SCOPE

Practical/Vocational nursing comprises the common core of nursing and, therefore, is a valid entry into the nursing profession.

Opportunities exist for practicing in a milieu where different professions unite their particular skills in a team effort for one common objective—to preserve or improve an individual patient's functioning.

Opportunities also exist for upward mobility within the profession through academic education and for lateral expansion of knowledge and expertise through both academic and continuing education.

STANDARDS

EDUCATION

The Licensed Practical/Vocational Nurse

1. Shall complete a formal education program in practical nursing approved by the appropriate nursing authority in a state.

2. Shall successfully pass the National Council Licensure Examination for Practical Nurses.

3. Shall participate in initial orientation within the employing institution.

LEGAL/ETHICAL STATUS

The Licensed Practical/Vocational Nurse

1. Shall hold a current license to practice nursing as an LP/VN in accordance with the law of the state wherein employed.

2. Shall know the scope of nursing practice authorized by the Nursing Practice Act in the state wherein employed.

3. Shall have a personal commitment to fulfill the legal responsibilities inherent in good nursing practice.

Table continued on the following page.

4. Shall take responsible actions in situations wherein there is unprofessional conduct by a peer or other health care provider.

5. Shall recognize and have a commitment to meet the ethical and moral obligations of the practice of nursing.

6. Shall not accept or perform professional responsibilities which the individual knows (s)he is not competent to perform.

PRACTICE

The Licensed Practical/Vocational Nurse

1. Shall accept assigned responsibilities as an accountable member of the health care team.

2. Shall function within the limits of educational preparation and experience as related to the assigned duties.

3. Shall function with other members of the health care team in promoting and maintaining health, preventing disease and disability, caring for and rehabilitating individuals who are experiencing an altered health state, and contributing to the ultimate quality of life until death.

4. Shall know and utilize the nursing process in planning (Assessing [data gathering]), implementing, and evaluating health services and nursing care for the individual patient or group.
   a. Planning (Assessing [data gathering]): The planning of nursing includes:
      1) assessment of health status of the individual patient, the family and community groups
      2) an analysis of the information gained from assessment
      3) the identification of health goals.
   b. Implementation: The plan for nursing care is put into practice to achieve the stated goals and includes:
      1) observing, recording and reporting significant changes which require intervention or different goals
      2) applying nursing knowledge and skills to promote and maintain health, to prevent disease and disability and to optimize functional capabilities of an individual patient
      3) assisting the patient and family with activities of daily living and encouraging self-care as appropriate
      4) carrying out therapeutic regimens and protocols prescribed by an RN, physician, or other persons authorized by state law.
   c. Evaluations: The plan for nursing care and its implementations are evaluated to measure the progress toward the stated goals and will include appropriate persons and/or groups to determine:
      1) the relevancy of current goals in relation to the progress of the individual patient
      2) the involvement of the recipients of care in the evaluation process
      3) the quality of the nursing action in the implementation of the plan
      4) a re-ordering of priorities or new goal setting in the care plan.

5. Shall participate in peer review and other evaluation processes.

6. Shall participate in the development of policies concerning the health and nursing needs of society and in the roles and functions of the LP/VN.

CONTINUING EDUCATION

The Licensed Practical/Vocational Nurse

1. Shall be responsible for maintaining the highest possible level of professional competence at all times.

2. Shall periodically reassess career goals and select continuing education activities which will help to achieve these goals.

3. Shall take advantage of continuing education opportunities which will lead to personal growth and professional development.

4. Shall seek and participate in continuing education activities which are approved for credit by appropriate organizations, such as the NFLPN.

From Nursing Practice Standards booklet. Raleigh, NC: National Federation of Licensed Practical Nurses (NFLPN).

Specialized Nursing Practice

Some of you will assume responsibility in a specialized nursing practice area. An example is to accept a leadership position in a nursing home or extended-care setting.

The NFLPN Nursing Practice Standards include standards for specialized nursing practice (see Table 19-4). Review your Board of Nursing criteria for specialized nursing practice before accepting a specialized nursing position.

PUTTING IT TOGETHER: VALUES, ETHICS, AND LEGAL ISSUES

As you read the following two situations, see yourself as the LPN who has to answer the following:

QUESTION: What will you do based on your values, nursing ethics, and legal issues involved?

How will your decision help you to maintain responsibility and accountability in nursing?

Situation #1

Amanda K. Havana, age 68, has experienced a hemorrhage, resulting in a significant loss of blood. She has been rushed from the nursing home to the hospital emergency room, and the physician determines that a blood transfusion is needed immediately in order to save her life. You have accompanied Mrs. Havana to the emergency room, and quickly inform the physician that Mrs. Havana adheres to the beliefs of the Jehovah's Witnesses (Watchtower Bible and

Table 19-4 NFLPN Specialized Nursing Practice Standards

The Licensed Practical/Vocational Nurse

1. Shall have had at least one year's experience in nursing at the staff level.

2. Shall present personal qualifications that are indicative of potential abilities for practice in the chosen specialized nursing area.

3. Shall present evidence of completion of a program or course that is approved by an appropriate agency to provide the knowledge and skills necessary for effective nursing services in the specialized field.

4. Shall meet all of the standards of practice as set forth in this document.

Tract Society). Mrs. Havana confirms this and further states that she does not want blood, and that if she dies for lack of it "so be it." Although the practical nurse does not usually administer blood, you need to be alert to the ethical and legal issues evoked by the patient's refusal to have a transfusion.

What belief holds Mrs. Havana firm to her refusal of a blood transfusion? First of all, she believes the Bible is God's word and the truth, and that all of God's laws presented in the Bible must be obeyed. Based on Genesis 9:3-4, Leviticus 17:10, and Acts 15:28-29, Jehovah's Witnesses equate blood with life and believe that taking blood into one's body through the mouth or veins is a violation of God's law (Anderson, 1983, p. 32). Mrs. Havana accepts her possible death due to refusal of a transfusion as dying for her beliefs, not as suicide. She is receptive to other options that do not violate her beliefs.

According to the *Emergency Nurse Legal Bulletin* (1982, p. 2), "treating a patient without consent is a battery whether or not the treatment is medically beneficial." The physician may attempt to get a court order for the transfusion. However, "when the patient is fully competent, is not pregnant and has no children, a court is unlikely to compel a life-saving blood transfusion over the patient's refusal." When faced with a similar situation, the practical nurse respects the patient's belief system and notifies the supervisor for further advice/interpretation.

Situation #2

You are employed in a pediatric unit. An infant admitted immediately after birth for emergency surgery is facing death. According to the parent's faith, the infant must be baptized. Since you are Baptist, you do not believe in infant baptism.

Look again at the questions presented to you prior to the situations. Discuss with your classmates the alternatives available to you that will fulfill the patient's and parent's needs without compromising your values, nursing ethics, and nursing standards of care.

Summary

Legal aspects of nursing refer to rules and regulations developed by society that help to control the practice of nursing. "Ethics are the rules or principles which govern right conduct. They deal with what is good or bad and with moral duty and obligations. Ethics are not unlike the law in that each deals with rules of conduct, that reflect underlying principles of right and wrong and codes of morality" (Kozier et al., 1991, p. 132).

You have the responsibility of knowing the law—the Nurse Practice Act of your state. It is a major resource for nursing standards of care. Nurses are held accountable for their nursing actions, and ignorance of the law is not accepted as an excuse for illegal or unethical practices.

Common areas of nursing liability most often can be avoided by following through on guidelines learned in basic nursing. Medication errors are number one on the list of recurring liabilities.

Guidelines for nursing ethics have been developed by the International Council of Nurses (ICN), the National Federation of Licensed Practical Nurses (NFLPN), and the National Association of Practical Nurse Education and Service (NAPNES) for practical/vocational nurses.

Evaluate your personal values and compare them with accepted codes of nursing ethics. Difficult decisions about topics such as AIDS, abortion, organ transplantations, confidentiality, maintenance of life through life-support systems, and refusal of treatment due to religious convictions are some of the many ethical/legal issues facing nurses today.

REFERENCES

Alexis A. Body searches and the right to privacy. J Psychosoc Nurs 1986; 24(11):21–25.

Anderson G. Medicine vs. religion: the case of Jehovah's Witnesses. Health Soc Work 1983.

Calloway SD. *Nursing and the Law.* Eau Claire, WI: Professional Education Systems, 1986.

Christenson BL, Kockrow EO. *Foundations of Nursing.* St Louis: CV Mosby, 1991.

Emergency Nurse Legal Bulletin. Westville, NJ: Med/Law Publishers, 1982.

Hurley ML. What Do the New JCAHO Standards Mean for You? RN 1991; 54(6):42–46.

Jones, I. Nurses and their religions three bearing witness. Nurs Times 1984; February 8:47–48.

Kendrick D, Wilber G. Seclusion: organizing safe and effective care. J Psychosoc Nurs 1986; 24(11):26–28.

Kozier B, Erb G, Oliveri R. *Fundamentals of Nursing.* Menlo Park, CA: Addison–Wesley, 1979.

Kozier B, Erb G, Oliveri R. *Fundamentals of Nursing.* Menlo Park, CA: Addison–Wesley, 1991.

Moss J. Membership Services, NFLPN; Raleigh, NC, 1992.

Muir R. Providing for the rights and safety of patients. J Psychosoc Nurs 1986; 24(11):29–31

NAPNES (National Association of Practical Nurse Education and Service), 1976, 1981.

Oriol M. Involuntary commitment and the right to refuse medication. J Psychosoc Nurs 1986; 24(11):15–20.

Scianfani M. Violence and behavior control. J Psychosoc Nurs 1986; 24(11):8–13.

CHAPTER
20
Preparing for NCLEX-PN

Learning Objectives

Upon completing this chapter, you will
1. Explain what is meant by NCLEX-PN.
2. Discuss the requirements of your state board of nursing for eligibility to take the licensing examination.
3. Define licensure through endorsement.
4. Differentiate between a temporary work permit and licensure.
5. Discuss minimum competency.
6. Practice exercises to reduce test-taking anxiety.

INTRODUCTION

Almost without exception, when student nurses are asked about their goal for the year, they respond by saying, "Pass Boards," meaning, pass the licensure examination. If you have begun to utilize the information offered you in previous chapters, you are on your way to attaining that goal. For example, in Chapter 4, "The Adult Learner," you were supported in the special needs of adult learners, meaning you, and encouraged to seek out areas of personal strengths and weaknesses. You learned about your rights and responsibilities as a learner, and were encouraged to participate actively in the learning process.

In Chapter 5, "Time Management," you learned about the value of managing your time. You had the opportunity, through specific planned activity, to develop a schedule for your individual needs—one that would allow for adequate time for study and clinical preparation.

Chapter 6 offered a unique opportunity in "Discovering Your Learning Style." It introduced you to ways of enhancing your primary learning style(s), so that you can make it work for you during this year. You also learned about the relationship of attitude and learning, and the difference between reactive and active learning.

Chapter 7 focused on "Learning How to Learn." Do you recall techniques to increase your personal degree of concentration in learning situations, improving personal listening skills, ways to enhance memory of information needed for practical nursing, and ways to increase speed of reading and degree of comprehension? That was a jam-packed chapter.

Chapter 8 provided "Hints for Using Learning Resources." Some of you learned for the first time about the PQRST method of textbook study. Practical suggestions were included on how to make the PQRST method work for you. You also learned how to gain the most from a variety of teaching methods used by instructors. Information on how to use library resources set the stage for locating assigned materials and, hopefully, set a lifelong pattern of using these valuable resources. The information

on test taking, if practiced faithfully, has already begun to make written evaluation a part of the educational process, rather than something to be feared. It has also begun to prepare you for the licensure examination, NCLEX-PN, made up of multiple-choice questions.

Chapter 9, "Personality Development," gave you pointers on maintaining a positive attitude during this new educational adventure. It focused on the need for positive self-talk as the basis for positive functioning, both personally and in your course of study.

Chapter 10, "Wellness And Personal Care," identified ways to keep your personal machinery in good repair. It challenged you to evaluate your current wellness and personal care and to make a realistic plan for change based on need. There is no doubt that good study habits, learning, and testing skills are put on hold when one does not feel physically or emotionally fit.

Chapter 11, "Assertiveness as a Nursing Responsibility," supported your need to advocate, not only for the patient, but also for yourself. It supported your right to let instructors know about your learning needs and for you to say "No" to unnecessary distractions that cut into preparation time at home.

Chapter 13 dealt with a major problem in the vocational domain—"Job-Related Communication." It offered ways for you to assess your communication style and ways to make sure that you are understood and that you understand the meaning of others.

Other chapters have been written to give you a sense of where you fit into nursing and, with your permission, a sense of belonging in nursing. Techniques, plus feeling good about your vocation enhance your ability to see NCLEX-PN as a step that you will be prepared for when the time comes. We intend for you to be successful in your pursuit of licensure in practical nursing. We further suggest that select chapters be reviewed throughout the year.

WHAT IS NCLEX-PN?

NCLEX-PN is the National Council Licensing Examination that graduate practical nurses take in order to practice nursing legally. This permits the nurse to use the title licensed practical nurse (LPN) or licensed vocational nurse (LVN). The purpose of a licensing examination is to protect the consumer of health care by ensuring minimal competency on the part of the practical nurse who is giving care. Statistics summarized by the testing service indicate that in 1990, over 42,000 graduates of practical nursing programs in U.S. jurisdictions took NCLEX-PN, and these test candidates had an 89% pass rate (Johnson, 1990, p. 5).

Changes in the nursing examination have occurred because of increasing concern that state board tests no longer reflected the actual knowledge base and responsibilities of the practical nurse in the workplace. In the early 1980s, the McGraw-Hill Publishing Company won a bid for item writers for the licensing examinations for registered and practical nurses. NCLEX-RN and NCLEX-PN were born!

Each state's Board of Nursing arranges for actual nurses to write items for the national boards. The same boards contract with NCLEX to arrange administration of the licensing examination. Items formulated for NCLEX-PN are based on job analysis of activities practical nurses perform in the workplace. The initial survey of practical nurses identified 180 workplace activities. These activities were validated and evaluated for frequency and criticality. Minimum competencies for safe practice were identified.

The purpose of a licensing examination in nursing is to ensure minimal competence on the part of the nurse in order to protect the consumer of health care. The 180 workplace activities identified are the basis for developing test items for NCLEX-PN.

During October, 1990 a three-year cycle for entry-level PN workplace analysis of activities plus an evaluation of the NCLEX-PN test plan was begun. The purpose of this is to keep the licensing examination reflective of current practice.

NCLEX-PN is currently administered twice a year, in April and October. The test is administered on the same day in each state. It is a one-day test with testing occurring two hours in the morning and two hours in the afternoon. There are approximately 200 items on the test that are used to test the writer's nursing competency.

The test also contains approximately 60 items that are being validated. They will not be calculated into your final score. Since a new test is used each time NCLEX-PN is administered, these validation questions may or not be on future tests.

In 1988, NCLEX-PN adopted a pass–fail method of informing test takers of their examination results. Each candidate receives an NCLEX Diagnostic Profile, which gives you the following information:

1. if you passed or failed

2. the approximate number of items you missed if you failed

3. your performance in each of the four phases of the nursing process

4. your performance in the four categories of client needs

The National Council of State Boards of Nursing, in the interest of public welfare, promotes policy that helps ensure safe and effective nursing practice. In 1989, an assembly of the National Council adopted a policy whereby the passing standard for the PN licensure examination will be evaluated every three years. This policy began in October 1990.

PREPARING FOR NCLEX-PN

To help erase some of the mystique that often surrounds the licensure examination, it is worth remembering that the examination tests minimum competency. This means that if you have met the requirements for attending a state-board–approved school of practical nursing and successfully complete all theory and clinical requirements, chances are excellent that you will pass NCLEX-PN.

Perhaps the biggest secret is to overstudy throughout the year. This means to continue to study after you think you know the information. Authorities suggest an additional 25% study time past the point of thinking you are adequately prepared. Review everything already studied with particular focus on the "shaky" areas.

Remember too, that normal anxiety is your friend. It is this "cause-and-effect" type of anxiety that actually makes you sharper and more alert during a test. It is only when anxiety overwhelms you that it becomes your enemy. Accept the energy resulting from normal anxiety as your partner. Total personal comfort is not the key. Normal anxiety leaves you somewhere between too much relaxation and too much tension: perfect for testing.

Make your daydreams and positive thinking work for you. Think about what you think about. Are you in the habit of seeing yourself failing or just squeaking by? Since everyone daydreams and sets the stage for their reality, it is a natural way to practice being confident and successful. Practice the following exercise on successive days. Find a time when you can visualize without interruption.

EXERCISE

PART 1

Close your eyes. See yourself walking to the door of a large room. Show your registration identification to the examining council monitor who is waiting at the door. Walk into the room; it is set up with tables and chairs—a well-lit room. Another examining council member will help you locate your assigned place. Sit down and watch as other practical nurses enter. Note that the atmosphere is formal, and yet very friendly. Let yourself experience some excitement in anticipation of this adventure. Listen to directions. You will find no problem in understanding and following them. A council member proctor distributes the test and makes note of your identification number and test number. You are told to fill in the required data on the front of the test. Now it is time to open the booklet and begin. A pleasant surprise: the situations and multiple-choice questions are easy to comprehend. Experience satisfaction as you complete the test. That is all for now.

PART 2

Place yourself in the same setting. Go through the test and answer all of the questions that are easy for you. Place a light mark beside each question that poses difficulty. Go back and think through answers to the questions that you were not able to answer immediately. Remember to erase the light mark you placed in the booklet. See yourself as being able to answer most of the questions. Remind yourself that the score is based on the number of correct answers. Leave the room knowing you have done well.

PART 3

Close your eyes and place yourself in the same setting. Remember to include the detail. This time, the examination seems really hard for you. Rather than giving up, you do your best on every question, focusing on the question rather than on the outcome of the test. Take all of the time permitted. When you get up to leave, remind yourself that you have done your best. Remember: your whole life doesn't depend on one test.

Continue to repeat the parts of the exercise in sequence until you find yourself less threatened by the idea of testing—any testing.

The director of your program or assigned instructor will distribute forms needed to apply for the licensure examination well in advance of the actual day. The forms and deadlines are explained verbally and written instructions are distributed. This is also a time to remind you that all course work and required certifications must be up to date. Information about temporary permits, in order to work as a practical nurse prior to licensure, is usually explained at this time. Pay attention to required fees that must accompany the application for licensure and temporary permit. Note also if your picture must accompany the application. All directions provided by your state board of nursing must be followed exactly.

Spend the evening before the licensing examination relaxing. Little will be accomplished by worrying or last-minute cramming. Read something light and entertaining, watch television, or do anything else that you already know will relax you.

Before going to bed, get your testing materials ready to take along in the morning. Use the information you received as your checklist. Usually, you are required to bring

Identification that verifies that you are registered to take the NCLEX-PN.

Personal photo (a requirement in most states) dated and signed by you and the director of your program.

No. 2 pencil, although these are usually furnished. If you are not sure, bring two pencils with erasers.

Directions for finding the testing center and room.

Anything else on your checklist.

Get a good night's sleep by going to bed at your usual time (whatever meets your sleep requirements). Going to bed extra early and not falling asleep may result in a new worry for you to contend with. Set your alarm so that you will have adequate time to get ready and to travel to the testing area.

Follow through with your usual morning habits. Although a balanced nourishing breakfast is recommended as a part of continuing personal care, the day of the licensing examination is not the time to initiate it. Stay with your usual breakfast habit and do not force your system to adjust to a new demand.

Casual neat attire is appropriate. Think of comfort for sitting and writing.

Test-Taking Tips

You will be presented with a nursing situation with data. Read the situation carefully. Refer back to it as necessary when reading the multiple-choice items that follow. Remember to pace yourself. Remember that some of the items are on the test for validation. You will not be penalized for not answering these items correctly. The only problem is, NCLEX will not identify these items as validation items. (*Hint 1:* Stay calm when you read a situation or item that you think you have never heard of. It could be a validation item. Or it could be a situation in which you could apply information from another area you know well.)

You can omit questions. If you find a question that is too difficult, go on to the next question. Come back to it later, if time permits. Remember that you get as much credit for answering easy questions correctly as you do for correctly answering difficult questions. Therefore, answer all the questions for which you know the answers before struggling with difficult questions.

"It will be to your advantage to answer every question because NCLEX-PN is scored by counting correct answers. Unlike some examinations, NCLEX-PN does not have a correction for guessing, which means that no points are subtracted for wrong answers. Even if you answer with a pure guess you will have a 25% chance of getting a right answer" (NCLEX-PN, 1989). Read all the distractors, and eliminate the obviously incorrect choices.

Mark your answers exactly as directed in the booklet. There is no separate answer sheet. Carefully erase all extra marks or changed answers. Since the tests are machine scored, the machine reads all marks, stray or otherwise, that it perceives as an answer. There is one test booklet for the morning session and one for the afternoon session.

Wear a watch to remind you not to spend too much time on any one question.

Expect that special requests such as leaving the room to go to the bathroom will mean being accompanied by a monitor. Periodically (and unfortunately), students arrive with the intent to cheat. This is why the examining council monitors and proctors move around the room during the test. Pretending to cheat may result in being expelled from the room and, of course, being unable to finish the examination—not funny and more expense for you when you apply to retest.

When you complete the test, raise your hand. The proctor will acknowledge you, check the test back in, and give you the assigned code that will permit you to leave the room.

Review the test-taking skills from Chapter 8.

*T*HE NCLEX-PN FORMAT

Nobody knows for sure what items are included on NCLEX-PN, because the tests are secure tests. However, a document entitled "Test Plan for the National Council Licensure Examination for Practical Nurses" is available for $3.00 through the National Council of State Boards of Nursing, Inc., 676 St. Clair St., Suite 550, Chicago, IL 60611-2921. It can be helpful in explaining the general content areas of the test. There are two major components of the test plan:

1. The nursing process
2. Client health needs

The test measures the PN's role in the nursing process as you have learned:

1. assisting in collecting data
2. contributing to the plan of care
3. performing basic therapeutic and preventive nursing measures
4. assisting in evaluating the outcomes of nursing intervention.

Table 20-1 contains the phases of the nursing process and the percent of items on the test plan for each of the phases.

Table 20-1 Percent of Items in Specific Phase of Nursing Process

PHASE OF THE NURSING PROCESS	PERCENT OF QUESTIONS ON NCLEX-PN
Assess	30%
Plan	20%
Implement	30%
Evaluate	20%

The health needs of clients are grouped under four broad categories. They are listed below with the percent of questions on the test plan in parenthesis.

1. Safe, effective care environment (24 to 30%)
2. Physiologic integrity (42 to 48%)
3. Psychosocial integrity (7 to 13%)
4. Health promotion/maintenance (15 to 21%)

An explanation of each client health need, along with the knowledge, skills, and abilities for each can be found in the above-mentioned document from the National Council. What follows is a listing of the four areas of client needs with the critical top five activities for each category. They were found by Kane and Colton's original survey of workplace activities (Kane & Colton, 1989). These were presented in an Instructor's Workshop explaining the NCLEX-PN format.

Safe, Clean Care Environment

1. Verfiy client's identity
2. Give shift report
3. Maintain asepsis
4. Label specimens for laboratory
5. Ask about allergies

Physiologic Integrity

1. Administer oral medications
2. Prevent respiratory complications
3. Give intramuscular or subcutaneous injections
4. Assess needs for prn medications
5. Report changes in consciousness

Psychosocial Integrity

1. Record behaviors indicating delusions
2. Assess potential for violence
3. Assess orientation
4. Assess environment of suicidal client
5. Plan to deal with anxiety from pain

Health Promotion and Maintenance

1. Help client with anxiety about dyspnea
2. Support terminally ill patients and family
3. Evaluate compliance with therapy
4. Teach to avoid infection
5. Help with activities of daily living

The encouragement and reminders you have received from your instructors in the area of understanding and applying information will pay off when you take your NCLEX-PN examination. The licensing examination will test you at the level of knowledge, comprehension (understanding), and application. "However, most items in the examination are at the comprehension and application levels" (NCLEX-PN Test Plan, 1989, p. 4).

Practice Settings and Age Ranges

The NCLEX-PN Test Plan document does not give the percent of questions that relate to specific practice settings and age ranges of clients. Most practical nurses are employed by acute-care hospitals and long-term–care facilities. It would make sense that when workplace activities were surveyed, sites frequently surveyed would be in acute care and long term care. One could deduce that many of the licensing examination items would be directed to acute care and extended care. The Test Plan document also mentions that the practical nurse should possess basic knowledge, skills, and abilities in reproduction, birthing and parenting, growth and development, and immunizations. Therefore, questions for Nursing of Children and Obstetric Nursing will be included on the licensing examination.

A WORD ABOUT REVIEW BOOKS/MOCK EXAMINATIONS

New review books based on the NCLEX-PN have been developed by the major medical publishing companies. Each review book basically includes an outline of practical nursing content, questions with explanations, and references for the answers. Questions are intended to simulate the NCLEX-PN. Please realize that the test items of the NCLEX-PN itself are highly guarded and confidential. Actual NCLEX-PN test items are not included in the book.

Review of content and test items are developed by instructors teaching in specific areas of practical nursing programs. The best preparation is to study faithfully from the beginning of the program to its conclusion and also on a regular basis until the examination. Do not put all your eggs in one basket and think that merely reading a review book, without studying, will help you pass boards.

Mock examinations are available for a fee. They offer practical nursing students the opportunity to assess their level of readiness for NCLEX-PN. These tests can be given according to the format of the actual licensing examination. A few weeks after taking some mock examinations, a student receives a readout of test performance. This includes

1. percentile score for each phase of the nursing process and category of client health needs
2. the items the student got wrong
3. a book listing correct answers, rationale, and explanations for correct answers and distractors for each item.

If students have an idea of strong and weak areas they can better focus study efforts. Be sure to check publishers' offerings of mock examinations. Choose the one that most closely resembles the actual format of the NCLEX-PN.

Note: In August, 1991, the Delegate Assembly of the National Council of State Boards of Nursing voted to implement computerized adaptive testing (CAT) as the future method for administering all NCLEX examinations. Implementation will occur "no sooner than November 1993" and will probably start with NCLEX-RN (National Council Adopts CAT for NCLEX Administration, 1991, 440).

Summary

Preparing for NCLEX-PN takes place throughout the course of your program. Follow the suggestions provided throughout the book on how to make the most of your abilities.

It is imperative that all course work be completed and that all grades be filed with the board of nursing. Forms for applying for licensure will be distributed and explained to you by the faculty. Follow directions carefully and submit all forms to the appropriate places according to the required time frame.

Plan in advance of actual testing so that you will remember to bring identification and materials required by the examining council.

Personal attitude and self-esteem play a significant role in successful testing. Do not permit a negative attitude to flunk you.

REFERENCES

Ference, H. *Practical Nurse Role Delineation and Validation Study for the National Council Licensure Examination for Practical Nurses.* Monterey, CA: CTB/McGraw-Hill, 1983.

Taking the SAT. Princeton, NJ: The College Board, 1986–87.

Gladstone W. *Preparation for the ACT.* New York: Monarch, 1985.

Johnson J. *National Council Licensure Examinations: Percent of Success Rate for Wisconsin Professional Nursing Programs and Practical Nursing Programs.* (Unpublished paper, 1990, pp. 1–5.)

Kane M, Colton D. Job Analysis of Newly Licensed Practical/Vocational Nurses 1986–87. Chicago: National Council of State Boards of Nursing, 1989.

Matassarin-Jacobs E. *Saunders Review of Practical Nursing for NCLEX-PN.* 2nd ed. Philadelphia: WB Saunders, 1992.

National Council Adopts CAT for NCLEX Administration. Nurs Health Care 1991; 12(8):440–41.

The National Council Licensure Examination For Practical Nurses. Chicago: National Council of State Boards of Nursing, October 1984.

NCLEX-PN Test Plan for the National Council Licensure Examination. Chicago: National Council of State Boards of Nursing, 1989.

Passing Standard Revised for NCLEX-PN: News Release. Chicago: National Council of State Boards of Nursing, July 27, 1990.

Rayfield S. Workshop: *Teaching Strategies/Test Development/NCLEX.* Green Bay, WI, October 25 and 26, 1990.

State of Wisconsin Department of Regulation and Licensing. Requirements for Licensure, 1985. Madison: Wisconsin Board of Nursing.

CHAPTER
21
Finding a Job

Revised by Michael S. Hill, MS, CRC QRC

Learning Objectives

Upon completing this chapter, you will
1. List employment opportunities available to LPNs.
2. Discuss how your nursing program offers a practical experience advantage.
3. Describe who is a part of your job-search network.
4. Explain how you can turn a community health agency visit into an informational interview.
5. Role play how to make an appointment for an interview on the phone.
6. Write a letter indicating interest in applying for a job.
7. Role play how to deal with common questions asked by an employer during an interview.
8. Explain why it is important to ask permission to use names for references.
9. Write a personal resume and a qualifications brief.
10. Write a cover letter and thank you, or a combination letter to an employer.
11. Write a letter of resignation.

INTRODUCTION

Concerned about your career opportunities after investing in your education? Upon graduation, you have become a member of one of the fastest-growing employment areas—health services. Practical nursing is bedside nursing and more. Employment opportunities vary according to geographic location and include

> Nursing homes and extended-care facilities as a staff or charge nurse
> Home health agencies
> Physicians' offices and clinics
> Pharmaceutical suppliers
> Weight-loss clinics
> Hospitals
> Insurance companies
> Private duty in homes
> State/federal prison systems
> Industry
> Veterinary clinics/hospitals
> Halfway houses for emotionally ill
> Residential treatment centers
> Military services

HOW TO BEGIN THE JOB SEARCH

Practical Experience

A common experience for nursing students is to identify any present clinical rotation, whatever it happens to be, as an area of major interest. This is healthy, since it helps to make employment opportunities limitless, rather than narrowed by select interests.

It is to your distinct advantage that your educational program includes actual nursing experience. Some educational programs do not include practical experience and therefore graduates should seek out internships and/or volunteer experiences in order to learn first-hand how to do the real work involved in the career/job. How fortunate you are to have an opportunity to do nursing, even though students complain because of the hours of clinical

work assigned to them. Think about it: A significant step of the job search is provided for you during your education. You have an opportunity to learn about and develop skills for the major nursing areas. The answers will emerge for the following:

QUESTIONS: 1. What population, that is, type of patient, do I find most rewarding to work with?
2. What kinds of nursing skills do I find most challenging and rewarding?

Networking

Think for a moment about the contacts you have both in the classroom and in the clinical areas. You have the unique opportunity of making contacts with nurses at all levels who can be instrumental in obtaining a job. This is what developing a job network is about—contacts for job openings and references. Consider, for example:

- Registering with your school's career services center

- Instructors who are willing to write a positive recommendation if your work warrants it. Be sure to ask for permission prior to bringing in a form and/or giving out his or her name. Do not assume that an instructor will give you a positive reference. Specifically ask, "May I list your name for a positive reference?"

- Unit managers, supervisors, team leaders, staff RNs, and LPNs are a source of information regarding job openings in their area, and can be approached for recommendations. Some students think that they are "invisible" in the eyes of regular facility staff. Not so. Frequently staff offer feedback to your instructors and to nurse managers regarding future employees. Listen carefully if this feedback is passed on to you. You often work directly with the primary nurses or team leaders. Identify the nurses whose work you admire, ask for their evaluation or suggestions regarding your work. Listen carefully to the feedback you receive. Before completing the rotation, ask select nurses if they are willing to write a positive reference letter for you. If the answer is "yes," write down her name (spelled correctly), title, address, and phone number. A brief courtesy letter at the time you begin your job search will remind her of you, and of her promise. The letter might be like the following examples.

May 1, 1993

Mr. Pat Bieser
Bieser's Family Restaurant
1212 Hackett Drive
Green Bay, Wisconsin 54302

Dear Mr. Bieser:

Thank you for agreeing to be a work reference. As we discussed, now that I have graduated from nursing school I am actively seeking employment. Knowing your busy schedule I have enclosed a possible reference letter for your review and signature. However, if you prefer to write your own letter you may wish to mention my ability to work under pressure, effective interactions with customers and staff, and work quality.

Your assistance in helping me to secure employment at a nursing organization is greatly appreciated. Please contact me if you have any questions or just want to catch up on my job search progress.

Sincerely,

Kavanaugh Jonjon
1234 Celonia Drive
Green Bay, Wisconsin 54303
(414) 555-4761
        555-2310 (messages)

May 14, 1993

Dear Employer:

Please accept this as a letter of recommendation for Kavanaugh Jonjon. While in our employ as a waitress we found her to display excellent interactions with customers and staff, a high degree of work quality, and scheduling flexibility.

We feel that Kavanaugh will make a positive contribution to any organization she may choose to work for. Should you have further questions about Kavanaugh's skills as a worker please feel free to contact me.

Sincerely,

Pat Bieser, Owner
Bieser's Family Restaurant
1212 Hackett Drive
Green Bay, Wisconsin 54302
(414) 555-0534

Be sure to remember other contacts you have made. For example, consider:

- Family and friend with nursing contacts. Let them know you are looking for work. Ask for job leads and names of contacts. Jobs are often located not by what you know as much as by whom you know.
- Former health-care-related employers. If interested in a nursing position, contact the employer.
- Newspapers, nursing journals, telephone yellow pages, the school career placement office, and state job service department.
- Call a prospective employer and ask "Are you currently hiring?" If the answer is "no," ask "Do you know of anyone else who is hiring?" If yes, also ask for the name of the contact person.

QUESTION: Who can you think of that is a part of your job network? List the individuals in the spaces below.

Name	Phone
_____	_____
_____	_____

Informational Interview

Chances are that at some time during your educational program, you will be asked to visit community health facilities. Your instructor will provide objectives/questions to help make the experience worthwhile. Objectives and/or questions may focus on the following areas:

- Purpose
- Staffing patterns
- Hours/shifts
- Facility specialty

Viewing this assignment as an informational interview will create an additional personal focus for you. The informational interview will allow you to find out how the facility works firsthand, assist you in determining if you would want to work there, and allow you to meet the employer prior to actually seeking a job. To obtain an informational interview with the employer it is important to practice with another individual prior to the telephone contact. Although it may be tempting to make the phone call and read without practicing in advance, remember, that is exactly how it will sound— Like you are reading! A telephone informational interview request would be as in the following example:

1. Hello, my name is ———.

2. Who is in charge of hiring? (Emphasis is on "who," *not* "May I speak to the person in charge of hiring?")

3. May I speak with Mr./Ms. ———.

4. Hello Mr./Ms. ———.
My name is ———.

5. I am a student nurse at ——— (school name).

6. As a part of my learning experience I would like to visit your facility for an informational interview.

7. Would it be possible to set up an informational interview on ——— (day) at 9:00 A.M. or 2:00 P.M. or another time?

— Great, I'll see you there!!!

There is usually no problem speaking directly to top nursing management during an informational interview. Management likes to get the word out as to what their facility really is about. However, do not make the mistake of turning this into a job interview. No one likes to be tricked, and management tends to have a long memory.

Look sharp during the informational interviews. These are not "T-shirt and jeans" side trips. Consider them future career opportunities. Keep a copy of the information, complete with name, address, and phone number, in a safe place, for the time your job search begins. Follow up the informational interviews with a thank you letter. A thank you letter might appear as below:

January 10, 1993

Ms. Barbara Bauer, Director of Nursing
Brown County Mental Health Center
2900 St. Anthony Drive
Green Bay, Wisconsin 54301

Re: Informational Interview

Dear Ms. Bauer:

Please accept my sincere appreciation for having the opportunity to meet with you on Wednesday, January 9, 1993. The informational interview was both valuable and interesting. I found the variety of programs offered progressive and individualized to meet the needs of the client. The tour that followed supported your comments about the positive interactions between staff and clients.

I can only hope to be fortunate enough to work at such a center following my graduation this May. Thank you again.

Cordially,

Kavanaugh Jonjon
1234 Celonia Drive
Green Bay, Wisconsin 54303

QUESTIONS: 1. With whom can you practice the informational interview telephone request? List three names: ———
———
———

2. What does "look sharp" mean? (*Clue:* Look around and identify people in all areas of work who look businesslike.)

Making Application

It is important to begin to make application for employment approximately two months prior to graduation if you expect to work shortly after graduation. If your graduation is in December do not fret. According to Challenger (1991), it is a myth that the November–December holiday season is the worst time to job hunt. The fact is that the holiday season is among the best times to look for a job.

You need to do some homework in preparation for seeking employment. Find out all you can about the facility at which you wish to work. Facilities often give away free pamphlets as part of their advertising. Remember also, the information that you have acquired and stashed away during school. Your nursing program director also has policies for the contract facilities; ask to see those manuals. It is very important to try to find out the name of the person who does the hiring or influences hiring. This is the person whom you will want to contact. You may be referred to another department, but there is a good chance that your name will be remembered later.

Ninety-five percent of available jobs are never advertised. Do not wait for an ad to appear in order to apply. Often a brief, to-the-point letter with a resume addressed to the director of nursing at the facility where you wish to apply is encouraged. Your cover letter might appear as the following examples.

March 23, 1993

Ms. Sandra Robertson, Director of Nursing
Lake View Memorial Hospital
1012 4th Avenue
DePere, Wisconsin 54300

Re: LPN Staff Nurse Position

Dear Ms. Robertson:

I will be graduating from the Northeastern Technical College practical nursing program.

While doing a medical nursing rotation at your hospital I was impressed by the quality of patient care, staff professionalism, and learning opportunities.

In addition to this rotation my work experiences include patient care planning, plan review, direct patient care, dispensing medications, and team participation.

I am interested in obtaining employment at your hospital and being able to work with your staff again. I will be contacting you on Tuesday March 30, 1993, to see if you have received my resume and to determine when we might arrange an interview. Should you wish to contact me prior to this I can be reached after 3:30 P.M.

Sincerely,

Kavanaugh Jonjon
1234 Celonia Drive
Green Bay, Wisconsin 54303
(414) 555-4761
        555-2310 (messages)

March 23, 1993

Ms. Sandra Robertson, Director of Nursing
Lake View Memorial Hospital
1012 4th Avenue
DePere, Wisconsin 54300

Re: LPN Staff Nurse Position

Dear Ms. Robertson:

On June 5, 1993, I will be graduating from the Northeastern Technical College practical nursing program. I am interested in obtaining a LPN staff nurse position at Lake View Memorial Hospital. My clinical work experience includes patient care planning, plan review, direct patient care, dispensing medications, and team participation. In addition, I have done volunteer work as a candy striper at Bellin Memorial Hospital in Green Bay, Wisconsin.

I will be contacting you on Tuesday, March 30, 1993, to see if you have received my resume and to determine when we might arrange an

interview. Should you wish to contact me prior
to this I can be reached after 3:30 P.M.

Sincerely,

Kavanaugh Jonjon
1234 Celonia Drive
Green Bay, Wisconsin 54303
(414) 555-4761
555-2310 (messages)

Do not include a personal reference list with
this letter. Retain the list for your interview and
provide it only on request. Do follow through
by calling for an interview on the day stated in
your letter. Mark the day on your calendar.
Those who wait to be contacted by employers
should prepare to be disappointed when it does
not happen.

If your resource for a job opening is through
the newspaper, call for an interview (unless the
directions specifically say to write). The reason
for doing this is because others are looking at
the same ad, and in this case, "he who hesitates
is lost." Request to speak to the person in
charge of hiring. Your conversation should reflect the following example.

1. Hello, my name is _____.

2. Who is in charge of hiring?

3. May I speak with Mr./Ms. _____.

4. Hello Mr./Ms. _____.
My name is _____.

5. I will be graduating from the practical nursing program at _____ in _____ (city).

6. Do you have any LPN staff positions open?

7. If yes—Would it be possible to set up an
interview on _____ (day) at 9:00 a.m. or 2:00
p.m. or another time _____ A.M. or P.M. Great,
I'll see you then!
If no—Do you know of anyone who might be
hiring?
If yes—Would you also know the contact person and/or have the telephone
number?

_____   _____   _____
(Facility) (Contact   (Telephone)
            person)

If no—"I appreciate your time. Thank
you."

or

If no—"Thank you for trying. Would it
be possible for me to come in for an informational interview?
If yes—see #7.
If no—Well, thanks again. Goodbye.

Defer the employer's questions until interview time because you do not want to be
"washed out" by a phone conversation. Should
the employer begin to ask you questions about
your background, education, or work experience you might respond, "I have the educational background and experience. I would like
the opportunity to discuss my qualifications
during our interview." See point #7. Say,
"Would it be possible to set up an interview
with you on Wednesday? etc."

The tone of your voice makes a significant
difference on the telephone. If you smile while
talking you will project a positive tone. Practice
the above suggested format with a friend in advance; write notes for yourself if necessary. Reread Chapter 11 on "Assertiveness as a Nursing
Responsibility."

Even if you are not ideally qualified for a job
opening, go ahead and apply if the job appeals
to you. Advertisements often describe the ideal
for the job, and the ideal is not always available.
At the interview you might inquire about in-
services and continuing education courses offered by the employer to prepare you for the
job.

You will be asked to fill out an application
either before or after the interview. It is important that you answer the questions truthfully. If
there are questions that you wish to defer until
the face-to-face interview write in, "N/A" (for
not-applicable), "Will explain," or leave the
space blank. Do not attempt to falsify information, because this will provide grounds for dismissal after being hired. You will note that some
applications may list optional questions, which
do not have to be answered because of personal
rights. For example, you do not have to answer
questions regarding age, religion, marital status,
children, physical data (unless it is a specific
requirement of the job), and criminal record
(unless it relates to security clearance, housing,

or perhaps employment in schools and child facilities).

An employer's eyes will naturally gravitate to any blank spaces. Therefore, answer all questions that you can even if they do not apply to you (e.g., military service). If the questions being asked are illegal you need to decide whether to answer them or leave them blank. Some employers view blanks or "Will explain" as an automatic screen for someone they do not want to employ. Should you choose to answer illegal questions the example below may be helpful.

QUESTION: Have you been hospitalized within the past five years?

ANSWER: I do not have any problems that would interfere with my work here (or for the position for which I am applying).

QUESTION: Have you ever been on worker's compensation?

ANSWER: Write in, "N/A" for not-applicable.
or
I did have a _____ injury in 19xx (year), but am fully rehabilitated and there is nothing to prevent me from doing the job for which I am applying.

Preparing for the Interview

During an interview, you are also interviewing the potential employer. If you have prepared adequately, you will be able to evaluate if your job skills match the objectives of the facility and if the values that you hold regarding patient care and treatment of staff are close enough to establish a positive working relationship.

Furthermore, you should consider that interviews are often stressful for the employer. Knowing that there are concerns on both sides—yours and the interviewer's—will help you to be less defensive. It will help you to understand the meaning of the questions that are asked and gain insight into answering them in an honest, reassuring way.

Often the first interview question is an "ice breaker." Take advantage of it, and let the interviewer know that you are a stable person and

plan to be around for a long time. Practice the "Sample Responses to Typical Interview Questions" below, as a part of your preparation for the interview. Do this as a role play with another person in the role of the interviewer. Ask the person to mix up the order of the questions to prepare you better.

Sample Responses to Typical Interview Questions

Tell Me About Yourself. I have a child, have lived here for several years, and plan on staying here for a long time.

Have You Ever Done this Kind of Work Before? Yes, in fact some of my experiences include. . . .

Why Do You Want to Work Here? The _____ (facility name) has the kind of job that I am good at and like to do.

Why Did You Leave Your Last Job? As you know, I am a recent graduate and am looking for employment in my field of study.

What Kind of Salary Do You Need? I know that you will pay as much as I am worth to you and can't ask for more than that.

Why Should We Hire You Instead of Someone Else? I think that my references can best answer that question, but I am sure that they will agree that I am hard working, dependable, and put in the time to get the job done right.

How Much Were You Absent from Work in Your Last Job? Very little, I have always been very healthy.

How Is Your Health? I do not have any health problems that would interfere with my work here.

When Are You Available for Work? Right away.

What Are Your Greatest Strengths? (1) _____, (2) _____, (3) _____, (4) _____, and (5) _____

What Are Your Weaknesses? If I make a mistake I have found that no one can be harder on me than myself because I want the job done right.

What Was Your Last Employer's Opinion of You? Great! I always had my work done and was willing to take on additional responsibility.

What Are Your Long-Range Goals? I am looking for a job like this in which I can continue to grow, and I don't see any reason why I would want to leave.

Can You Work Under Pressure? Yes, I've had to do this throughout the years and know that working under pressure is a part of nursing.

Are There Any Questions You Have? No, you seem to have done a good job of describing the job, and it looks like we would be a good match. My only question is how soon can I start?

Presenting Yourself

The kind of person that you are is an additional concern, and that impression includes everything that has been previously discussed, plus your personal appearance and habits during the interview. Suggestions for all nurses include:

- Personal hygiene—Bathe. Hair should be clean and in a moderate style. Men's hair and beard should be neatly trimmed. Nails clean and nicely manicured (avoid bright polish). If you are a smoker, yellow finger stains may be removed with bleach and water. Deodorant. Recent mouth care to remove bad breath (remember not to have indulged recently in food or drink with a heavy unpleasant odor). Brush your teeth, tongue, palate, and cheeks with a soft toothbrush. Use a breath freshener. Easy on the aftershave or perfume. Limit yourself to light makeup (a "clean" look goes a long way).

- Clothing—Dress conservatively. Men should wear a white shirt, dark suit, and solid-colored tie and wear black leather shoes. Women should choose a dark or solid-colored dress or suit with closed-toe shoes cleaned and polished. Wear plain simple jewelry or none at all. Never wear a topcoat into an interview. The coat detracts from your appearances and makes it appear that you are anxious to

leave. Reality is that a student may not always be able to afford the ideal. You can look your best with clothes clean and ironed and shoes polished. Check out thrift stores as they are resources waiting to be discovered.

- Posture—Walk tall, sit erect but not entirely at the back of the chair. Both feet resting on the floor and your head upright. Arms and hands in an open position and not crossed (remember you have nothing to hide). Keep your hands inactive. If you must fidget consider bringing a paper clip in with you to the interview.

- Manner—Assured. Do not interrupt the interviewer. Pause to think as needed, then answer without hesitating. Ask for explanations or repetitions of questions that you do not understand. Eye contact is needed, especially when answering questions. If you are uncomfortable with eye contact, two techniques are available. Looking at the employer's nose or the space between the eyebrows gives an illusion of eye contact. Remember to look away periodically. Avoid negative statements regarding school, former jobs, and/or personal problems.

- Courtesy—When meeting the employer, smile and extend your hand for a firm handshake. (*Hint:* If your palms tend to sweat rub your hand along your thigh when standing up. It will remove the moisture while appearing very natural.) Then say "Mr./Ms. _____, my name is _____." Similarly, when the interview is over, stand up, look the person in the eyes, and offer your hand for a firm handshake. Address the employer by surname—"Mr./Ms. _____, thank you for the opportunity to interview with you. Based on what I have learned here today I know that I can do the job. I would like to call you in four days to see if you have made a decision. Would that be okay? Is it better to call in the morning or afternoon?" If you want the job, give the employer a list of your work references and/or letters of recommendation.

- Habits—Do not chew gum or smoke. Politely refuse an offer for coffee/tea or cigarette if offered. In addition, do not read any materials on the employer's desk.

References and Personal Data

Potential employers will be more interested in some work references than in others. A hierarchy exists when considering which references are more credible than others. Consider the hierarchy when asking individuals to become references and when developing your reference list. When determining most to least important think about:

1. Current/former supervisors, unit managers, teachers

2. Coworkers who have seen your work

3. Personal references and/or friends

Include name, job title, and address of that person. Three is the usual number of references requested, so pick and choose from your list for maximum impression.

The statement "References on request" can be stated at the end of your resume. It is a matter of personal choice. References can be listed separately and given to the interviewer if requested. References are "treasures," do not give them out if you are not interested in the position.

Development of a resume is a must! It focuses on your work skills, experiences, and qualifications. Resumes are not to be used as a confession or personal "tell-all" script. Haack (1984, p. 28) recommends omitting such items as reasons for leaving past jobs, salary requirements, personal photographs, hobbies (unless work-related), and personal data such as marital status, race, religion, height, weight, or number/age of children.

Unfortunately, many resumes are never read. The initial impression makes a significant difference. Basics to be considered include:

- Length—Maximum of two pages. One page preferred.

- Paper—Quality bond. Stay with colors such as white, cream, beige or gray. Use matching paper for the cover letter and envelope.

- Typing—Absolutely no errors or extra marks. If possible, type your resume on a computer. Corrections can be made painlessly, and updating the resume may be performed quickly. It is worth going to a quick print shop to run resume copies, as standard copy machines provide poor quality.

- Balance and space—Uncluttered balanced design so the resume is easy to read.

- Emphasis—Depends on whether you have a strong or limited work history.

A suggested format follows and may be varied according to the job you are seeking. Remember, you want to let the employer know that you can fill the job without having met you.

- Personal data—Include your legal name, address, phone number, and/or message phone.

- Employment objective—Clearly state the kind of job you are seeking.

- Work history—Organize by most recent job and/or duties. List the job title, employer's name, and duration or years. A statement about the tasks performed and any special equipment including computer, medical devices, or typing. If you wish eventually to become a charge nurse at a nursing home mention any management responsibility, no matter how minor. Also list any accomplishments, such as quality assurance committee member.

  Homemakers: Remember you have several valuable skills that need to be commented on. Skills include bookkeeping, scheduling, transportation, home management, inventory, quality control, supervision, and payroll.

- Education—List diploma, certificates, licensure, honors, scholarships, continuing education classes, or memberships in professional organizations.
- Military service

Two sample resumes and a work reference sheet have been provided below to give you an idea of how to put the above suggestions to work for you.

KAVANAUGH JONJON

1234 Celonia Drive
Green Bay, WI 54303
(414) 555-4761
(414) 555-2310 (messages)

JOB GOAL

To obtain a medical LPN staff position in which I may use my skills and abilities for quality patient care.

WORK HISTORY

Medical Nursing St. Mary's Hospital	3-month rotation

Responsibilities for this nursing school rotation included assisting with patient assessment, performance/charting of vital signs, dispensing medication, patient care planning, patient care and other duties as assigned.

Domestic Manager	12 years

Duties included money management, budgeting, bookkeeping, inventory control, liaison to community resources, transportation, purchasing food/clothing and related products, health care, and TLC.

Waitress Bieser's Family Restaurant	2 years

These job duties included greeting customers, taking food/beverage orders, transferring orders to cooks, assisting in food preparation, serving food/beverages, accepting payment, making change, bussing, and table cleaning.

EDUCATION

Northeast Wisconsin Technical College—Practical Nursing Green Bay, Wisconsin	Diploma 1993
Green Bay West Senior High Green Bay, Wisconsin	Diploma 1979

*** References on Request ***

(Form recommended by the American Disabilities Act—1990 to avoid discrimination).

KAVANAUGH JONJON

1234 Celonia Drive
Green Bay, WI 54303
(414) 555-4761
(414) 555-2310 (messages)

JOB GOAL

To obtain a geriatric LPN staff position in which I may use my work experiences and abilities to assure quality patient care. In addition, to participate in learning opportunities to enhance my work skills.

WORK SKILLS

* Direct patient care   * Communications
* Flexibility   * Injury prevention
* Family support   * Charting/reporting

WORK HISTORY

St. George Nursing Home   Nurse Aide
De Pere, Wisconsin   1991–1992

Responsibilities for this position included providing support to families, assisting physicians, charting vital signs, injury prevention, quality patient care, including toileting, feeding, and hygiene. In addition, worked with family members and assisted with recreational activities.

EDUCATION

Northeast Wisconsin Tech. College—Practical Nursing   Diploma
Green Bay, Wisconsin   (in progress)

Green Bay West Senior High   GED
Green Bay, Wisconsin   1990

*** References on Request ***

KAVANAUGH JONJON

1234 Celonia Drive
Green Bay, WI 54303
(414) 555-4761
(414) 555-2310 (messages)

WORK REFERENCES

Ms. Jenny Franks,
Nursing Supervisor
St. Mary's Hospital
2543 North Green Street
Green Bay, Wisconsin 54303
(Work) (414) 555-7326

Mr. Pat Bieser, Owner
Bieser's Family Restaurant
1212 Hackett Drive
Green Bay, Wisconsin 54302
(Work) (414) 555-0534

Ms. Marla May, Nurse Aide
St. George Nursing Home
P.O. Box 30
De Pere, Wisconsin 54300
(Work) (414) 555-7125
(Home) (414) 555-3456

A cover letter needs to accompany the resume. The content will vary according to your reason for sending the resume. Variations are necessary depending on whether you are answering an ad, are following up an unsolicited telephone call to the employer, or are pursuing a personal contact. Neatness and correct spelling are essential. A sample cover letter to an employer whom was contacted through an unsolicited telephone call would appear as in the example below.

March 23, 1993

Ms. Mary L. Gmur, Director of Nursing
Lake View Memorial Hospital
1012 4th Avenue
DePere, Wisconsin 54300

Re: LPN Staff Nurse Position

Dear Ms. Gmur:

Thank you for taking the time to talk with me about the practical nurse staff position. As we discussed, I have enclosed my resume for your review. My clinical work experience includes patient care planning, plan review, direct patient care, dispensing medications, and team participation. In addition, I have done volunteer work as a candy striper at Bellin Memorial Hospital in Green Bay, Wisconsin.

I will be contacting you on Tuesday, March 30, 1993, to see if you have received my resume and determine when we might arrange an interview. Should you wish to contact me prior to this I can be reached after 3:30 P.M.

Sincerely,

Kavanaugh Jonjon
1234 Celonia Drive
Green Bay, Wisconsin 54303
(414) 555-4761
555-2310 (messages)

Following a job interview an essential courtesy is to follow each interview with a thank-you note. Do it that very day, whether you want the job or not. Remember, the more times the employer sees or hears your name the greater are your chances of getting hired over the person who waits for the employer to call. A thank-you letter may be as simple as in the following example.

April 2, 1993

Ms. Mary L. Gmur, Director of Nursing
Lake View Memorial Hospital
1012 4th Avenue
DePere, Wisconsin 54300

Re: LPN Staff Nurse Position

Dear Ms. Gmur:

Please accept my sincere appreciation for the opportunity to interview for the LPN staff nurse position on Thursday, April 1, 1993. Following our discussion about the job duties and subsequent tour I feel that my skills are a good match.

I remain interested in the position and will be contacting you on Monday, April 5, 1993, to see if you have made a decision. Thank you again!

Sincerely,

Kavanaugh Jonjon
1234 Celonia Drive
Green Bay, Wisconsin 54303
(414) 555-4761
        555-2310 (messages)

Resignation

An important responsibility is the way in which you leave a job. It is important that an employer be given written notice of your intention to leave, with adequate time to hire a replacement. It is expensive for an employer to provide the orientation that it takes for you to become fully productive on the job. Workplace policies identify the amount of time for giving notice; the usual is two weeks.

Use a business format and plain paper and type. Even if you are leaving because of unhappy circumstances on the job, do not vent these feelings in the letter. You may need a work reference from this employer for your next job, and blasting an employer will usually guarantee a negative reference. Since the resignation is a part of your permanent record it provides you with an opportunity to recap your accomplishments or special recognition. The employer may refer to the letter when contacted by employers with whom you are seeking employment. See the following example of a resignation letter.

February 14, 1995

Ms. Elsie Berts, Director of Nursing
Parkland Nursing Home
1001 Wentworth Drive
Green Bay, Wisconsin 54303

Dear Ms. Berts:

Please accept my resignation as Charge Nurse on Unit 3 to be effective February 28, 1995. My association with the Parkland Nursing Home has been rewarding both professionally and personally. It is satisfying to have been able to contribute to the positive reputation of client care.

I am especially pleased to have been part of the nursing team that established patient care plans for shift and individualized reporting. In addition, I remain appreciative of having been honored as "Employee of the Month." Please accept my thank you for the support you have provided through the past 1 1/2 years of employment.

Sincerely,

Kavanaugh Jonjon, LPN

Summary

To be successful in your job search, it is vital that the research itself be treated like a job. The more time you can devote to it, the more it will improve your chances of finding a job. The most effective way to find a job is to meet face to face with prospective employers. This method is more effective than sending resumes, sending letters, or answering ads. However, you are encouraged to try all methods that are available and that appeal to you. In preparation for a job search, review the knowledge and skills that you presently hold, that is, inventory yourself. Furthermore, do some homework on a facility prior to applying for work.

Do contact facilities you have contacted before. However, there is a difference between being persistent and being annoying; know the difference.

Apply for jobs that you may not be exactly qualified for if the work sounds interesting. Employers do not always know just what the qualifications for a position should be or may have other job opportunities.

Continue to let your network know that you are looking. Take time on the same day as the interview to send a thank-you note to everyone that helped you with that interview.

Look sharp. Be sharp. And contrary to what you may believe—no one owes you a job. Get out there and find the job you really want. Attitude and effort go hand in hand.

*R*EFERENCES

Allen J, Gorkin J. *Finding the Right Job at Midlife.* New York: Simon & Schuster, 1985.

Barlow L. *How to Sell Yourself.* Lakeside, CA: VCA Publication, 1981.

Bolles R. *The 1986 What Color is Your Parachute?* Berkeley, CA: Ten Speed Press, 1992.

Bostwick B. *Resume Writing.* 4th ed. New York, Wiley, 1990.

Challenger J. *The Job Hunt Myths and Facts About Jobs.* St Paul, MN: Saint Paul Pioneer Press, December 1, 1991.

Falvey J. *After College: The Business of Getting Jobs.* Charlotte, VT: Williamson Publishing, 1986.

Haack C. *Points, Plugs and a Roadmap.* Blaine, MN: Carol Haack, 1984.

Haas C. *What Color is Your Parody?* Los Angeles: Price Stern Sloan, 1984.

Lander J. *How to Get Hired Faster, for More Money.* Laverne, CA: Exponent, 1980.

Leape M, Vacca S. *The Harvard Guide to Careers.* Cambridge, MA: Harvard University Press, 1987.

Lipman B. *The Professional Job Search Program: How to Market Yourself.* New York: Wiley, 1983.

Appendixes

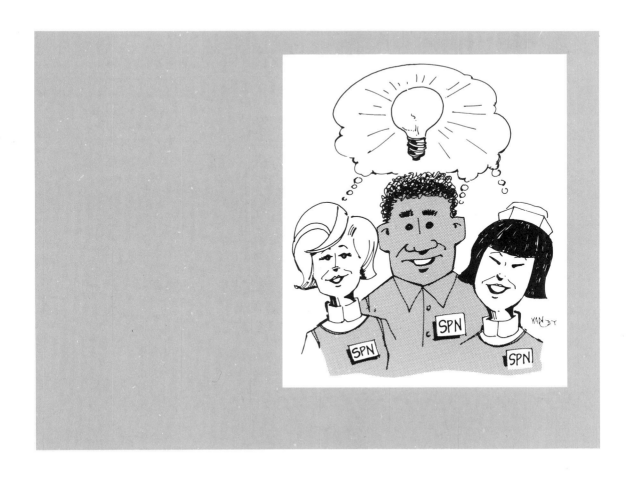

APPENDIX A

State Boards of Nursing

Alabama

Alabama Board of Nursing
500 Eastern Blvd., Suite 203
Montgomery, AL 36117
(205) 261-4060

Alaska

Alaska Board of Licensing
P.O. Box D–LIC
Juneau, AK 99811-0800
(907) 465-2544

American Samoa

American Samoa Health Service Regulatory
   Board
Pago Pago, American Samoa 96799
(684) 633-1222 ext. 206

Arizona

Arizona State Board of Nursing
5050 N. 19th Ave.
Phoenix, AZ 85015
(602) 255-5092

Arkansas

Arkansas State Board of Nursing
University Towers Bldg.
Suite 800 1123 S. University Ave.
Little Rock, AR 72204
(501) 371-2751

California

California Board of Vocational Nurse and
   Psychiatric Technician Examiners
1414 K St.
Sacramento, CA 95814
(916) 323-2167

Colorado

Colorado Board of Nursing
State Services Bldg., Room 132
1525 Sherman St.
Denver, CO 80203
(303) 866-2871

Connecticut

Connecticut Board of Examiners for
   Nursing
150 Washington St.
Hartford, CT 06106
(203) 566-1041

Delaware

Delaware Board of Nursing
Margaret O'Neill Bldg.
Federal and Court Sts.
Dover, DE 19901
(302) 736-4522

District of Columbia

District of Columbia Board of Nursing
614 H St., N.W.

Washington, DC 20001
(202) 727-7468

Florida

Florida Board of Nursing
111 Coastline Dr., Suite 504
Jacksonville, FL 32202
(904) 359-6331

Georgia

Georgia State Board of Licensed Practical
  Nurses
166 Pryor St., S.W.
Atlanta, GA 30303
(404) 656-3921

Guam

Guam Board of Nurse Examiners
Department of Public Health and Social
  Services
P.O. Box 2816
Agana, Guam 96910
(671) 734-4813

Hawaii

State of Hawaii Board of Nursing
Box 3469
Honolulu, HI 96801
(808) 548-3086

Idaho

Idaho Board of Nursing
500 S. 10th St.
Suite 102
Boise, ID 83720
(208) 334-3110

Illinois

Illinois Department of Registration and
  Education
320 W. Washington St.
3rd Floor
Springfield, IL 62786
(217) 785-0800

Indiana

Indiana State Board of Nursing, Health
  Professions Bureau
One American Square

Suite 1020, Box 82067
Indianapolis, IN 46282-0004
(317) 232-2960

Iowa

Iowa Board of Nursing
1223 East Ct.
Des Moines, IA 50319
(515) 281-3255

Kansas

Kansas Board of Nursing
Landon State Office Building
900 S.W. Jackson, Room 551
Topeka, KS 66612-1256
(913) 296-4929

Kentucky

Kentucky Board of Nursing
4010 Dupont Circle, Suite 430
Louisville, KY 40207
(502) 897-5143

Louisiana

Louisiana State Board of Practical Nurse
  Examiners
1440 Canal St., Suite 2010
New Orleans, LA 70112
(504) 568-6480

Maine

Maine Board of Nursing
295 Water St.
Augusta, ME 04330
(207) 289-5324

Maryland

Maryland Board of Examiners of Nurses
201 W. Preston St.
Baltimore, MD 21201
(301) 225-5880

Massachusetts

Massachusetts Board of Registration in
  Nursing
100 Cambridge St.
Room 1519
Boston, MA 02202
(617) 727-7393

Michigan

Michigan Board of Nursing
P.O. Box 30018
Lansing, MI 48909
(517) 373-1600

Minnesota

Minnesota Board of Nursing
2700 University Ave. W., #108
St. Paul, MN 55114
(612) 642-0567

Mississippi

Mississippi Board of Nursing
239 N. Lamar
Suite 401
Jackson, MS 39201
(601) 359-6170

Missouri

Missouri Board of Nursing
P.O. Box 656
3523 N. Ten Mile Dr.
Jefferson City, MO 65102
(314) 751-2334

Montana

Montana State Board of Nursing
Department of Commerce
1424 9th Ave.
Helena, MT 59620-0407
(406) 444-4279

Nebraska

Nebraska Board of Nursing
P.O. Box 95007
Lincoln, NE 68509
(402) 471-2001/4358

Nevada

Nevada Board of Nursing
1281 Terminal Way, Suite 116
Reno, NV 89502
(702) 786-2778

New Hampshire

New Hampshire Board of Nursing
Division of Public Health Services
Health and Welfare Bldg.
6 Hazen Dr.
Concord, NH 03301-6527
(603) 271-2323

New Jersey

New Jersey Board of Nursing
1100 Raymond Blvd.
Room 319
Newark, NJ 07102
(201) 648-2490

New Mexico

New Mexico Regulation and Licensing
    Department/Nursing
4125 Carlisle N.E.
Albuquerque, NM 87107
(505) 841-6524

New York

New York Board for Nursing
State Education Department
Cultural Education Center
Albany, NY 12230
(518) 474-3843

North Carolina

North Carolina Board of Nursing
P.O. Box 2129
Raleigh, NC 27602
(919) 828-0740

North Dakota

North Dakota Board of Nursing
919 S. 9th St.
Suite 504
Bismarck, ND 58501
(701) 224-2974

Ohio

Ohio Board of Nursing Education & Nurse
    Registration
65 S. Front St., Suite 509
Columbus, OH 43266-0316
(614) 466-3947

Oklahoma

Oklahoma Board of Nurse Registration and
    Nursing Education

2915 N. Classen Blvd., Suite 524
Oklahoma City, OK 73106
(405) 525-2076

Oregon

Oregon Board of Nursing
1400 S.W. Fifth Ave., Room 904
Portland, OR 97201
(503) 229-5653

Pennsylvania

Pennsylvania Board of Nursing
P.O. Box 2649
Harrisburg, PA 17105-2649
(717) 787-7146

Rhode Island

Rhode Island Board of Nurse Registration
   & Nurse Education
Cannon Health Bldg.
75 Davis St., Room 104
Providence, RI 02908-2488
(401) 277-2827

South Carolina

South Carolina Board of Nursing
1777 St. Julian Pl., Suite 102
Columbia, SC 29204-2488
(803) 737-6594

South Dakota

South Dakota Board of Nursing
304 S. Phillips Ave., Suite 205
Sioux Falls, SD 57102
(605) 334-1243

Tennessee

Tennessee Board of Nursing
Bureau of Manpower and Facilities
283 Plus Park Blvd.
Nashville, TN 37219-5401
(615) 367-6232

Texas

Texas Board of Nurse Examiners
1300 E. Anderson Ln.

Bldg. C, Suite 225
Austin, TX 78752
(512) 835-4880

Utah

Utah Division of Occupational and
   Professional Licensing Board of Nursing
Heber Wells Bldg., 4th Floor
160 East 300 South
P.O. Box 45802
Salt Lake City, UT 84145
(801) 530-6733

Vermont

Vermont Board of Nursing
Redstone Bldg.
26 Terrace St.
Montpelier, VT 05602
(802) 828-2396

Virgin Islands

Virgin Islands Board of Nurse Licensure
P.O. Box 7309
St. Thomas, VI 00801
(809) 774-9000 ext. 132

Virginia

Virginia Board of Nursing
1601 Rolling Hills Dr.
Richmond, VA 23229-5005
(804) 662-9909

Washington

Washington Board of Nursing Licensing
   Information
P.O. Box 9649
Olympia, WA 98504
(206) 586-1923

West Virginia

West Virginia Board of Examiners for
   Practical Nurses
922 Quarrier St.
Embleton Bldg., Suite 506
Charleston, WV 25301
(304) 348-3572

Wisconsin

Wisconsin Board of Nursing
Room 174
P.O. Box 8935
Madison, WI 53708
(608) 266-3735

Wyoming

Wyoming Board of Nursing
Barrett Bldg., Suite One
2301 Central Ave.
Cheyenne, WY 82002
(307) 777-7601

APPENDIX
B
Learning Exercises for Chapter 5

Time Management: Sample Personal Roles and Activities

Below is an example of one person's listing of personal roles and activities. Using the blank page provided on the next page, list your personal roles and activities for each category. (Explanations for notations appear below.*)

SCHOOL

A Be at school 40 hours per week.
A Be prepared to teach three courses each week (total of 25 hours in class and clinical).

COMMUNITY

Ⓐ Lector at church.
Ⓑ Member of library board.
Ⓑ Member of homemaker's group.

RECREATION

A Write a book.
A Attend symphony five times per year.
A Attend Civic Music five times per year.
B Periodically attend movies and watch television
B Night out with husband.
A "Special" activities with son.
Ⓑ Selected activities that come up in community during year.

JOB

A School is my job.

FAMILY

A Principal organizer for family of three.
Ⓐ Spend time with son.
Ⓐ Prepare dinner seven evenings per week.
Ⓑ Prepare one special breakfast on weekend.
Ⓐ Do one load of laundry per day.
Ⓐ Do several loads of laundry on weekend.
Ⓐ Food shop several times a week.
B Major housecleaning one time per year.
Ⓐ Daily straightening up of house.
Ⓐ Perform errands as necessary.
Ⓑ Attend PTA.
Ⓑ Attend Boy Scout activities.

---

*A = priority items (These items *have* to be done.);
B = nonpriority items (These items *do not have* to be done.);
Circled items = delegated items.

My Personal Roles and Activities

SCHOOL	JOB	FAMILY	COMMUNITY	RECREATION

Use of Personal Time

In order to record personal time most accurately, be sure to pick a school day that includes usual activities. A blank page has been provided on p. 294 so you can record your activities in chronologic order. When you total up the minutes spent in each activity, they should total 1440, the number found in each 24-hour day. A sample day's activity log has been provided below. This example does not reflect how you actually spend your time. It merely reflects one person's use of time in a 24-hour period. You will see as many different one-day logs as there are students in your personal issues class.

Sample Personal Time and Activity Log for Monday
<u>(Day)</u>

TIME SPAN	ACTIVITY	TOTAL TIME
5:45– 6:00 A.M.	Shampoo and blow dry hair	15 minutes
6:00– 6:30 A.M.	Breakfast and make "to do" list	30 minutes
6:30– 6:45 A.M.	Dress	15 minutes
6:45– 7:05 A.M.	Drive to school	20 minutes
7:05– 7:30 A.M.	Prepare for first class	25 minutes
7:30– 9:00 A.M.	Class	90 minutes
9:00– 9:20 A.M.	Break	20 minutes
9:20–10:20 A.M.	Class	60 minutes
10:20–10:30 A.M.	Break	10 minutes
10:30–11:20 A.M.	Class	50 minutes
11:20–12:30 P.M.	Lunch	70 minutes
12:30– 1:20 P.M.	Class	50 minutes
1:20– 1:30 P.M.	Break	10 minutes
1:30– 2:20 P.M.	Class	50 minutes
2:20– 2:30 P.M.	Break	10 minutes
2:30– 3:30 P.M.	Study	60 minutes
3:30– 3:50 P.M.	Drive home	20 minutes
3:50– 4:30 P.M.	Start laundry, dinner, "pick up" house	40 minutes
4:30– 5:45 P.M.	Talk to son, study	75 minutes
5:45– 6:15 P.M.	Dinner	30 minutes
6:15– 8:00 P.M.	Study	105 minutes
8:00– 8:30 P.M.	Bathe, set out clothes for tomorrow.	30 minutes
8:30– 9:45 P.M.	Watch TV/study	75 minutes
9:45– 5:45 A.M.	Sleep	480 minutes
		1440 minutes

Personal Time and Activity Log for _____

(Day/Date)

TIME SPAN	ACTIVITY	TOTAL TIME

Setting Personal Priorities

Review all the activities you have listed on page 292 of Appendix B under the five categories of roles you play in everyday life, and rank them according to the following directions:

1. Place an "A" beside the activities you have to do without question. Remember, "A" activities are those you HAVE to do, not necessarily WANT to do. These are your priority activities. For example, you might not want to get up on rainy mornings and go to school, but you have to if you want to graduate.
2. Place a "B" beside those activities that DO NOT have to be done. These are nonpriority items as far as your long-term goal and your well-being are concerned. You might want to do these activities, but you don't have to do them.

Many of you came to the practical nursing program while filling a variety of roles in your family and community. As much as you hate the idea, you will not be able to do everything you did before starting school. Are all the "A" activities really "A" activities? Can some of them be moved to the "B" category while you are in school? This is like moving them to the back burner for now. Take a few minutes and review the "A" and "B" status of the roles you have listed. The sample roles and activity list on page 291 has examples of setting priorities with activities.

Delegating Activities

Review your list of personal activities on page 292 of Appendix B with the goal of determining if the activity can be delegated to someone else while you are a student, and make the following notations:

1. Read over all your "A" activities (your "have-to" activities).
2. Circle the activities that can realistically be delegated while you go to school.

Are the "B" activities still on your mind? Can any of these be delegated while you go to school? If so, circle them also. The "Sample Personal Roles and Activities" on page 291 also has examples of activities that were chosen to be delegated. The only thing left to do is to contact the appropriate person to ask about delegating or assigning an activity.

Time Management: Weekly Schedule

TIME	SUN	MON	TUE	WED	THUR	FRI	SAT
6–7:00 A.M.							
7–8:00 A.M.							
8–9:00 A.M.							
9–10:00 A.M.							
10–11:00 A.M.							
11–12:00 A.M.							
1–2:00 P.M.							
2–3:00 P.M.							
3–4:00 P.M.							
4–5:00 P.M.							
5–6:00 P.M.							
6–7:00 P.M.							
7–8:00 P.M.							
8–9:00 P.M.							
9–10:00 P.M.							
10–11:00 P.M.							

APPENDIX C
Specialists

Allergist A doctor who diagnoses and treats allergies.

Anesthesiologist A doctor who administers anesthetics (drugs that decrease sensation to pain) and observes patients while they are under the effects of these drugs.

Cardiologist A doctor who diagnoses and treats diseases of the heart.

Dermatologist A doctor who diagnoses and treats diseases of the skin.

Endocrinologist A doctor who diagnoses and treats diseases of the pituitary gland, thyroid gland, pancreas, adrenals, parathyroids, pineal gland, thymus, ovaries, and testes.

Gynecologist A doctor who diagnoses and treats diseases of the reproductive organs in women.

Hematologist A doctor who diagnoses and treats diseases of the blood and blood-forming tissues.

Obstetrician A doctor who treats women while they are pregnant, in labor, and after the baby is born.

Oncologist A doctor who treats patients with cancer.

Opthalmologist A doctor who diagnoses and treats diseases of the eye.

Otolaryngologist A doctor who diagnoses and treats diseases of the ear, nose, and throat.

Neonatologist A doctor who diagnoses and treats diseases of newborns.

Neurologist A doctor who diagnoses and treats diseases of the nervous system.

Pediatrician A doctor who diagnoses and treats diseases in children.

Psychiatrist A doctor who diagnoses and treats mental illness.

Radiologist A doctor who uses x-rays and radioactive substances to diagnose and treat disease.

Surgeon A doctor who treats diseases and injuries using surgery.

Urologist A doctor who diagnoses and treats diseases of the urinary tract.

APPENDIX D

The Howlett Style of Nursing Leadership

The idea for this management style was found in the *One Minute Manager* and *Putting the One Minute Manager to Work* and was originally written as *The Howlett Theory of Management for Nursing Instructors.*

1. Never assume employees know what is expected of them. Employees are informed of what is expected of them in their job descriptions. They are held accountable for these expectations. Expected performance needs to be stated objectively. This will make employees aware of the appropriate behavior to reach the institution's goals.

2. Reward employees for their "good" behavior (doing what is expected or for going beyond the call of duty). This will encourage them to repeat good behavior. But do not ignore bad performance; to do so will have a negative effect. Most employees know what it is like to be caught doing something "bad." Surprise the heck out of them and catch them doing something good. Let them know how you feel about the "good" behavior. Praise them in some way (name on bulletin board, note indicating you caught them doing something "good," and list the behavior).

3. Employees, being human beings, will sometimes make mistakes, for example, they may not follow rules/policies, etc. When these situations arise, determine if it involves something the employee *cannot* or something she *will not* do. If the employee *cannot* do something, it is a training problem. Skill development is the suggested way of handling the situation. If the employee *will not* do something, it is an attitude problem. A reprimand may be in order, according to the policies of your institution. See #6.

4. Employees who feel good about themselves produce good results. Let your employees know they are the best group in the world to work with because . . . (identify reason). Wear an apron that says you work with the best staff in the world.

5. Written and oral feedback about behavior and its consequences, whether positive or negative, needs to be objective. Unemotionally, indicate what they did. Relate feedback as closely as possible to the event. Do not save feedback until clinical performance evaluation time. Point out the consequences of positive and negative behavior. For positive behavior, give praise in measurable terms so the behavior can be repeated. Blanchard and Johnson suggest reprimanding negative behavior in such a way that the person will think about the *reprimand* after the episode and *not* the manner in which it was delivered. Offer praise at the end of a reprimand so that the reprimand is heard more clearly and does not ruin the impact of the praising. Focus reprimands on behaviors, not on the individual.

6. Sometimes employees do not respond to support or assistance and need to be disciplined or terminated. Refer to the policies of your institution.

APPENDIX
E
Problem-Solving
Leadership Scenarios

Scenario 1*: Wayne, a nursing assistant, is a full-time employee on the evening shift of his local nursing home. He has missed five out of twenty scheduled shifts this month. When questioned about his absences, Wayne states he has personal problems. Frequent absences have been a problem since Wayne was first employed.

ASSESSMENT	PROBLEM	INTERVENTION	EVALUATION
Absent on 9/12, 9/13, 9/20, 9/22, and 9/30. Scheduled to work evenings on these dates. States he has personal problems.	Five absences in one month. States he has personal problems.	1. Meet in private with Wayne for oral warning. 2. Review attendance record for month. 3. Review attendance and sick leave policy. 4. Review existence of the Employee Assistance program for help with personal problems. 5. Set limits. Waynes's attendance will be documented for one month. Absences will be recorded for inclusion in a written warning and placed in his file. 6. Schedule meeting for the end of October to review attendance.	Evaluate Wayne's compliance with set limits.
Absent on 10/14, 10/15, 10/19, 10/20, 10/25, and 10/26. States he has personal problems. Has not made arrangements to see Employee Assistance.	Continues to be absent from assigned shift (six absences since last meeting) for personal reasons.	1. Objectively document absences in writing. 2. In private, discuss written warning with Wayne. Have Wayne write his comments on warning and sign it, indicating he has read the written warning.	Evaluate Wayne's compliance with set limits.

4. Distribute copies of written warning to supervisor and employee. Keep a copy in your file.
5. Set date, in writing, for desired change in behavior (attend when scheduled).
6. Refer situation to supervisor and discuss appropriate actions if Wayne is not present.

---

*The interventions presented are an example of suggested actions in this situation. Actual handling of the situation depends on the established policies of the health care institution and experience of the first-line nursing leader. This scenario presents one legal way of handling an absentee problem.

Scenario 2*: Ceil completed her nursing assistant training four months ago and has been employed at a nursing home since she became registered. Since completing her orientation at the nursing home, she has had continuing problems getting her assignment completed in an acceptable time frame. Ceil states her patient load is too heavy and is impossible to complete. The other nursing assistants have helped Ceil with her patients, but they tell you they are tired of carrying her load because she can frequently be seen sitting at the desk making personal phone calls.

ASSESSMENT	PROBLEM	INTERVENTION	EVALUATION
9/14—employed in May after being registered as a nursing assistant. Unable to finish patient load since orientation. States her patient load is too heavy.	Unable to finish patient assignment. Possible problem with time management.	1. Review patient load as to number of residents assigned and degree of need for assistance and compare to assignments of peers. 2. In private, discuss findings with Ceil. 3. Ask Ceil for suggestions for improving her performance.	Assignment equal to peers in number and degree of need for assistance.

		Interventions	Evaluation
		4. Suggest that Ceil observe and assist a successful peer to learn how to prioritize care and complete assignment for one week.	
		5. After observing and assisting for one week try Ceil with patient assignment.	Is able to get assignment completed.
9/28—Resident A states he did not receive oral hygiene or his bath today. Was assigned to Ceil. 9/29 and 9/30—Resident B states her bed was not made and she was not helped to bathroom when asked. Assigned to Ceil. From 9/28 to 9/30 Ceil was observed sitting at nurse's desk frequently.	Possible lack of skill development versus attitude problem.	1. Document dates and complaints from residents. 2. Document time sitting at desk. 3. Meet privately with Ceil, and present written documentation. 4. Through discussion, determine if problem is due to lack of skills or an attitude problem. 5. If problem is due to lack of skills, TRAIN. 6. If problem is due to attitude problem, proceed according to policies of institution.	Determine through discussion if problem is due to lack of skills or an attitude problem.

*The interventions presented are an example of suggested actions in this situation and reflect one legal way of handling a problem dealing with inability to complete assignments. Actual handling of this situation depends on the established policies of the health care institution and experience of the first-line manager.

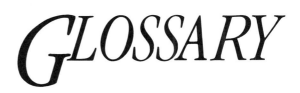

GLOSSARY

Accountability   Obligation to answer for your actions.

Acculturate   To adopt the culture of a different group.

Active learner   Takes charge of his or her own education.

Active listener   A person who hears sounds and searches for relevant information in those sounds so that the sounds may be understood.

Affirmations   Positive statements to oneself that set the stage for changing negative images and behaviors.

Aggressiveness   Attacking type of behavior that occurs in response to frustration and hostile feelings.

Answer   Response by the defendant to the plaintiff after the formal charge has been made.

Appeal   Request for another trial.

Assault   An unjustified attempt or threat to touch someone.

Assertiveness   A way of accepting responsibility for oneself by expressing thoughts and feelings directly and honestly without blaming oneself or others.

Assessment   Step 1 of the nursing process. Gathering as much significant information about a patient as is possible.

Assessment   The act of making a judgment based on gathered data.

Assisting   Maintaining a dependent role under supervision of RN.

Associate Degree nurse   A registered nurse who has received his or her education in a two-year community-college or technical-school program.

Attitude   How you project yourself to others; described as being either positive or negative. Expressed both verbally and nonverbally.

Audiovisual materials   Films and videotapes.

Auditory learner   Talks to himself or herself or hears sounds when he or she thinks.

Baccalaureate nurse   A registered nurse who has received his or her education in a four-year college or university program.

Barton, Clara   Founder of the American Red Cross.

Basic daily needs   The physical, social, and emotional aspects of all persons.

Battery   Actual physical harm to someone.

Bilingual   Using or ability to use two languages fluently.

Body language   Nonverbal communication of one's thoughts and feelings.

Burial society   A group of persons affiliated with a synagogue who prepare the dead for burial.

CAI   Abbreviation for computer-aided instruction.

Case nursing   A method of patient care in which one nurse is assigned to give total care to one patient.

Civil action   Related to individual rights, that is, relationships between people.

Clinical area   An area, such as a hospital or nursing home, where nursing students can apply classroom learning.

Clinical evaluation   The task, shared by instructor and student, of identifying positive behaviors and behaviors that need to be modified as they relate to meeting your goal.

Clustering   An unstructured method of mapping.

Common law   Judge-made law. Has its origins in the courts.

Communication   Conveying a thought or idea from a sender to a receiver or one person to another.

Compensation   A coping/mental mechanism whereby the individual is covering for real or imagined inadequacy by developing or exaggerating what some consider a desirable trait.

Concentration   Ability to keep the mind completely on the task at hand.

Confidence   The ability to look at yourself and respect what you see, projected in a positive manner through verbalization and body language.

Confidentiality   A patient's right to privacy.

Criminal action   Involves persons and society as a whole, for example, murder.

Cultural bias   Prejudice.

Culture   The total of all the ideas, beliefs, values, attitudes and objects that a group of persons possesses. Culture includes ways of doing things.

Custom   Unwritten, usually acceptable way of giving nursing care.

Customs   Ways of doing things that are common to a group of people of the same culture.

Data   Information.

Defamation   Damage to someone's reputation through false or unprivileged communication.

Defendant   Individual whom the plaintiff claims is at fault.

Despair   Absence of hope.

Diploma nurse   A registered nurse who has received her education in a three-year hospital-based program.

Discipline   Internal source of control for one's behavior.

Discovery period   Pretrial period during which defendant and plaintiff attempt to get all the facts.

Distraction   Anything that draws attention away from the task at hand.

Dix, Dorothea Lynnde   Advocate for the mentally ill. Through her efforts the first hospital for the mentally ill was established.

Eastern Orthodox Churches   Christian churches in the East that do not recognize the Pope, the Bishop of Rome, as their spiritual leader.

Effectiveness   Setting priorities among tasks that have a high priority.

Efficiency   Getting tasks done in the shortest time possible.

Endorsement   An agreement between some State Boards of Nursing to accept an LPN for licensure in that state, without written examination, if the LPN's score is at or above the score established by the board of nursing in the state to which application is made.

Ethics   Rules or principles that govern right conduct.

Ethnocentrism   The belief that your own culture is best; the belief that your way of doing things is best.

Evaluation   Step 5 of the nursing process. Involves taking a critical look at the effectiveness of nursing action.

Extended family   The nuclear family plus all other relatives.

Facilitators   Those who assist you in your learning.

False imprisonment   Keeping someone detained against their will without cause.

Functional nursing   A method of patient care that is task-oriented and involves dividing the tasks to be done among staff members, according to abilities.

Gamp, Sairey   A fictitious character developed by Charles Dickens in his 1849 novel *Martin Chuzzlewit*. She characterized the ignorant, gin-soaked hospital nurse of that time.

Generalizations   Broad, sweeping statements made about a group.

Genes   Structures in the body cells that pass on inherited traits.

Goals   Realistic, measurable, time-limited statements of resolution of a problem/need.

Health care setting   An agency or facility that provides health care and to which the patient goes for care.

Health care team   The various individuals who provide the services needed for the comprehensive care of patients.

High-priority task   A task of importance.

Hippocrates   Considered the "Father of Modern Medicine."

Hispanic Americans   U.S. residents whose country of origin is Mexico, Cuba, Puerto Rico, or Central or South America.

Holistic   The adjective for holism, a philosophy that looks at a person as a complete unit.

Idea sketch   Representing a verbal concept with a picture.

Imagery   A way deliberately to "picture" future encounters.

Immersion   Baptism by dipping under water.

Impaired nurse   One who is addicted to alcohol and/or to other drugs.

Implied consent   Assumed permission given by patient by entering an institution for certain routine treatments. Patient retains the right verbally to refuse any treatment and may leave the institution when he or she chooses, unless he or she is there for court-ordered treatment.

Implementation   Step 4 of the nursing process. Using the patient-care plan as a guideline for daily care, and carrying out planned activities.

Incongruous   Inconsistent with expected behavior.

Interaction   An action between two or more persons.

Internship   A program of clinical experiences to complete the requirements for licensure as a practicing physician.

Kinesthetic (tactual) learner   Experiences feelings in regard to what is being thought about.

Learning   The active process of acquiring new knowledge and skills.

Left-brain dominant   More ordered, logical, reads and writes well, and excels at analytical thinking.

Liabilities   Drawbacks.

Liability   Legal responsibility of a person to account for wrongful acts by making financial restitution.

Liability insurance   Insurance to protect the nurse from the consequences of negligent acts and from malpractice costs.

Libel   Damage to someone's reputation through written communication or pictures.

Long-term goal   A general realistic statement of what you hope to attain.

Long-term memory   A function of the brain that allows you to store information over time, for example, knowledge of what you wore on your first date (synonym—permanent memory).

LRC   Abbreviation for the learning resource center.

Malpractice   A part of negligence that relates to lack of skill or misconduct by professional persons.

Mandatory licensure   Licensing required to practice nursing.

Mapping   A form of notemaking in which information and its relationships are put in a visual pattern.

Medical asepsis   Being free from germs and infection.

Medical school   A program that provides the basic knowledge and skills needed to be a medical doctor.

Message   Idea being conveyed or the question being asked.

Minimum competency   The least amount of knowledge and skill needed to attain something.

Motivation   An internal push that makes you do what needs to be done.

Muscle tone   Muscle resistance or firmness.

NCLEX-PN   National Council Licensing Examination—Practical Nursing

Negligence   Conduct that falls below the standard of care established by law for the protection of others, and involves an unreasonable risk of harm to the patient.

Neural trace   A record of information in the brain.

Nightingale, Florence   Founder of Modern Nursing. Often known as "The Lady with the Lamp" because of her after-hours rounds with her lamp during the Crimean War.

No-code order   Written order by physician not to resuscitate patient.

Nonverbal communication   Sending or receiving information by facial expressions or body language.

Norm   A standard by which to measure something; the expected way to do things.

Notemaking   The act of condensing the words of a speaker or narrator into the main ideas presented.

Note taking   The act of trying to capture every word of a speaker or narrator.

Nuclear family   Mother, father, and children.

Nurse Practice Act   Governs the practice of nursing. Developed by each state and provincial board of nursing.

Nursing   The diagnosis and treatment of human responses to actual or potential health problems (ANA definition). Assisting sick or well individuals in performing activities that contribute to health or its recovery (Kron's definition).

Nursing process   RN's orderly way of developing a plan of care for the individual client. Usually broken down into five steps: assessment, nursing diagnosis, planning, implementation, and evaluation.

Nursing team   The individuals who carry out the patient's plan of care 24 hours a day, seven days a week. Includes registered and practical nurses, nursing assistants, ward clerks, and unit managers.

Optimism   The ability to see problems as challenges with solutions that can be arrived at through problem solving.

Passive (nonassertive) behavior   Dishonest, self-defeating behavior, which is an attempt to avoid conflict by not dealing with issues.

Passive listener   A person who receives sounds with little recognition or personal involvement.

Pastoral care team   Members of the health team who assist nurses in meeting the spiritual needs of patients.

Permissive licensure   May practice nursing without a license, but cannot use title of LPN.

Philosophy of individual worth   The belief in the uniqueness and value of each individual.

Plaintiff   Individual who claims to have had his or her legal rights violated.

Planning   Step 3 of the nursing process. Involves setting priorities, establishing goals, determining approaches to achieve the goals, and documentation of plan of care. A blueprint for action.

PQRST   A method of reading to increase understanding by developing comprehension.

Practical nurse   A person who performs, for compensation, any simple acts in the care of convalescent, subacutely or chronically ill, injured, or infirm persons, or of any act or procedure in the care of the acutely ill, injured, or infirm under the specific direction of a registered nurse, physician, podiatrist, or dentist. The individual on the nursing team who functions dependently regarding decision making in nursing care.

Prejudice   An opinion a person has about something, even though facts dispute the opinion.

Presenting complaint   The health care problem or symptom for which the patient is seeking care.

Primary-care nursing   A method of patient care in which one nurse is responsible and accountable for care given to patients on all shifts from admission to discharge. Primary-care nursing places emphasis on meeting the total needs of patients.

Procrastination   Putting off tasks that must be done.

Projection   A coping/mental mechanism whereby an individual attributes his own weaknesses to others.

Punishment   External source of control provided by others, circumstances, or events.

Rapport   A harmonious relationship.

Rationalization   A coping/mental mechanism in which the individual offers a logical, but untrue reason as an excuse for his behavior.

Reactive learner   Expects to be taught.

Reading efficiency   Rate of speed and degree of comprehension.

Receiver   Person receiving the message, idea, or question.

Registered nurse   A member of the nursing team who has gone to nursing school for two, three, or four years and has passed an exam to be registered. The person on the nursing team who functions independently in decision making regarding nursing care of patients.

Religious denomination   An organized group of persons with a philosophy that supports their particular concept of God.

Representational   As used in this textbook, refers to system corresponding to the three senses—vision, hearing, and feeling—in which people think.

Residency   A program for medical doctors, to prepare them for practice in a medical specialty.

Responsible   Reliable and trustworthy.

Resume   Summary of what you have accomplished—work, education, and sometimes personal achievements. Used to persuade an employer that you are the right person for the job; submitted with your job application.

Returning adult learner   A learner in the age bracket of mid-20s or older who has entered an educational program and has not experienced formal education for a period of time.

Revocation of license   Nursing license taken away because of illegal or unethical nursing actions.

Right brain dominant   More creative; exhibits ability in the fine arts and fantasy.

Rite   A system of ceremonies.

Ritual   A solemn act.

Role identification   How one sees one's role regarding work, family, and other societal positions.

Script   Dialogue or self-talk.

Self-esteem   Confidence or satisfaction with oneself.

Self-image   Way you view personal strengths and weaknesses.

Self-talk   The constant talk that goes on in your head, thought to be as high as 1200 words per minute.

Semmelweis, Ignaz Phillip   Developed the first method and use of antisepsis in care of obstetric patients. Dramatically reduced deaths due to childbed fever.

Sender   Person conveying an idea or asking a question.

Short-term goal   A smaller, more reasonable and manageable unit of a long-term goal, that is, the small step toward attaining a long-term goal.

Short-term memory   A function of the brain that allows you to store information for a short time, for example, a telephone number (synonym—temporary memory).

Slander   Damage to someone's reputation by verbalizing untrue or confidential information.

Social class   A person's standing in society that sociologists base on economic level and educational background. Ancestry is also sometimes used as a criterion for social class standing.

Socialization   Learning the ways of a group.

Spiritual   Pertaining to the soul; pertaining to the immaterial.

Spiritual needs   Requirements that arise out of human beings' desire to find meaning in life, suffering, and death.

Standard of care   How an ordinary prudent nurse would perform in the same or a similar situation.

Statutory law   Law developed by the legislative branch of state and federal governments.

Steepled position   Resembling a steeple.

Stereotyping   The fixed notion that all individuals in a cultural group are the same.

Study skills   Techniques that help you learn.

Team nursing   A method of patient care in which small teams of nursing personnel are assigned to give total care to groups of patients.

Temporary work permit   Permission to practice nursing during the interval between graduation and when results of the NCLEX-PN are received. Permit is revoked if licensure is unsuccessful.

Therapeutic   Having healing properties; results of treatment.

Time management   The effective use of time to meet goals.

Tort   Wrong or injury done to someone, which violates his or her rights.

Traditional adult learner   Learner who comes to an educational program directly from high school or another program of study, usually in late teens or early 20s.

Uniate Churches   Churches of the East that recognize the Pope, the Bishop of Rome, as their spiritual leader.

Validation study   Investigation to show sound reasoning for what is being done.

Values   Personal beliefs learned from family and significant others that influences one's perception of right and wrong.

Verbal communication   Using words or language to convey messages, written or spoken.

Verdict   Decision reached by judge or jury after a trial is over.

Visual learner   Generates visual images, that is, thinks primarily in pictures.

Wald, Lillian   Founder of Public Health Nursing. Established the Henry Street Settlement in New York in 1893.

Index

Note: Page numbers in *italics* refer to figures. Page numbers followed by the letter t refer to tables.